PRAISE FOR *THE GREAT CHOLESTEROL MYTH* ...

"*The Great Cholesterol Myth* goes far beyond the standard information and advice for anyone worried about heart disease. The style is breezy and easy to read, but the information is solid and will surprise many readers. A must for anyone who needs to combat heart problems."

–JOE GRAEDON, M.S., AND TERESA GRAEDON, PH.D., *New York Times* best-selling authors of *The People's Pharmacy*

"The simplistic view that dietary and serum cholesterol are the primary causes of heart disease and heart attack is no longer tenable. Doctors Sinatra and Bowden provide all of us with a persuasive, fact-based interpretation and vision of the true role of cholesterol in cardiovascular illnesses."

–MARK HOUSTON M.D., M.S., F.A.C.P., F.A.H.A., F.A.S.H., F.A.C.N., director, Hypertension Institute, Saint Thomas Hospital, Nashville, TN, and author of *What Your Doctor May Not Tell You About Heart Disease*

"*The Great Cholesterol Myth* is a remarkable book that will revolutionize the way in which heart disease is prevented, detected, and treated in this country."

–ANN LOUISE GITTLEMAN, PH.D., C.N.S., best-selling author of *The Fat Flush Plan*

"This book clearly explains the tragic and harmful cholesterol and statin myths, and gives readers insight into those factors that really do promote a healthy heart."

–PETER H. LANGSJOEN, M.D., F.A.C.C., founding member, Executive Committee, International CoEnzyme Q_{10} Association

"Full of useful facts, backed up by the research literature, this book is entertaining and accessible to just about anybody who cares about their health. A must-read for those who are worried about their cholesterol levels and on the fence with statin therapy."

–STEPHANIE SENEFF, B.S., M.S., E.E., PH.D., senior research scientist, Massachusetts Institute of Technology

"Increasingly, doctors are questioning assertions that cholesterol is responsible for arterial disease, and that effective management requires lowering of cholesterol levels, especially with statins. At the same time, the noxious properties of the latter are being appreciated. It is therefore timely that Bowden and Sinatra provide this very readable explanation of why they think the way they do. Many readers will be persuaded."

–HYWEL DAVIES, M.D., F.R.C.P., F.A.C.P., F.A.C.C., former chief of cardiology at the Denver VA Hospital

"[The authors] demonstrate with compelling logic backed by scientific studies that doctors are doing more harm than good by prescribing statins as if they were after-dinner mints, with the false hope that a lower cholesterol level will prevent heart disease when underlying inflammation and oxidative stress are the real root causes of heart disease."

—**TODD LEPINE, M.D.,** The UltraWellness Center

"Dr. Bowden and Dr. Sinatra do an outstanding job providing a deep dive into all the causes of heart disease, while clarifying the role cholesterol plays. I would encourage this book to be required reading for all health science students, nutritionists, and physicians who treat patients!"

—**COLETTE HEIMOWITZ, M.SC.,** vice president of nutrition and education, Atkins Nutritionals, Inc.

"If you're concerned about your cholesterol level and are thinking of taking a statin drug, this book is a must-read! It will change the way you think about heart disease—and it may save your life!"

—**PRUDENCE HALL, M.D.,** founder and medical director, The Hall Center

"Be ready to be surprised, entertained, and to become healthy."

—**LARRY MCCLEARY, M.D.,** best-selling author of *Feed Your Brain, Lose Your Belly*

"This book is well written with excellent scientific references and from extremely knowledgeable authors. Read this book so you can be armed with the knowledge you need to make an informed decision before you treat your high cholesterol!"

—**JENNIFER LANDA, M.D.,** chief medical officer of BodyLogicMD, author of *The Sex Drive Solution for Women*

"Jonny Bowden and Stephen Sinatra set the record straight on decades of bad science [and] put forth a far better solution about the true culprits that rob you of longevity: processed carbohydrates, insufficient vegetables, excess omega 6, and too many trans fats. Masterly, readable, and life-altering."

—**SARA GOTTFRIED, M.D.,** author of *The Hormone Cure*

"The authors have done their homework, and rather than rotely 'following the leader' they have dug into the extensive research and correlated it with their wide clinical experience to reveal the truth. This book can save many lives, including your own!"

—**HYLA CASS, M.D.,** author of *8 Weeks to Vibrant Health*

"Thanks to the extensive scientific evidence provided by Bowden and Sinatra, the truth about cholesterol will hopefully end the utter madness that has plagued our society for far too long. Don't even think about taking another statin drug, cutting your fat and cholesterol intake, or other 'heart-healthy' measures until you read *The Great Cholesterol Myth.*"

—JIMMY MOORE, author of *Livin' La Vida Low Carb* and *A Patient's Guide to Understanding Your Cholesterol Test Results*

"This powerful new book will help the cholesterol test get the rest it deserves."

—ALAN CHRISTIANSON, N.M.D., co-author, *The Complete Idiot's Guide to Thyroid Disease*

"If you want to know the truth about cholesterol, and what you absolutely must do to improve your heart health, this is the book for you. Jonny Bowden and Dr. Stephen Sinatra reveal the facts in a compelling and insightful way. This invaluable book belongs on the bookshelf of anyone who cares about the truth in medicine and healing."

—DANIEL AMEN, M.D., CEO, Amen Clinics, Inc., author of *Use Your Brain to Change Your Age*

"Got high cholesterol or heart disease? Get this book!"

—JACOB TEITELBAUM, M.D., author of *Beat Sugar Addiction Now!* and *From Fatigued to Fantastic!*

"Finally! This timely book, written by the eminently qualified dream team of Dr. Jonny Bowden and Dr. Stephen Sinatra, exposes and unravels the great American cholesterol scam. Statin drugs sell in the U.S. for over $30 billion per year, but do they really prevent heart disease? No! This must-read book will tell you how to really prevent heart disease and live a longer, healthier, leaner, fuller life."

—DEAN RAFFELOCK, D.C., DIPL.AC., D.A.A.I.M., D.I.B.A.K., D.A.C.B.N.,C.C.N., author of *A Natural Guide to Pregnancy and Postpartum Health*

"The book you're holding is dangerous, and may even upset you. That's because everything you know about cholesterol is probably wrong. Doctors Jonny Bowden and Stephen Sinatra provide both the science to vindicate this unfairly demonized molecule and a plan of action so you can attain optimal health."

—JJ VIRGIN, best-selling author of *The Virgin Diet*

PRAISE FOR *THE GREAT CHOLESTEROL MYTH COOKBOOK* ...

"You owe it to yourself, your heart, and your family to read this book, but more importantly, follow the program!"

— **ROBB WOLF**, best-selling author of The Paleo Solution

"Take it from the trusted experts in this book and learn to enjoy the best foods for your heart, mind, and body!"

— **LARRY MCCLEARY, M.D.**, author of Feed Your Brain, Lose Your Belly and The Fracture Cure

"This team is a powerhouse of complementary skills and experience: Jonny Bowden is one of the world's leading authorities on functional foods. Stephen Sinatra is the first voice of metabolic cardiology. Deirdre Rawlings is an inspiring life coach."

— **LEO GALLAND, M.D.**, best-selling author of The Fat Resistance Diet

"[The authors'] conclusions are contrary to conventional medical thinking—and in line with the best research out there! I find myself giving my patients the same message daily. I appreciate being able to back it up with this well-considered, beautifully written book, which then provides recipes that are both practical and delicious. Let them eat fat!"

— **HYLA CASS, M.D.**, author of 8 Weeks to Vibrant Health

"[The authors'] arguments are based on scientific research published in peer-reviewed journals, which makes them difficult to refute. Tenets such as limit sugar, limit grains, no need to avoid saturated fat, and minimize processed foods, will go a long way in reversing risk factors for heart disease."

— **COLETTE HEIMOWITZ**, vice president of Atkins Nutritionals, Inc.

"The dietary recommendations [the authors] make are right on target, and they are going to surprise you."

— **JENNIFER LANDA, M.D.**, chief medical officer of BodyLogicMD, author of The Sex Drive Solution for Women

"You can trust [the authors'] collective wisdom, which tends to go against everything you've ever heard from conventional wisdom sources—it's spot-on! You won't go wrong heeding the advice they're sharing. In fact, it very well could save your life!"

— **JIMMY MOORE**, author of Cholesterol Clarity: What the HDL Is Wrong with My Numbers?

THE
GREAT CHOLESTEROL
MYTH

THE

NOW INCLUDES **100 RECIPES**
FOR PREVENTING AND REVERSING HEART DISEASE
FROM *THE GREAT CHOLESTEROL MYTH COOKBOOK*

GREAT CHOLESTEROL

MYTH

WHY LOWERING YOUR CHOLESTEROL WON'T PREVENT HEART DISEASE—
AND THE STATIN-FREE PLAN THAT WILL

JONNY BOWDEN, PH.D.
BESTSELLING AUTHOR OF
THE 150 HEALTHIEST FOODS ON EARTH

STEPHEN SINATRA, M.D.
BESTSELLING AUTHOR OF
THE SINATRA SOLUTION: METABOLIC CARDIOLOGY

RECIPES BY DEIRDRE RAWLINGS, PH.D., N.D.

Fair Winds Press
100 Cummings Center, Suite 406L
Beverly, MA 01915

FAIR WINDS

fairwindspress.com • bodymindbeautyhealth.com

First published in the USA in 2015 by Fair Winds Press, a member of
Quarto Publishing Group USA Inc.
100 Cummings Center
Suite 406-L
Beverly, MA 01915-6101
www.fairwindspress.com

Visit www.bodymindbeautyhealth.com. It's your personal guide to a happy, healthy, and extraordinary life!

19 18 17 16 15   1 2 3 4 5

ISBN: 978-1-59233-712-5

Digital edition published in 2015
eISBN: 978-1-62788-786-1

The content for this book was originally published in *The Great Cholesterol Myth* (Fair Winds Press 2012) and *The Great Cholesterol Myth Cookbook* (Fair Winds Press 2014)

Printed and bound in USA

The information in this book is for educational purposes only. It is not intended to replace the advice of a physician or medical practitioner. Please see your health care provider before beginning any new health program.

CONTENTS

"The mind is like a parachute—it only works if it's open."
–Anthony J. D'Angelo

"Never underestimate the convictions of the conventional,
particularly in medicine."
–William Davis, M.D.

· SECTION 1 ·

Revealing the Truth about Heart Health

FOREWORD

TWO HUNDRED YEARS AGO physicians routinely bled, purged, and plastered their patients. Bloodletting was the standard treatment for a host of diseases and had been so since the time of the philosopher-physician Galen almost 2,000 years before. The theory was that there were four humors—blood, phlegm, black bile, and yellow bile. Blood was dominant, requiring the most balancing for returning an ill patient to health.

Every doctor's kit was equipped with a variety of lancets, brutal-looking scarificators, and, starting in the early nineteenth century, leeches. In fact, the latter were used so often that physicians were themselves commonly referred to as leeches. Learned physicians conferred on the best veins to tap for given diseases and the optimal placement of leeches for the most therapeutic value, and countless protocols dictated the proper amount of blood to be let or number of leeches to be applied. Doctors wrote lengthy papers describing their own bleeding techniques and presented them at august medical conferences.

The whole idea was nonsense, of course, and has been shown to be so in the early 1600s by William Harvey, the discoverer of how the circulatory system actually works. But the fact that the "scientific" basis for bloodletting was nonexistent didn't give pause to physicians 200 years ago, some of whom applied as many as fifty leeches to a single patient and, in the case of George Washington, relieved him of almost two quarts of blood in an effort to treat the throat infection that, coupled with the physician-caused anemia, ultimately killed him.

We look back today and can only shake our heads. And be thankful we, ourselves, don't have to worry about getting bled by lancet or leech or that with today's modern, truly science-based medicine, we would ever be exposed to such nebulously grounded treatments. Surely with all the scientific studies performed in great institutions the world over, today's doctors would never ignore the actual evidence and pursue unnecessary and possibly even harmful treatments. Would they?

Sadly, many doctors today have the same herd mentality as those doctors of yore. By the tens of thousands, they treat a nonexistent disease with drugs that are far from benign. And they do so based not on any hard scientific data, but because they, like

> Cholesterol is an essential molecule without which there would be no life, so important that virtually every cell in the body is capable of synthesizing it.

their colleagues of 200 years ago, are firmly in the grip of group think. What is the nonexistent disease? Elevated cholesterol.

The vast majority of laypeople have been bombarded with so much misinformation about cholesterol that most take it as a given that cholesterol is a bad thing and that the less they have the better. The reality is that nothing could be further from the truth.

Cholesterol is an essential molecule without which there would be no life, so important that virtually every cell in the body is capable of synthesizing it. Among its other duties, cholesterol is a major structural molecule, a framework on which other critical substances are made. Were we able to somehow remove all its cholesterol, the body, would, in the words of Shakespeare, "melt, thaw and resolve itself into a dew." And that's not to mention that we wouldn't have bile acids, vitamin D, or steroid hormones (including sex hormones), all of which are cholesterol-based.

Despite the essential nature of cholesterol, doctors the world over administer billions of dollars' worth of drugs to try to prevent its natural synthesis. The fact that only a tiny minority of patients actually extend their lives by taking these drugs is lost on the multitude prescribing them, but not, of course, on the pharmaceutical industry making and selling them. How did we come to this sorry state?

Sixty years ago a researcher, little known outside of academic circles, singlehandedly set us on this path of cholesterol paranoia: Ancel Keys, Ph.D., a proponent of what has become known as the lipid hypothesis, concluded that excess cholesterol caused heart disease. He started out thinking that dietary fat in general drove cholesterol levels up, but as the years went by, he came to believe that saturated fat was the true cholesterol-raising villain. (This idea of saturated fat as villain is so ingrained in the minds of health writers that the words "saturated fat" are almost never written alone but always as "artery-clogging saturated fat.") Which is more or less the basis for the lipid hypothesis: saturated fat runs up cholesterol levels, and elevated cholesterol leads to heart disease. Nice and simple, but not true. It has never been proven, which is why it is still called the lipid *hypothesis*.

Because of Keys's influence, researchers for the past five decades have been beavering away in labs the world over, desperate to find enough actual proof to convert the lipid hypothesis into the lipid fact. But so far, they've fallen way short. In the process, however, they have vastly expanded our knowledge of the bio-chemistry and physiology of the cholesterol molecule. Thanks to their efforts, we now know that cholesterol is transported in the blood attached to carrier proteins, and that these protein-cholesterol complexes are called lipoproteins. Their densities now describe these lipo-proteins: HDL (high-density lipoprotein), LDL (low-density lipoprotein), VLDL (very-low-density lipoprotein), and a number of others. Some of these lipoproteins are considered good (HDL) and others bad (LDL). And, of course, the drug companies have developed medica-tions purported to increase the former while decreasing the latter.

But they jumped the gun. Researchers have discovered a type of lipoprotein called small, dense (or type B) LDL that may actually end up being a true risk factor for heart disease. Problem is, this small, dense type B LDL is worsened by the very diet those promoting the lipid hypothesis have hailed for decades as the best diet to prevent heart disease: the low-fat, high-carbohydrate diet. Turns out that fat, especially saturated fat, decreases the amount of these small, dense LDL particles while the widely recommended low-fat diet increases their number. The opposite of the small dense LDL are large fluffy LDL particles, which are not only *not* harmful but are actually healthful. But the LDL-lowering drugs lower those, too.

Cracks should have appeared in the firm entrench-ment of the lipid hypothesis (that now basically posits that elevated LDL causes heart disease) when a recent study showed that of almost 140,000 patients admitted to the hospital for heart disease, almost half of them had LDL levels *under* 100 mg/dL (100 mg/dL has been the therapeutic target for LDL for the past few years). Instead of stepping back, scratching their heads, and thinking, *Hmmm, maybe we're on the wrong track here,* the authors of this study concluded that maybe a therapeutic level of 100 mg/dL for LDL is still too high and needs to be even lower. Such is their lipo-phobic herd mentality.

Nutritionist Jonny Bowden, Ph.D., and cardiologist Stephen Sinatra, M.D., have teamed up in this book to slash through the tall thicket of misinformation surrounding cholesterol, lipoproteins, and the lipid hypothesis. They wrote their fact-based book using easy-to-understand terminology, and present a much more valid hypothesis of what really causes heart disease and a host of other diseases such as diabetes, high blood pressure, and obesity, that will open your eyes to the emperor's state of undress. If you are worried about your cholesterol level or contemplating taking a choles-terol-lowering drug, we urge you to read this book! This book will put the facts in your hands to make a more informed decision. And we're confident you will enjoy their book as much as we did.

Michael R. Eades, M.D.
Mary Dan Eades, M.D.
May 2012
Incline Village, Nevada

CHAPTER 1

WHY YOU SHOULD BE SKEPTICAL OF CHOLESTEROL AS AN INDICATOR OF HEART DISEASE

THE TWO OF US CAME TOGETHER TO WRITE THIS BOOK because we believe that you have been completely misled, misinformed, and in some cases, directly lied to about cholesterol.

We believe that a weird admixture of misinformation, scientifically questionable studies, corporate greed, and deceptive marketing has conspired to create one of the most indestructible and damaging myths in medical history: that cholesterol causes heart disease.

The millions of marketing dollars spent on perpetuating this myth have successfully kept us focused on a relatively minor character in the heart disease story, and created a market for cholesterol-lowering drugs worth more than $30 billion a year. The real tragedy is that by putting all of our attention on cholesterol, we've virtually ignored the *real* causes of heart disease: inflammation, oxidation, sugar, and stress.

In fact, as you'll learn in this book, cholesterol numbers are a pretty poor predictor of heart disease; more than half the people hospitalized with heart attacks have perfectly normal cholesterol levels, and about half the people with elevated cholesterol levels have perfectly normal, healthy tickers.

Many of the general dietary guidelines accepted and promoted by the government and by major health organizations such as the American Heart Association are either directly or indirectly related to cholesterol phobia. These standard guidelines warn us to limit the amount of cholesterol we eat, despite the fact that for at least 95 percent of the population, cholesterol in the *diet* has virtually no effect on cholesterol in the *blood*.

These guidelines warn us of the dangers of saturated fat, despite the fact that the relationship between saturated fat in the diet and heart disease has never been convincingly demonstrated, and despite the fact that research shows that replacing saturated fat in the diet with carbohydrates actually *increases* the risk for heart disease.

Both of us became skeptical of the cholesterol theory at different points in our careers, traveling different pathways to arrive at the same conclusion: Cholesterol does not cause heart disease.

We also believe that, unlike trans fat, for example, saturated fat is *not* the dietary equivalent of Satan's spawn (and we'll show you why). Finally, and most important, we strongly believe that our national obsession with lowering cholesterol has come at a considerable price. Cholesterolmania has caused us to focus all our energy around a fairly innocuous molecule with a marginal relationship to heart disease, while ignoring the *real* causes of heart disease.

We're each going to tell you in our own words how we became cholesterol skeptics and why we fervently believe the information contained in this book could save your life.

◄ **WHAT YOU NEED TO KNOW**

- Cholesterol is a minor player in heart disease.
- Cholesterol levels are a poor predictor of heart attacks.
- Half the people with heart disease have normal cholesterol.
- Half the people with elevated cholesterol have healthy hearts.
- Lowering cholesterol has extremely limited benefits.

DR. JONNY

Before I became a nutritionist and ultimately an author, I was a personal trainer. I worked at Equinox Fitness Clubs in New York City, and the vast majority of my clients were there for one thing: to lose weight. It was 1990. Fat was considered dietary enemy number one, and saturated fat was considered *especially* bad because we all "knew" it clogged your arteries, raised your cholesterol, and led to heart disease. So, like most trainers, I put my clients on low-fat diets and encouraged them to do a ton of aerobics plus a little bit of weight training.

Which worked.

*Some*times.

More often than not, the strategy bombed.

Take Al, for example. Al was an incredibly successful, powerful businessman in his early sixties with a huge belly he just couldn't get rid of. He was eating a very low-fat diet, doing a ton of aerobics on the treadmill in his house, and yet his weight was hardly budging. If everything I had been taught as a personal trainer was right, that shouldn't have been happening.

But it was.

Then Al decided to do something I didn't approve of. He went on the Atkins diet.

Remember, those were the days when all of us were taught that fat, especially saturated fat, was pure evil. We had been taught that we "need" carbo-hydrates for energy and survival (we don't, but that's a discussion for another book). We had been taught that high-protein diets such as the Atkins diet were dangerous and damaging, largely because all that

saturated fat would clog your arteries, raise your cholesterol, and lead to a heart attack.

So I was pretty sure Al was headed for disaster.

Except he wasn't.

Not only did he start shedding weight and losing his substantial "apple-shaped" belly, but he also had more energy and was feeling better than he had in decades. I, meanwhile, was impressed with Al's results, but I was convinced he was paying a huge price and that once he got the blood test results from his annual physical, I would be vindicated.

I wasn't.

Al's triglycerides—a type of fat found in the bloodstream and elsewhere—had dropped, his blood pressure had gone down, and his cholesterol had risen slightly, but his "good" cholesterol (HDL) had gone up more than his "bad" cholesterol (LDL), so overall his doc was pretty happy.

Right around this time, a biochemist named Barry Sears came to New York City to give a workshop at Equinox, which, of course, I eagerly attended. Sears, whose Zone diet books have sold millions, had a novel approach that can be summed up in four words: *eat fat, lose weight*. (If Sears had been anything but an MIT-trained biochemist, he probably would have been laughed out of the room. But given his credentials and remarkable knowledge of the human body, he was pretty hard to dismiss.)

Now Sears wasn't the first one to embrace fat and protein in the diet and recommend that we eat fewer carbs. Atkins, whose original diet was the one Al had tried so successfully, had been saying similar things since 1972. But the whole rap against Atkins was that

What if the whole theory that cholesterol causes heart disease was wrong in the first place?

his diet was high in saturated fat and would therefore likely cause heart disease. So even though many people grudgingly admitted that you could lose weight easily following his program, everyone (including me) believed that the cost would include a hugely increased risk for heart disease.

Meanwhile, my eyes were telling me something very different, and it wasn't just because of what I had seen happen with Al. It was happening with other clients as well. Sick of not getting results on low-fat, high-carb diets, they threw caution to the wind and embraced the Atkins diet and the Protein Power diet and other protein- and fat-friendly diets. They were eating more fat—even more saturated fat—but nothing bad was happening at all, unless, of course, you count feeling better and getting slimmer as nothing.

Which got me thinking.

Why weren't we seeing consistent results with our clients who were faithfully following low-fat diets and getting plenty of aerobic exercise? Conversely, why were our clients who were going on low-carb diets getting such high marks on their blood tests and astonishing their doctors? What if everything we'd been told about the danger of saturated fat wasn't exactly correct? And—if what we'd been taught about saturated fat wasn't the complete truth—what

about this relationship between fat and cholesterol? Was it really all as simple as I'd been taught?

After all, even back in the early '90s when people only talked about "good" and "bad" cholesterol, it was still obvious that, overall, saturated fat had a positive effect on Al's cholesterol, as it did on the cholesterol levels of so many of my other clients. Saturated fat raised their HDL much more than it did their LDL. Could this whole cholesterol issue be a little more complicated than I and everyone else had previously believed?

Eventually, I thought—going way out on a limb here—what if the whole theory that cholesterol causes heart disease was wrong in the first place? If that were the case, the effect of saturated fat on cholesterol would be pretty much irrelevant, wouldn't it?

Then I began reading the studies.

The Lyon Diet Heart Study[1] found that certain dietary and lifestyle changes were able to reduce deaths by 70 percent and reduce cardiovascular deaths by an even more impressive 76 percent, all without making as much as a dent in cholesterol levels. The Nurses' Health Study[2] found that 82 percent of coronary events were attributable to five factors, none of which had anything to do with lowering cholesterol. And that was just the tip of the evergrowing iceberg.

Contrary to what everyone thought, study after study on high-protein, low-carb diets, including those rich in saturated fat, showed that the blood tests of people on these diets were similar to Al's. Their health actually *improved* on these diets. Triglycerides went down. Other measures that indicated heart disease risk also improved.

In the mid-'90s I went back to school for nutrition, ultimately earning a C.N. (certified nutritionist) designation and later a Ph.D. in holistic nutrition and a C.N.S. (certified nutrition specialist) certification from the Certification Board for Nutrition Specialists, which is associated with the American College of Nutrition. During my studies, I learned that I wasn't the only one questioning the links among saturated fat, cholesterol, and heart disease. I talked to many other health professionals who shared my concerns, including one of the top lipid biochemists in the country, Mary Enig, Ph.D., whose entire academic career has been spent studying fat and who believes that we have nothing to fear whatsoever from saturated fat. (Enig, by the way, did some of the early research on trans fats and fervently believes that it is trans fats, not saturated fats, that are the real villains in the American diet; I wholeheartedly agree.)

Enig is hardly alone in thinking that we have been collectively brainwashed on the subject of saturated fat and cholesterol. She has pointed out that when Americans were consuming whole, full-fat foods such as cream, butter, pasture-raised meats, raw milk, and other traditional foods, the rate of heart disease was a fraction of what it is now. She had wondered aloud, as so many have since, whether it was indeed a coincidence that the twin global pandemics of obesity and diabetes just happened to occur around the time we collectively banished these foods because of the phobia about cholesterol and saturated fat in the diet and began to replace them with vegetable oils, processed carbs, and, ultimately, trans fats.

Enig was very active in a group for which I have come to have great respect: The Weston A. Price Foundation. Named after a pioneering researcher in the fields of diet and health, the foundation is an outspoken advocate for "traditional" unprocessed foods, including butter, raw milk, grass-fed meat, and other foods that have been demonized by the cholesterol establishment because of their relatively high saturated fat content. The foundation has also called much-needed attention to the fact that when Americans ate these foods regularly—for example, in the early part of the twentieth century—heart disease was much less common than it is now.

In my career, I have examined the strategies that seemed to work for the healthiest, longest-living people on earth and found that lowering cholesterol has almost *nothing* to do with reducing heart disease, and definitely nothing to do with extending life. Study after study, including the Lyon Diet Heart Study, mentioned above, has shown that lowering the risk for heart disease has just about nothing to do with lowering cholesterol.

And more and more studies and reports were coming out demonstrating that the real initiators of damage in the arteries were oxidation and inflammation, with cholesterol more or less in the role of innocent bystander. Oxidation and inflammation,

One of the greatest frustrations I experienced was trying to reassure my clients that not only would they not die if they went on higher-protein, higher-fat diets, but they'd also see significant improvements in their weights and the health of their hearts.

along with sugar and stress (more on that in chapters 4 and 8), were clearly what aged the human body the most. It seemed to me then—and it seems to me even more now—that *these* were the culprits we should be focused on, not on a fairly innocent molecule that is utterly essential to human health.

By now, I was pretty convinced that we had been massively misled about the role of cholesterol in heart disease, and we had been misled about the dangers of saturated fat as well. One of the greatest frustrations I experienced during this time was trying to reassure my clients that not only would they not die if they went on higher-protein, higher-fat diets, but they'd also see significant improvements in their weights and the health of their hearts. But I was constantly butting heads with my clients' doctors, who completely bought into the myth that saturated fat will kill you by clogging your arteries, raising your cholesterol, and ultimately leading to heart disease.

Fast-forward to 2010.

In 2010, Fair Winds Press—my publisher for thirteen books over the course of seven years—came to

me with an idea. "How about a book on how to lower cholesterol with food and supplements?" they asked.

To which I replied, "I'm probably not the guy to write that one. I don't think lowering cholesterol matters very much."

As you can imagine, that was met with a collective startle. My publishers were more than a little curious. "How can lowering cholesterol *not* be important?" they wanted to know. "Don't doctors believe high cholesterol is the cause of heart disease? Don't they believe that lowering it is the most important thing you can do when it comes to preventing heart attacks?"

"They do indeed," I replied, "and they're wrong."

Intrigued, my publishers asked me for more information. I suggested they start by exploring the website of The International Network of Cholesterol Skeptics, www.thincs.org. I sent them a number of peer-reviewed studies that cast doubt on the relationship between saturated fat and heart disease. And I sent them the impeccable investigative work of award-winning science writer Gary Taubes, whose exhaustive investigations of the role of fat in heart disease (beginning with his seminal *New York Times* article, "What If It's All Been a Big Fat Lie?") has been so instrumental in calling attention to the profound weaknesses in the saturated fat-cholesterol-heart disease connection.

My friend Steve Sinatra is not only a board-certified cardiologist but also a trained psychotherapist and nutritionist. Like me, he's also a member of the American College of Nutrition. And Steve has long believed that we've been sold a bill of goods on cholesterol. The story of how he came to the same conclusion that I did is fascinating and includes his own personal experience as a lecturer/educator for some of the biggest pharmaceutical companies on earth.

Steve promoted statin drugs and fully bought into the cholesterol-causes-heart-disease mythology that both of us have since abandoned.

Listen to his story in his own words, and you will begin to appreciate why we are both so passionate about revealing the truth about cholesterol and heart disease.

DR. SINATRA

Most doctors today will recommend that you take a statin drug—they might even nag you to do so—if your cholesterol numbers are high. They will do so whether or not you have evidence of arterial disease and are a man or woman, and despite your age. In their minds, you prevent heart disease by lowering cholesterol.

Once upon a time I used to believe that, too. It made sense, based on the research and information that was promoted to doctors. I believed it to the extent that I even lectured on behalf of drug makers. I was a paid consultant to some of the biggest manufacturers of statin drugs, lecturing for hefty honorariums. I became a cholesterol choirboy, singing the refrain of high cholesterol as the big, bad villain of heart disease. Beat it down with a drug, and you cut your risks. My thinking changed years ago when I began seeing conflicting evidence among my own patients. I saw, for instance, many patients with low total cholesterol—as low as 150 mg/dL!—develop heart disease.

In those days we pushed patients to undergo angiograms (invasive arterial catheterization imaging) if they had sufficient symptoms of chest pain, border-line exercise tests, and especially cholesterol readings of greater than 280 mg/dL. We did this because our profession believed that all people with high cholesterol were in danger of having a heart attack.

We did the imaging to see how bad their arteries were. And, indeed, sometimes we found diseased arteries. But just as often we didn't. Many arteries were perfectly healthy. These results were telling me something different than the establishment message—that it wasn't just a simple cholesterol story.

Faced with these discrepancies I began questioning and investigating conventional thinking about cholesterol and looking at the cholesterol research more closely. I found other doctors who had made similar discoveries on their own and heard about how study findings were being manipulated. For example, bio-chemist George Mann, M.D., of Vanderbilt University, who participated in the development of the world-famous Framingham Heart Study, later described the cholesterol-as-an-indicator-of-heart-disease hypothesis as "the greatest scam ever perpetrated on the American public."

These and other dissenting voices were drowned out by the cholesterol chorus. To this day, practically all of what has been published—and receives media attention—supports the cholesterol paradigm and appears to have the backing of the pharmaceutical and low-fat industries along with leading regulatory agencies and medical organizations.

However, I stopped being a choirboy for cholesterol. I stopped believing. Here's why:

I found that life can't go on without cholesterol, a basic raw material made by your liver, brain, and almost every cell in your body. Enzymes convert it into vitamin D, steroid hormones (such as our sex hormones—estrogen, progesterone, and testosterone—and stress hormones), and bile salts for digesting and absorbing fats. It makes up a major part of the membranes surrounding cells and the structures within them.

The brain is particularly rich in cholesterol and accounts for about a quarter of all the cholesterol we have in our bodies. The fatty myelin sheath that coats every nerve cell and fiber is about one-fifth cholesterol. Neuronal communication depends on cholesterol. It is not surprising that a connection has been found between naturally occurring cholesterol and mental function. Lower levels are linked to poorer cognitive performance.

I remember one patient—a federal judge I'll call Silvio—who came to see me. He was taking a statin drug and complained that his memory had gone to pot, so much so that he voluntarily took himself off the bench. His LDL level was down to 65 mg/dL. I took him off the statin, told him to eat a lot of organic, cholesterol-rich eggs, and within a month got his LDL level up above 100 mg/dL. His memory came roaring back. (Memory loss is one potential side effect of cholesterol-lowering drugs.)

Some researchers suggest that doctors should be extremely cautious about prescribing statin drugs to the elderly, particularly those who are frail. I totally agree. I have seen frail individuals become even frailer and much more prone to infections. Though that surprised me at the time, it no longer does. Cholesterol plays a big role in helping fight bacteria

Life can't go on without cholesterol, a basic raw material made by your liver, brain, and almost every cell in your body.

and infections. A study that included 100,000 healthy participants in San Francisco over a fifteen-year period found that those with low cholesterol values were much more likely to be admitted to hospitals with infectious diseases.[3]

Many such patients told me afterward that their strength, energy, appetite, and vitality returned after going off statin drugs. They obviously needed their cholesterol.

In addition to being a board-certified cardiologist, I've had a lifelong interest in nutrition. I'd been using nutritional supplements in my practice since the early 1980s, particularly coenzyme Q_{10} (CoQ$_{10}$), an absolutely vital nutrient that is made in every cell in the body and is a major chemical participant in the production of cellular energy. CoQ$_{10}$ is critically important for the strong pumping action of the heart, which gobbles the stuff up. And in the early '90s I discovered something that shook my belief in statin drugs to the core—they depleted the body of CoQ$_{10}$.

That fact is widely known now, but it wasn't then. And it certainly gave me pause. How could these miracle drugs that were believed to be the answer to heart disease be good for you in the long run if they depleted the very nutrient upon which the heart depends?

Even today, many doctors aren't aware of the effect that statin drugs have on CoQ$_{10}$ levels. How ironic that the very drug they prescribe to reduce the likelihood of a heart attack actually deprives the heart of the fuel it needs to perform properly? No wonder fatigue, low energy, and muscle pain are such frequent accompaniments to statin drug use.

It wasn't until the mid-1990s that statin drugs really took off, but prior to then physicians had other go-to drugs for lowering cholesterol. Many research studies were conducted using these drugs, and in 1996 the U.S. Government Accountability Office evaluated these trials in a publication titled *Cholesterol Treatment: A Review of the Clinical Trials Evidence*. The report explained that though some trials showed a reduction in cardiovascular-related deaths (primarily among those who entered the studies with existing heart disease), there was a corresponding *increase* in *non*-cardiovascular-related deaths across the trials. "This finding, that cholesterol treatment has not lowered the number of deaths overall, has been worrisome to many researchers and is at the core of much of the controversy on cholesterol policy," the authors wrote.

It was also quite clear from the report that those who benefited the most from lowering their cholesterol levels were middle-aged men who already had heart disease. "The trials focused predominantly on middle-aged white men considered to be at high risk of coronary heart disease," the report stated. "They provide very little information on women, minority men and women, and elderly men and women."

It's been more than a decade since that report was written, but it remains true that lowering cholesterol has a very limited benefit in populations other than middle-aged men with a history of heart disease. Yet doctors continue to prescribe statin drugs for women and the elderly, and, shockingly, many are arguing for treating children with statins as well.

Lowering cholesterol has a very limited benefit in populations other than middle-aged men with a history of heart disease.

By now my conversion from cholesterol true believer to cholesterol skeptic is complete. I still prescribe statins—but only on occasion, and almost exclusively to middle-aged men who've already had a first heart attack, coronary intervention (e.g., bypass, stent, angioplasty), or coronary artery disease.

I've come to believe that cholesterol is a minor player in the development of heart disease and that whatever good statin drugs accomplish has very little to do with their cholesterol-lowering ability. (We discuss this at great length in chapter 6, "The Statin Scam.") Statin drugs are anti-inflammatory, and their power to reduce inflammation is much more important than their ability to lower cholesterol. But we can lower inflammation (and the risk for heart disease) with natural supplements, a better diet, and lifestyle changes such as managing stress. Best of all, none of these come with the growing laundry list of troubling symptoms and side effects associated with statin drugs and cholesterol lowering.

LIKE DEAD MEN WALKING

So there you have it. Two individuals with very different journeys arriving at the same conclusion.

And because that conclusion may be pretty hard to swallow if you've been brainwashed by the cholesterol establishment—and who hasn't?—it might be helpful to take a moment and talk about a study we alluded to earlier—the Lyon Diet Heart Study.

In the early 1990s, French researchers decided to run an experiment—known as the Lyon Diet Heart Study—to test the effect of different diets on heart disease.[4]

They took 605 men and women who were prime candidates for heart attacks. These folks had every risk factor imaginable. All of them had already survived a first heart attack. Their cholesterol levels were through the roof, they smoked, they ate junk food, they didn't exercise, and they had high levels of stress. People like this give insurance underwriters nightmares. To be frank, these folks were "dead men walking."

The researchers divided the participants into two groups. The first group was counseled (by the research cardiologist and the dietician during a one-hour session) to eat a Mediterranean-type diet which emhasizes fresh fruit and vegetables, whole grains, legumes, nuts, healthy fats like olive oil, and seafood. The second group was the control group and received no dietary advice from the investigators but was advised, nonetheless, to follow a *prudent diet* by their attending physicians.

What was this prudent diet, you ask? Pretty much the standard (and, as we shall see, useless) diet that doctors have been recommending for decades: Eat no more than 30 percent of your calories from fat, no more than 10 percent from saturated fat, and no more than 300 mg of cholesterol a day (about the amount in two eggs). So what happened with the study?

Actually, it was stopped.

Why? Because the reduction in heart attacks in the Mediterranean diet group was so pronounced that the researchers decided it was unethical to continue. To be precise, the Mediterranean diet group had a whopping 70 percent reduction in deaths and an even more impressive 76 percent reduction in cardiovascular deaths. What's more, angina, pulmonary embolism, heart failure, and stroke were also much lower in the intervention group. A huge victory for the Mediterranean diet and a big dunkin' for the prudent diet.

So what happened to these folks' cholesterol levels? Gosh, you'd imagine they dropped like crazy, because so few of them were dying of heart disease.

Um, not so much.

Their cholesterol levels *didn't budge.*

Let's repeat that one more time: a 76 percent reduction in deaths from heart disease but not a whit of change in cholesterol levels. Neither in their *total* cholesterol levels *nor* in their levels of LDL (the so-called "bad" cholesterol). You'd think this would shake up the cholesterol establishment a bit, wouldn't you?

Think again. The prestigious *New England Journal of Medicine* refused to publish the study. (It was eventually published in another highly regarded medical journal, *The Lancet.*) We have a hunch that the reason the *New England Journal of Medicine* didn't publish the study was precisely because there was no difference in cholesterol levels between the two groups of people, the ones who did so well and the ones who did not. The American medical establishment is so firmly locked into the notion that cholesterol and fat cause heart disease that any inconvenient evidence to the contrary—and there is a massive amount of it, as you will soon find out—has to be ignored or explained away.

Lower heart disease rates? And no movement in cholesterol numbers?

Something has to be wrong!

Actually something *was* wrong, but not with the study. What was—and is—wrong is the blind belief that cholesterol simply makes a huge difference.

An Inconvenient Fact

Not convinced? Fast-forward to a drug study completed in 2006, the widely publicized ENHANCE trial.[5] If you were following the news in 2008 you couldn't have missed this one, because it made the front pages of the newspapers and all of the television news shows. Here's what happened.

A combination cholesterol-lowering medication called Vytorin had been the subject of a huge research project, the results of which were finally coming to light and receiving an enormous amount of negative attention. One of the many reasons for this negative attention was the fact that the companies jointly making the drug (Merck and Schering-Plough, who've since merged) waited almost two years before releasing it.

No wonder. The results stunk. Which was the *other* reason this drug test made the front pages.

The new "wonder" drug lowered cholesterol just fine. In fact, it lowered it *better* than a standard statin drug. So you'd think everyone would be jumping for joy, right? Lower cholesterol, lower heart disease, let's have a party for the shareholders.

Um, not quite. Although the people taking Vytorin saw their cholesterol levels plummet, they actually had *more* plaque growth than the people taking the standard cholesterol drug. The patients on Vytorin had almost twice as great an increase in the thickness of their arterial walls, a result you definitely don't want to see if you're trying to prevent heart disease.

So their cholesterol was wonderfully lowered and their risk for heart disease went up—shades of "the operation was a success but the patient died."

There are countless other examples, many of which we'll discuss later on, but let's just mention one of them right now. It's known as the Nurses' Health Study, and it's one of the longest-running studies of diet and disease ever undertaken. Conducted by Harvard University, the study has followed more than 120,000 females since the mid-1970s to determine risk factors for cancer and heart disease.[6] In an exhaustive analysis of 84,129 of these women, published in the *New England Journal of Medicine*,[7] five factors were identified that significantly lowered the risk for heart disease. In fact, wrote the authors,

"Eighty-two percent of coronary events in the study . . . could be attributed to lack of adherence to (these five factors)."

Are you ready for the five factors?

1. Don't smoke.
2. Drink alcohol in moderation.
3. Engage in moderate-to-vigorous exercise for at least half an hour a day on average.
4. Maintain a healthy weight (BMI under 25).
5. Eat a wholesome, low-glycemic (low-sugar) diet with plenty of omega-3 fats and fiber.

Wait, didn't they miss something? Where's the part about lowering cholesterol?

Oh. It's not there. Never mind.

Of course, there's not roughly $30 billion plus a year to be made peddling that advice (a number that represents the gross revenue from statin drugs alone), and popping a pill is a lot easier than changing your lifestyle, but there it is. The inconvenient fact that lowering cholesterol has almost *no effect* on extending life is simply ignored by the special interests that profit enormously from keeping you in the dark.

As the writer Upton Sinclair said, "It is very difficult to get a man to understand something, when his salary depends upon his not understanding it."

CHAPTER 2

"CHOLESTEROL IS HARMLESS!"

NOW LET'S TALK ABOUT YOU FOR A MOMENT.

Unless you're just an information junkie, there's a good chance that you're reading this book because you have something at stake here. Let us guess: You're concerned about *your* cholesterol.

Maybe you're a woman whose doctor has read you the riot act because your cholesterol is approaching 300 mg/dL, and your doc has convinced you that you'll drop dead of a heart attack if you don't go on medication right away.

Maybe you're a middle-aged man who has already had a heart attack, and your doctor is adamant about putting you on a cholesterol-lowering drug.

Or maybe you're a fit guy in your sixties whose cholesterol is 240 mg/dL and whose doctor is "worried" about that number.

However, only *one* of the three hypothetical cases listed above has any business being on a cholesterol-lowering drug. Can you guess which one? Don't worry: By the time you finish this book, you'll not only know the answer, you'll also know a heck of a lot more about cholesterol than most doctors in America. And, no, we don't make that statement lightly.

CHOLESTEROL BASICS

Cholesterol is a waxy substance–technically a *sterol*–that is an important constituent of cell membranes. The vast majority of cholesterol in the body is made in the liver, while the rest is absorbed from the diet.

Cholesterol is the basic raw material that your body uses to make vitamin D; sex hormones such as estrogen, progesterone, and testosterone; and the bile acids needed for digestion. Cholesterol travels in particles called lipoproteins, the most common of which are high-density lipoproteins (HDL) and low-density lipoproteins (LDL).

Below we address the long-held, conventional views on cholesterol basics that we believe to be outdated.

WHAT IS HDL?

Old School

HDL is considered "good" cholesterol because it helps remove so-called "bad" cholesterol, LDL. When measured, HDL levels should be as high as possible, preferably 60 milligrams per deciliter of blood (mg/dL) and above. Maintaining a healthy weight, physical activity, and a diet that includes healthy fats like olive oil are believed to keep HDL levels high.

New School

HDL is much more tightly controlled by genetics than LDL. A 2011 study from the National Institutes of Health, AIM-HIGH, found that raising HDL did nothing to protect against heart attacks, strokes, or death. And all HDL is not the same. HDL-2 particles are large and buoyant and the most protective. HDL-3 particles, on the other hand, are small and dense and may be inflammatory. HDL-2 is anti-inflammatory and anti-atherogenic (atherosclerosis being the condition in which an artery wall thickens from the accumulation of fatty materials, called plaque, induced by inflammation, inhibiting blood flow from the heart). HDL-3, on the other hand, is poorly understood. You want to have higher levels of HDL-2 than HDL-3.

The "New School" generally agrees that higher levels of HDL are desirable, but research is concentrating on the *function* of HDL subtypes rather than the total amount. Daniel Rader, M.D., director of preventive cardiology at the University of Pennsylvania, wrote in the *New England*

(continued on page 30)

Journal of Medicine, "Recent scientific findings have directed increasing interest toward the concept that measures of the function of HDL, rather than simply its level in the blood, might be more important to assessing cardiovascular risk and evaluating new HDL-targeting therapies."

WHAT IS LDL?

Old School

LDL is "bad" cholesterol because it can build up in the arteries, impeding blood flow. Its levels should be kept low. Current standards are 100 to 129 mg/dL, with lower than 100 being the target for those at risk for heart disease, and lower than 70 being the target for people at very high risk. Too much saturated fat in the diet, inactivity, and being overweight are considered to raise LDL levels.

New School

All LDL is not the same. LDL-A is a buoyant, fluffy molecule that does no harm whatsoever as long as it is not damaged by oxidation (a process caused by free radicals that enables cholesterol to form plaque). LDL-B is a small, hard, dense, molecule that promotes atherosclerosis. A pattern of high LDL-A is the most beneficial. Blood tests today can also measure the number of LDL-A and LDL-B particles.

The most important cholesterol particle of all, which conventional tests do not focus on, is Lp(a). Lp(a) is a very small, highly inflammatory particle that is thrombogenic (blood clotting). Dr. Sinatra calls it "the alpha wolf" of cholesterol particles. In a healthy body, low Lp(a) levels aren't much of a problem. Lp(a) circulates and carries out repair and restoration work on damaged blood vessels. However, the more repairs you need on your arteries, the more Lp(a) is utilized. Lp(a) concentrates at the site of damage, binds with a couple of amino acids within the wall of a damaged blood vessel, dumps its LDL cargo, and starts to promote the deposition of oxidized LDL into the wall, leading to more inflammation and ultimately to plaque.

Also, Lp(a) promotes the formation of blood clots on top of the newly formed plaque, which narrows the blood vessels further.

HOW CHOLESTEROL IS MEASURED

Old School

A standard blood test will tell you your total cholesterol level and your HDL and LDL levels.

New School

Measure cholesterol with the newer particle tests, which tell you how much of your LDL is type A and how much of your LDL is type B (see chapter 9 for more information). Measure the *number* of actual particles, and the amount of the potentially dangerous Lp(a). That is the only information that matters.

DIETARY ADVICE

Old School

Eat less 300 mg of cholesterol a day and eat less than 10 percent of calories as saturated fat.

New School

According to the Framingham Heart Study, people who consumed the most cholesterol in their diets did not have any higher blood cholesterol levels than those who consumed the least amount. The effect of dietary cholesterol on blood (serum) cholesterol is very variable and individual, and for most people—though not all—the effect of dietary cholesterol on serum cholesterol is insignificant.

In any case, because cholesterol is not as important a risk factor for heart disease as once believed, it doesn't matter very much. Saturated fat raises cholesterol, but it raises overall HDL cholesterol and the *good* part of LDL cholesterol (LDL-A) far more than it raises the bad part of LDL cholesterol (LDL-B). There is no evidence that supports a *direct* relationship between saturated fat and heart disease.

RELATIONSHIP TO HEART DISEASE

Old School

High levels of cholesterol are an important risk factor for heart disease because cholesterol builds up in the arteries, inhibiting blood flow from the heart.

New School

Cholesterol is a relatively minor player in heart disease and a poor predictor of heart attacks. More than half of all people who are hospitalized with heart attacks have perfectly normal cholesterol levels.

When the National Cholesterol Education Program lowered the "optimal" cholesterol levels in 2004, eight out of nine people on the panel had financial ties to the pharmaceutical industry.

Besides the fact that you're concerned about your cholesterol, there are two other things we can assume. One, you don't tend to blindly follow recommendations without doing your own research. (If you did, you'd simply be following your doctor's orders and have no interest in reading this book.)

The second thing we're pretty sure about you is that you're smarter than the average reader.

Here's why:

To understand the cholesterol myth—and to fully appreciate how the health advice that follows from the myth is obsolete—you'll need to know a lot more about cholesterol than the average person knows. But reading—and understanding—the full story of cholesterol, including the myths, misconceptions, outright lies, and misguided medical practices, doesn't make for easy reading. It'll take quite a bit more intelligence, motivation, and perseverance than, say, reading the latest romance paperback.

The cholesterol story touches on not only medicine and research but also politics, economics, psychology, and sociology. It's got a cast of characters ranging from the obnoxious and egotistical to the well-meaning and misguided.

It has heroes and villains, mavericks and tradition-alists, all engaged in a battle that, sadly, has little to do with saving lives (though it may have started out that way). It involves staggering amounts of money, the politics of publication, the sociology of belief (why bad ideas continue to survive past their expiration dates), and the revolving door that exists between government advisory committees and the industries they're supposed to police. (Example: When the National Cholesterol Education Program lowered the "optimal" cholesterol levels in 2004, eight out of nine people on the panel had financial ties to the pharmaceutical industry, most of them to the manufacturers of cholesterol-lowering drugs who would subsequently reap immediate benefits from these same recommendations.)

By now it should be pretty clear that neither of us buys into the myth that cholesterol is the proper target for the prevention of heart disease. But how did the myth get started in the first place? How, exactly, did cholesterol and saturated fat come to be branded as the twin demons of heart disease?

To answer that question, we need to go back to 1953, when a young, ambitious biologist named Ancel Keys proposed the then-radical theory that heart disease was caused by too much fat in the diet.

THE BIRTH OF THE DIET-HEART HYPOTHESIS

It's hard to imagine that this theory was radical given how widespread its acceptance is today, but at the time the prevailing wisdom was that diet had little to do with heart disease. But Keys felt he was on to something.

Previous research by Russian scientists had shown that when you fed rabbits large amounts of cholesterol and then dissected them later on, their arteries were filled with cholesterol-containing plaque and looked suspiciously like the arteries of people who died of heart disease. Never mind the inconvenient fact that rabbits are herbivores. The amount of cholesterol they normally get in their diets is pretty close to zero. Other animals, such as rats and baboons, do *not* react in the same way as rabbits to a high-cholesterol diet, and they metabolize cholesterol very differently. Even Keys himself understood that cholesterol in the diet was of no importance. In 1997, he stated, "There's no connection whatsoever between cholesterol in food and cholesterol in blood. And we've known that all along. Cholesterol in the diet doesn't matter at all unless you happen to be a chicken or a rabbit."

Yet the admonition to eat "no more than 300 mg of cholesterol" a day remains the advice of every major health organization to this day, despite the fact that even the scientist most responsible for popularizing the diet-heart hypothesis thought it was ridiculous.

Inconvenient facts to the contrary, excess cholesterol in the *blood*, not the diet, seemed to Keys to be a likely culprit in the development of heart disease.

Since fat in the diet and cholesterol in the blood were believed to be linked, this led Keys to investigate fat in the diet and its connection to heart disease. He looked at data on fat consumption and heart disease from various countries and published the results of his famous study, the Seven Countries Study, which supposedly demonstrated a clear link between the amount of dietary fat consumed and the incidence of heart disease. Those countries eating the most fat also had the highest rates of heart disease. Sounds like an open-and-shut case against dietary fat, doesn't it?

Except it was anything but. When Keys published the results of his study, he actually had available to him reliable food consumption data from twenty-two countries, but he used only seven. By hand-selecting the seven countries that supported his preconceived hypothesis, Keys was able to make a convincing case that there was a direct connection between dietary fat and heart disease.

The fact that Keys had chosen to include only seven countries and ignored the other fifteen didn't exactly go unnoticed. Many researchers criticized Keys for conveniently omitting data that didn't support his theory. Researchers analyzing the data from all twenty-two countries found that the correlation between fat, cholesterol, and heart disease literally vanished.

One of the researchers who questioned Keys was a British doctor named John Yudkin from the University of London. He found that there were countries where the intake of fat was virtually the same, but the rates of cardiovascular disease were vastly different. For example, Finland was one of the

> Yudkin's much more comprehensive data showed that the single dietary factor that had the strongest association with coronary heart disease was—wait for it—*sugar.*

countries used by Keys to make his case, because Finland had a high per capita fat intake and a high rate of heart disease. But Yudkin found that the people of West Germany ate the exact same amount of fat as the people of Finland, but they had about one-third the rate of heart disease. The paradox was even more pronounced in the Netherlands and Switzerland, which also had only one-third the rate of heart disease seen in Finland, even though the Dutch and Swiss consumed even *more* fat than the Finns.

Yudkin did a far more extensive analysis of dietary factors than Keys did. He looked at fat as a percentage of calories. He looked at different types of fats. He even looked at the roles of carbohydrates and protein. And instead of confirming Keys's hypothesis, Yudkin's much more comprehensive data showed that the single dietary factor that had the strongest association with coronary heart disease was—wait for it—*sugar.*

So back to Keys. By all accounts, Keys was a very smart and well-liked man who just happened to be dead wrong on the cholesterol and fat issue. But he was hardly without ambition and ego. Known for being blunt and biting, he presented his theory on fat, cholesterol, and heart disease to a distinguished audience in 1954, when the World Health Organization

(WHO) held its first expert committee on the pathogenesis of atherosclerosis. One of his longtime collaborators, Henry Blackburn, recalled that Keys was stunned to find that his ideas were not accepted on the spot. One participant asked him to cite the principle piece of evidence for his diet-heart theory, and he was caught, to put it mildly, off guard. "Ancel fell into a trap, he made a mistake," Blackburn said. "He cited a piece of evidence, and they were able to destroy it. He got up from being knocked to the ground and went out saying, 'I'll show those guys,' and designed the Seven Countries Study."[3]

The Seven Countries Study[4] is actually the cornerstone of current cholesterol and fat recommendations and official government policy, so it's worth looking at in some detail. Keys examined saturated fat consumption in seven countries, and, lo and behold, he found a straight-line relationship between heart disease, cholesterol levels, and saturated fat intake—exactly what he had hoped to find.

The seven countries were Italy, Greece, the former Yugoslavia, the Netherlands, Finland, the United States, and Japan. It hardly went unnoticed that Keys chose only the countries that fit his hypothesis. He easily could have chosen a different group of countries and proven a completely different hypothesis.

In fact, British physician Malcolm Kendrick, M.D., did exactly that. Kendrick used the same data available to Keys and quickly discovered that if you simply chose different countries, you could easily prove that the *more* saturated fat and cholesterol people consumed, the *lower* their risk of heart disease.[5]

Anticipating a challenge to his "proof" by defenders of the cholesterol hypothesis, Kendrick pointed out that he was merely doing exactly what Keys did—hand-selecting data that would prove his theory. "What do you mean I can't choose my own countries?" he asked sarcastically. "That's not fair. Keys did!"[6]

Cherry-picking the countries that proved this theory was only one of the many problems with the Seven Countries Study. There were tremendous variations in heart mortality within these countries, even though saturated fat consumption was identical. In Finland, for example, the intake of saturated fat was almost identical in two population groups from Turku and North Karelia. But heart mortality was three times higher in North Karelia. Similarly, saturated fat intake was also equal on two Greek islands, Crete and Corfu. But heart mortality was a whopping seventeen times higher on Corfu than it was on Crete.[7]

How did Keys explain these facts, which were clearly present in his data?

Simple. He ignored them.

Keys was a member of the nutrition advisory committee of the American Heart Association, so despite the flaws in his study, he managed to get his theories officially incorporated into the 1961 American Heart Association dietary guidelines,[8] where they have influenced government policy on heart disease, fat consumption, and cholesterol for decades.

At the time, Keys's theories about fat and cholesterol weren't exactly widely known outside scientific circles, and the whole theoretical fight between the advocates of the "sugar" hypothesis and the advocates of the "fat" hypothesis was all so much ivory-tower name-calling, well out of the earshot of the general public. But all that was about to change.

And the man who was indirectly responsible for that change was, interestingly, not a scientist at all but a politician named George McGovern.

The Politics of Science

McGovern, chairman of the Senate Select Committee on Nutrition and Human Needs, practically changed the national policy on nutrition in this country. And they were directly responsible for transforming the idea that dietary fat causes heart disease from a not-so-solid hypothesis into solidified dogma.

McGovern's committee instituted a wonderful series of landmark federal food assistance programs, but its work on malnutrition started to wind down around the mid-1970s. McGovern's committee staffers, notably its general counsel, Marshall Matz, and staff director, Alan Stone, both lawyers, decided to go for broke and take on the reverse side of the malnutrition coin: *overnutrition*. "It was a casual endeavor," Matz said. "We really were totally naive, a bunch of kids who just thought, 'Hell, we should say something on this subject before we go out of business.'"[9]

The committee listened to two days of expert testimony in 1976 and then assigned a young writer

◀ **WHAT YOU NEED TO KNOW**

- The theory that fat and cholesterol cause heart disease became widely accepted *despite* much evidence to the contrary. This evidence deserves to be reexamined. The case needs to be reopened.
- Many doctors did *not* agree with the cholesterol myth and questioned the science upon which it was based.
- The studies upon which the cholesterol myth was based were later found to be problematic.
- The adoption of the cholesterol myth by mainstream organizations and the government had a strong political component to it.

named Nick Mottern to write the whole thing up. The only problem was that Mottern didn't know anything about nutrition and health and had no science writing background to boot. So he did what any smart young writer would do: He went to the experts for guidance.

Except in this case, Mottern didn't actually go to the "experts"; he went to one *particular* expert, Mark Hegsted, a Harvard nutritionist, and relied almost exclusively on Hegsted's interpretation of the testimony, as well as on Hegsted's own personal recommendations.

Hegsted was a fervent believer in the emerging theory that low-fat diets would prevent heart disease and that fat and cholesterol were the spawn of Satan.

Whoops.

So Mottern wrote up the committee's recommendations with Hegsted as the final authority—no more than 30 percent of calories from fat, no more than 10 percent of calories from saturated fat—and in 1977 the committee disbanded. But right around that time, a newly appointed assistant secretary at the U.S. Department of Agriculture (USDA) named Carol Tucker Foreman decided that the USDA ought to *do* something with these recommendations. Like make them official policy! The only problem was that she needed some good scientific cover.

Fair enough. Foreman wasn't a scientist herself, but she sure had access to some good ones. So she went to the president of the National Academy of Sciences (NAS), Philip Handler, a distinguished expert in human metabolism.

Want to know what he told her?

The anti-fat dietary goals written by Mottern were utter and complete nonsense.

Well.

So Foreman did what other good officials would do when they don't like the advice they're getting. She went to someone else.

Can you guess whom she went to?

Hegsted. The champion of the low-fat, low-cholesterol eating plan who had practically written the guidelines in the first place.

Not surprisingly, Hegsted had an entirely different opinion from Handler. With cover from Hegsted, the USDA was able to release *Using the Dietary Guidelines for Americans*, a low-fat, low-cholesterol manifesto that echoed exactly the same anti-fat, anti-cholesterol sentiments written in the original Mottern–Hegsted document put out by the McGovern committee.

What happened next makes the backstabbing antics of the television show *Survivor* look like child's play.

The National Academy of Sciences Food and Nutrition Board, not happy with the USDA report, issued its own set of guidelines titled *Toward Healthful Diets*. Here's the *Reader's Digest* condensed version of what it said: "Don't worry about fat."

This pretty much directly contradicted the report of the USDA, which had recommended very specific fat intakes: less than 30 percent of total calories from fat and less than 10 percent from saturated fat.

The USDA didn't take this slap in the face sitting down and leaked reports to the press saying that the chairman of the NAS Food and Nutrition Board and one of the board's members had financial ties to the food industry, as if this were enough to explain why the board as a whole didn't endorse the USDA recommendations to avoid fat. The beef and dairy industries went nuts and lobbied with all their might against the recommendations, calling them unjustified by science. But the die had been cast. In the current political climate, the "fat cat" cattle ranchers reminded folks of the tobacco industry, which had responded in much the same way when cigarettes first came under attack. Meanwhile, the grain lobbyists, as you can imagine, were in heaven.

The media had a field day, and they were not kind to the NAS. Mainstream apologist Jane Brody, who has written about food and nutrition for the *New York Times* for decades, accused the NAS board members of being "all in the pockets of the industries being hurt."[10] And because everyone on both sides of the argument had enormous amounts of money at stake, the debate between the beef industry and the grain industry was hardly a model of scientific objectivity. It was far more about image and public relations: The fat cat ranchers were portrayed as peddling unhealthy, "high-fat," "artery-clogging" foods, while the grain farmers were seen as the "good guys," on the side of science, health, granola, and the well-being of the American people. High-carb, low-fat cereals became the new health food, while high-fat meats were seen as poison, peddled by greedy cattle ranchers indifferent to the health of America. Basically, the anti-fat movement didn't evolve out of science at all, but instead was a grassroots movement fueled by a distrust of the "establishment"–Big Food, Big Medicine, and Big Ranchers. It was also fueled by the countercultural bias against excessive consumption, represented in this case by big, fatty steaks and bacon and eggs.

We all know who won that public relations battle.

Think it's a coincidence that the obesity and diabetes epidemics went into overdrive around the same time that we started pushing low-fat, high-carb diets as an alternative to those containing more fat and protein? We don't.

The Snackwell Phenomenon

Low-fat had become the new mantra of the times, something we like to call the "Snackwell Phenomenon." Food companies rushed to create low-fat versions of every food imaginable, all marketed as "heart-healthy," with no cholesterol. (No one seemed to notice that manufacturers *replaced* the missing fat with tons of sugar and processed carbs, both of which are far more dangerous to our hearts than fat ever was.)

Butter was demonized and replaced with margarine, one of the most supremely stupid nutritional swap-outs in recent memory. Only much later did we discover that the supposedly healthier margarine was laden with trans fats, a really bad kind of fat created by using a kind of turkey baster to inject hydrogen atoms into a liquid (unsaturated) fat, making it more solid and giving it a longer shelf life. (Any time you read "partially hydrogenated oil" or "hydrogenated oil" in a list of ingredients, that means the food in question contains trans fats.) Unlike saturated fats from whole foods such as butter, trans fats (at least the manmade kind) actually *do* increase the risk for heart disease and strokes!

About 80 percent of trans fats in the American diet come from factory-produced partially hydrogenated vegetable oil.[11] Yet vegetable oils were (and are!) aggressively promoted as the healthy alternative to saturated fats, even though most of these oils are highly processed, pro-inflammatory, and easily damaged when reheated over and over again, which is standard procedure in many restaurants.

Think it's a coincidence that the obesity and diabetes epidemics went into overdrive around the same time that we started pushing low-fat, high-carb diets as an alternative to those containing more fat and protein? We don't.

But by now, fat—and, by extension, cholesterol—had become the new bogeyman of the American diet, defended only by people who clearly had a horse in the race (e.g., the dairy and meat industries), and low-fat had become the new religion of the masses. Now it was left for the science to catch up. The National Institutes of Health (NIH) funded half a dozen studies that were published between 1980 and 1984, hoping it would find persuasive evidence that low-fat diets prolonged lives.

Did they?

Not exactly.

Let's Go to the Videotape

The first four of these trials compared heart disease rates and diets in four locations: Honolulu, Puerto Rico, Chicago, and, most famously, Framingham, Massachusetts. Not *one* of these trials showed the slightest evidence that men who ate low-fat diets lived any longer, or had fewer heart attacks, than those who ate high-fat diets.

The fifth trial was the MRFIT study, a research project that cost $115 million and involved twenty-eight medical centers and 250 researchers. In the MRFIT study, 360,000 men, aged thirty-five to fifty-seven, from eighteen different U.S. cities were screened between 1973 and 1977, and eventually about 13,000 middle-aged, healthy men who were considered especially prone to heart disease were selected to participate. These 13,000 men were randomly assigned to one of two groups. The control group received no special instructions about diet or lifestyle and just continued on with whatever general medical care they received from their doctors. The intervention group, however, was urged to avoid eating fat, to quit smoking, to exercise, and to lower their blood pressure.

After seven years of follow-up, the intervention group had slightly lower blood pressure and cholesterol than the control group, but there was *no difference* in either cardiovascular mortality or all-cause mortality (scientific lingo for "total number of deaths no matter what the reason"). The intervention group had 17.9 deaths per one thousand men from cardiovascular disease, and the control group had 19.3 deaths per one thousand men, a variation that did not amount to what researchers call *statistical significance*, meaning it was likely due to chance.[12]

In addition, the data on overall mortality—death from any cause—was troubling. There were actually *more* deaths in the intervention group—from any cause—than there were in the control group! Remember, the real reason we want to avoid heart disease is so we can live longer; avoiding heart disease isn't much of a victory if it means you die early from some other disease!

The researchers themselves described the results as "disappointing." The only *real* reduction in overall mortality was seen with the people who stopped smoking, regardless of the group they were in.[13]

Leaping to the Wrong Conclusion

The sixth of the NIH-funded trials, the Lipid Research Clinics Coronary Primary Prevention Trial (LRC-CPPT), which was initiated in 1973, is worth mentioning because of an interesting leap of faith made by the investigators based on virtually no evidence. But this leap of faith became the cornerstone of anti-fat policy for decades to come. Here's what happened.

Researchers from the National Heart, Lung, and Blood Institute measured cholesterol in almost one-third of a million middle-aged men and chose only those with the highest cholesterol levels for the study (about 4,000 men). They gave half of them a new cholesterol-lowering drug (cholestyramine), while the other half got a placebo. The medicine did indeed lower cholesterol levels in the men who had abnormally high levels to begin with, and it modestly reduced heart disease rates in the process. (The

WHAT THE FRAMINGHAM HEART STUDY FOUND

One study mentioned most often by the defenders of the cholesterol theory is the Framingham Heart Study. This long-running research study started back in 1948 and monitored heart disease in more than 5,000 residents of Framingham, Massachusetts. After following up for sixteen years, the researchers claimed to find a direct correlation between heart disease and cholesterol levels.

But God is in the details. As it turned out, the group of Framingham residents who developed heart disease and the group of Framingham residents who didn't had similar ranges of cholesterol levels. In fact, the *average* cholesterol level of the heart disease group was only 11 percent higher than that of the group *without* heart disease. Cardiovascular disease struck people with cholesterol levels as low as 150 mg/dL. Low cholesterol, according to this study, was hardly a guarantee of a healthy heart.

It gets better (or worse, depending on your position). When researchers went back and looked at the Framingham data thirty years after the project started, they found that once men passed the age of forty-seven, it didn't make a whit of difference whether their cholesterol was low or high.[14] Those with high cholesterol at age forty-eight lived just as long as, or *longer* than, those who had low cholesterol. So if cholesterol is important only for the relatively few who have had a heart attack before the age of forty-eight, why are the rest of us worried about high-fat food and cholesterol levels?

The question is hardly academic. In 1992, forty-four years after the Framingham project began, study director William Castelli, M.D., wrote the following in an editorial in the *Archives of Internal Medicine*:

"In Framingham, Mass., the *more* saturated fat one ate, the *more* cholesterol one ate, the *more* calories one ate, the *lower* the person's serum cholesterol . . . we found that people who ate the *most* cholesterol, ate the *most* saturated fat, [and] ate the *most* calories weighed the least and were the most physically active [italics ours]."[15]

probability of suffering a heart attack during the seven to eight years of the study went from 8.6 percent in the placebo group to 7 percent in the group treated with cholestyramine, while the probability of dying from a heart attack dropped from 2 to 1.6 percent, not exactly jaw-dropping numbers.[16])

Okay, cholesterol goes down, heart disease drops by a thimble, and the researchers conclude that lowering cholesterol lowers the risk of heart disease. But remember, this was a *drug* trial, not a *diet* trial. The researchers made a huge leap of faith by assuming that if lowering cholesterol is "good" (i.e., it reduces the risk of heart disease), it shouldn't much matter *how* you lower it. Lowering it through diet should get you the same "good" result (if you can call the miniscule drop in heart disease that may or may not be related to the drop in cholesterol a "good" result). Their leap of faith was that we should recommend low-fat diets because they will achieve the same result as the drug—cholesterol will go down and everyone will live happily ever after.

But drugs often have many effects in addition to their main purpose. (Remember, Viagra was originally designed as a blood pressure medication!) The drug used in the LRC-CPPT might also have had some good effects, such as lowering inflammation, for example. Assuming that lowering cholesterol with a low-fat diet was identical to lowering it with a multifaceted medication that could in fact have had unintended benefits was a complete leap of faith and led to the wholesale recommendation of a low-fat diet for the prevention of heart disease.

That same year, the NIH held what's called a "consensus conference" to basically justify the LRC-CPPT and the dietary recommendations that came out of it, yet it was anything but a consensus. Several experts pointed to significant defects in the studies and even called into question their accuracy. But you'd never know it from the final report, which made it seem like everyone had unquestioningly hitched their collective stars to the low-fat bandwagon.

Well, not exactly everyone.

CONSENSUS? NOT EXACTLY

George Mann, M.D., associate professor of biochemistry at Vanderbilt University College of Medicine and a participating researcher in the Framingham Heart Study, was one of the doubters.

The diet-heart idea is the "greatest scam" in the history of medicine, he said. "[Researchers] have held repeated press conferences bragging about this cataclysmic breakthrough, which the study directors claim shows that lowering cholesterol lowers the frequency of coronary disease. They have manipulated the data to reach the wrong conclusions."[17]

Mann also declared that NIH managers "used Madison Avenue hype to sell this failed trial in the way that media people sell an underarm deodorant!"[18]

Michael Oliver, a highly respected British cardiologist, concurred. "The panel of jurists . . . was selected to include experts who would, predictably, say that . . . all levels of blood cholesterol in the United States are too high and should be lowered. Of course, this is exactly what was said."[19]

But the dissenting voices met with radio silence. With pompous certainty, the committee made clear in its final report that low-fat diets would afford significant protection against coronary heart disease for men, women, and children over two years old. "The evidence justifies . . . the reduction of calories from fat . . . to 30 percent, calories from saturated fat to 10 percent or less, and dietary cholesterol to no more than 250 to 300 mg daily," it declared.[20]

As Dr. Phil might ask, "And how's that workin' for you?"

One study that attempted to answer this hypothetical question was the Women's Health Initiative, the same program that has suggested that hormone therapy after menopause has more risks than benefits. This $415-million NIH study involved close to 49,000 people, aged fifty to seventy-nine, who were followed for eight years in an attempt to answer the question, "Does a low-fat diet reduce the risk of getting heart disease or cancer?"[21]

They got their answer.

"The largest study ever to ask whether a low-fat diet reduces the risk of getting cancer or heart disease has found that the diet has no effect," the New York Times reported in 2006.[22]

"These studies are revolutionary," said Jules Hirsch, M.D., physician-in-chief emeritus at the Rockefeller University in New York City and an expert on how diets influence weight and health. The studies "should put a stop to this era of thinking that we have all the information we need to change the whole national diet and make everybody healthy."[23]

Of course, none of these questionable findings stopped the cholesterol-lowering, fat-avoiding juggernaut that went into full swing in the late 1970s and continues, albeit bruised and battered, to this day. And we have to give the misguided researchers kudos for their motives—by reducing cholesterol levels, they sincerely believed they would be reducing heart disease. As Dwight Lundell, M.D., author of *The Cure for Heart Disease*, wryly put it, "They were taking the bull by the horn—but it was the wrong bull."[24]

When we first met about this project, Steve brought to the meeting a series of papers by one of the most respected researchers in the world, Michel de Lorgeril, M.D., a French cardiologist and researcher at the prestigious National Centre for Scientific Research, the largest public organization for scientific research in France.

De Lorgeril has authored dozens of papers in peer-reviewed journals, and he was the lead researcher for the Lyon Diet Heart Study. The following quotation comes from his only book written in English, and it's a perfect way to end this chapter:

"We can summarize . . . in one sentence: *Cholesterol is harmless* [italics ours]!"[25]

CHAPTER 3

INFLAMMATION: THE TRUE CAUSE OF HEART DISEASE

SO IF CHOLESTEROL *ISN'T* THE CAUSE OF HEART DISEASE, what is?

We know you don't want to wait any longer, so here's the short answer: The primary cause of heart disease is *inflammation*.

The subject of inflammation will be a running theme throughout this book for reasons that will soon be made clear, but the first thing you need to know about inflammation is this: It comes in two flavors. You're probably already familiar with one of them, but it's the one you're *less* familiar with that's at the core of heart disease.

Let us explain.

Almost all of us have experience with *acute* inflammation. It happens every time you stub your toe, bang your knee, or get a splinter in your finger. When you complain about your aching back, an abscess in your mouth, or a rash on your skin, that's acute inflammation. It's visible and uncomfortable, if not downright painful. The redness on your skin is a result of blood that's rushed to the affected area. The swelling you experience is the result of an army of specialized cells (with names like *phagocytes* and *lymphocytes)* dispatched by the immune system to mend the injured area. (The job of these immune system cells is to surround the site of the injury and neutralize nasty invaders such as microbes, preventing the spread of potential infection.) The swelling, redness, and soreness you experience as a result of acute inflammation are all natural accompaniments to the healing process.

So we all know about acute inflammation, most of us from personal experience. But the *other* flavor of inflammation, *chronic* inflammation, well, that's a whole different ball game.

Acute inflammation hurts, but chronic inflammation kills.

WHY YOU SHOULD CARE ABOUT CHRONIC INFLAMMATION, NOT CHOLESTEROL

Chronic inflammation flies beneath the pain radar. Much like high blood pressure, it has no obvious symptoms. Yet chronic inflammation is a significant component of virtually every single degenerative condition, including Alzheimer's, diabetes, obesity, arthritis, cancer, neurodegenerative diseases, chronic lower respiratory disease, influenza and pneumonia, chronic liver and kidney diseases, and, most especially, heart disease.

A BETTER WAY TO PREDICT HEART DISEASE

Want a much better way to tell whether you're at risk? Look at these two line items on your blood test: triglycerides and HDL (the so-called "good" cholesterol).

Now if you're not too freaked out about doing a bit of math, calculate the ratio of your triglycerides to your HDL. If, for example, your triglycerides are 150 mg/dL and your HDL is 50 mg/dL, you have a ratio of 3 (150:50). If your triglycerides are 100 mg/dL and your HDL is 50 mg/dL, you have a ratio of 2 (100:50).

This ratio is a far better predictor of heart disease than cholesterol ever was. In one study out of Harvard published in *Circulation*, a journal published by the American Heart Association, those who had the highest triglyceride-to-HDL ratios had a whopping sixteen times the risk of developing heart disease as those with the lowest ratios.[1] If you have a ratio of around 2, you should be happy, indeed, regardless of your cholesterol levels. (A ratio of 5, however, is problematic.)

When chronic inflammation exists unchecked in the cardiovascular system, it usually spells big trouble for the heart.

And inflammation is rarely a local phenomenon. For instance, women with rheumatoid arthritis, a highly inflammatory condition that primarily affects the joints, wind up having double the risk of a heart attack when compared to women without it. Microbes that cause problems in one part of the body can easily migrate to other areas and cause inflammatory damage there. An infection that starts in the gums, for example, can easily leak bacteria into the bloodstream, bacteria that may then find fertile ground in a weakened arterial wall and fan the fires of inflammation there.

So how exactly does inflammation happen, and, more importantly, what can we do about it?

OXIDATION:
THE INITIATOR OF INFLAMMATION

In *The Most Effective Ways to Live Longer*, Dr. Jonny introduced the concept of the "Four Horsemen of Aging." These Four Horsemen all contribute mightily to heart disease, and we'll go over all of them in the pages that follow. For those of you who just have to know *right now* what they are, here's the list: oxidation, inflammation, sugar, and stress. In this chapter, we'll concentrate on the first two.

One of the prime initiators of inflammation is *oxidation*. If you've ever seen rust on metal, you're familiar with oxidation (also known as *oxidative damage*), even if you didn't know the technical name for

it. You're also familiar with oxidation if you've ever left apple slices out on a picnic table where they were exposed to the air. They turned brown, didn't they? *That's* oxidative damage.

For those of you who don't remember high school chemistry (or would understandably prefer to forget it), electrons travel in pairs and orbit around atoms. Every so often one of those electrons gets "loose," and pandemonium ensues. The atom with the unpaired electron—known as a *free radical*—starts running around like a headless chicken trying to find its head. Free radicals are like college sophomores on spring break—temporarily free from the constraints of dormitory living, they basically go nuts and will "mate" with anyone! Free radicals "hit" on existing, stable pairs of electrons thousands of times a day, trying to find an electron they can pair-bond with and meanwhile, inflicting enormous damage upon your cells and DNA.

The free radicals that come from oxygen (known, not surprisingly, as *oxygen free radicals*) are the most deadly and damaging. (Now you know what the term "*anti*oxidants" means—it's a class of substances, including certain vitamins, minerals, and many plant chemicals, that helps neutralize free radicals, soaking them up like little sponges, thus limiting the damage they can do to your body. The reason cut apple slices don't turn brown so quickly when you squirt lemon juice on them is because lemon juice contains a fair amount of vitamin C, a powerful antioxidant.)

Free radicals are so important that in the mid-1950s a scientist named Denham Harman, M.D., Ph.D., put forth a theory called the Free Radical Theory of

Aging that remains popular to this day.[2] In it he basically proposes that aging is a kind of "rusting from within," largely due to the damage caused by oxygen free radicals.

Okay, hold that thought. We're going to come back to it. But before we go any further, let's look at the arteries, or more specifically the arterial walls, because that's where the damage starts.

Ground Zero for Damage: Introducing the Endothelium

The arterial walls are anything but hard and firm. They're composed of smooth muscle that expands and contracts like a mini accordion; they respond to the rhythm of the heart and accommodate the pulsing of the blood. These arteries—far from being a static system of tubes and pipes—are a living, breathing, *very* dynamic organ. And the innermost layer of the artery walls—the "interface," if you will, between the blood inside the arteries and the walls that contain it—is a central player in our little drama. This layer is called the *endothelium*—and it's the starting point for the damage that can ultimately lead to a heart attack.

Big word, endothelium, yes, not often bandied about in cocktail party chatter about heart disease, but it's one of the most important places in the arteries for

---

◀ WHAT YOU NEED TO KNOW

- Cholesterol is the parent molecule for sex hormones (estrogen, progesterone, and testosterone) as well as vitamin D and bile acids needed for digestion.
- The only time cholesterol is a problem is if it's *oxidized* (damaged).
- Damaged or oxidized LDL cholesterol sticks to the lining of the arteries and begins the process of inflammation.
- The true cause of heart disease is inflammation.
- Inflammation is initiated by damage from free radicals (oxidative stress).
- The concept of "good" and "bad" cholesterol is outdated.
- There are several types of LDL ("bad") cholesterol and several types of HDL ("good") cholesterol.
- It is far more important to know whether you have a pattern A or pattern B LDL cholesterol profile than to know your total amount of LDLs.
- A cholesterol level of 160 mg/dL or less has been linked to depression, aggression, cerebral hemorrhages, and loss of sex drive.

FOR MEN ONLY

Note to the men reading this: Endothelial dysfunction has the same acronym (ED) as another condition you may be familiar with or concerned about: erectile dysfunction. They're not unrelated. Our friend Mark Houston, M.D., director of the Hypertension Institute and an associate professor of medicine at Vanderbilt University, wryly commented, "I've never seen a case of ED (erectile dysfunction) that didn't also have ED (endothelial dysfunction)."

Bottom line: A healthy functioning endothelium is essential for . . . more things than just the heart!

you to know about because *that's* where the damage to your arteries starts. The endothelium is only one cell thick, but it's where a tremendous amount of biochemical activity takes place. There's even a name for the pathological state in which damage to that innermost layer exists—it's called *endothelial dysfunction*, and it's a key event in the development of heart disease.

Okay, we've introduced two important concepts here—oxidative damage and inflammation—and one important structure—the endothelium. Now we need to take a look at what cholesterol is and see how it fits into the whole picture. Once we do, we will return to the interaction among oxidation, inflammation, and the arterial walls.

"GOOD" AND "BAD" CHOLESTEROL: A COMPLETELY OUTDATED CONCEPT

Contrary to cholesterol's negative reputation, your body simply can't function without it. It's found in every single cell and is so essential that the lion's share of the cholesterol in your body is actually *made* by your body, specifically by the liver, which produces this fatty, waxy substance precisely *because* it is so essential to the health of your cells.

The cholesterol you eat has a minimal effect on your blood levels of cholesterol, which is why the admonition to eat less of it and the prominent listing of cholesterol on food nutrition labels are not as significant as we are led to believe they are. If you eat *less* cholesterol,

> Cholesterol's ability to fight toxins may be one reason why it's found at the site of arterial injuries caused by inflammation. But blaming cholesterol for those injuries is a little like blaming firemen for fire.

your liver will simply take up the slack and make more. If you eat *more* of it, the liver makes *less*. It is primarily, overwhelmingly made in the liver, though small amounts are made in other locations. For all intents and purposes, "manufacturing central" is the liver, and this is what responds to the "eat more/make less, eat less/make more" seesaw. The Framingham Heart Study found that there was virtually *no difference* in the amount of cholesterol consumed on a daily basis by those who went on to develop cardiovascular disease and those who did not. Egg-white omelet eaters, take note!

As we said earlier, cholesterol is the basic raw material that your body makes into vitamin D; sex hormones such as estrogen, progesterone, and testosterone; and the bile acids needed for digestion. The emphasis on lowering cholesterol as much as possible is not only misguided but also dangerous. Studies show that those at the lowest end of the cholesterol spectrum have a *significantly* increased risk of death from myriad conditions and situations unrelated to heart disease, including, but not limited to, cancer, suicide, and accidents.

Accidents and suicides? Really? Yes. Here's the connection: You need cholesterol to make brain cells.

A cholesterol level too low (around 160 mg/dL) has, in fact, been linked to depression, aggression, and cerebral hemorrhages. (The connection to sex drive will be discussed later in chapter 6—it's a doosey!)

The membranes of your cells contain a ton of cholesterol because it helps maintain their integrity and also facilitates cellular communication. The consistency of the cell membrane has to be just right—hard enough to act as a barrier to all sorts of molecular riff-raff but pliable and soft enough to allow access to the molecules that need to get inside. Essentially, you *need* cholesterol for memory. Lower cholesterol too much and it can easily promote a kind of global amnesia; with too little cholesterol in the cell membranes, nerve transmission can be affected. It's no surprise to us that Duane Graveline, M.D.–a former flight surgeon and astronaut who received international recognition for his research on zero gravity deconditioning–gave his book about the memory loss he experienced after taking statin drugs the ominous title *Lipitor: Thief of Memory*.

Cholesterol is also one of the important weapons your body uses to fight infections. It helps neutralize toxins produced by bacteria that swarm into the bloodstream from the gut when the immune system is weakened. When you have an infection, the total blood level of cholesterol goes up, but HDL (which we'll define in a moment) falls because it's being used up in the fight. Cholesterol's ability to fight toxins may be one reason why it's found at the site of arterial injuries caused by inflammation. But blaming cholesterol for those injuries is a little like blaming firemen for the fire.

Now here's an interesting fact of which you might not have been aware: It's actually impossible to measure cholesterol directly in the bloodstream. Being a fatty substance, cholesterol is not soluble in water or blood. So how does it get in the bloodstream? Simple. Your liver coats it with a "protein wrapper" and bundles it with a few other substances (such as triglycerides); packaging it in this protective shell allows it to enter your circulatory system, much like stones would float in the ocean if they were contained in a buoyant, waterproof container. In our case, the protein wrapper acts like a passport, allowing cholesterol to travel throughout your bloodstream. It's these packages, known as *lipoproteins*, that we actually measure when we measure our cholesterol levels.

We know these cholesterol-protein combinations as HDL (*high-density lipoprotein*) and LDL (*low-density lipoprotein*). Both contain cholesterol and triglycerides, but the percentages are different, and the two types of lipoproteins have different functions in the body. LDL, known as "bad" cholesterol, carries cholesterol to the cells that need it, while HDL, known as "good" cholesterol, picks up the excess and carries it back to the liver.

But this old idea of "good" and "bad" cholesterol is a wholly outdated concept.

We now know that there are many different "subtypes" of both HDL and LDL, and they do very different things. LDL, the imprecisely named "bad" cholesterol, has several different subtypes, and not all of them are bad at all—quite the contrary.

The most important subtypes of LDL are subtype A and subtype B. When most of your LDL is of the "A" type, you're said to have a *pattern A* cholesterol profile. When most of your LDL is of the "B" type, you're said to have a *pattern B* cholesterol profile. Simple, right? And absolutely essential to know for reasons soon to be made clear.

Subtype A is a big, fluffy molecule that looks like a cotton ball and does just about as much damage, which is to say none. Subtype B, however, is small, hard, and dense, like a BB gun pellet. It's the real bad actor in the system, because it's the one that becomes oxidized, sticks to the arterial walls, and starts the cascade of damage. Subtype B particles (what we might call the "bad" bad cholesterol) are atherogenic, meaning that they contribute significantly to heart disease. As we've already noted, big, fluffy LDL particles (the "good" bad cholesterol) are pretty much benign. Knowing you have a "high" LDL level is pretty much a useless piece of information *unless* you know how *much* of that LDL is the small, dense kind (harmful) and how much is the big, fluffy kind (not harmful in the least). Both of us would be totally comfortable having a high LDL number if the bulk of it was composed of the big, harmless, cotton ball-type molecules (the pattern A distribution). That's much more preferable than having a *lower* LDL number mostly composed of the BB gun pellet-type molecules (the pattern B distribution).

Unfortunately, most doctors are behind the times on this one. They look at that total LDL number—not the size and type—and if that number is even slightly higher than the lab says it should be, out comes the prescription pad. Pharmaceutical companies love when advisory committees—which are often heavily stacked with doctors who have financial ties to the pharmaceutical companies—recommend that we maintain lower and lower LDL levels, because that means a bigger and bigger market for cholesterol-lowering drugs. Sadly, most doctors do not perform the easily available tests—often covered by insurance—that determine your LDL.

You may recall from the first chapter that present-day health recommendations to reduce cholesterol by any means possible started with the Framingham Heart Study. In 1948, when the study began, cholesterol was only measured as "total" cholesterol. If you knew what your cholesterol was, you knew one specific number (200 mg/dL or 220 mg/dL, for example). As recently as 1961 we didn't have the technology to distinguish between "good" and "bad" cholesterol (HDL and LDL), much less the newer technology that allows us to zero in on different subtypes of the so-called "bad" cholesterol, which, as you can see, is far from being all "bad" after all.

Even HDL, the so-called "good" cholesterol, isn't *all* good. A study published in the December 2008 issue of the *FASEB Journal*, produced by the Federation of American Societies for Experimental Biology, challenged the conventional wisdom that simply having high levels of good cholesterol (HDL) and low levels of bad cholesterol (LDL) is necessary for good health. The researchers showed that even *good* cholesterol has varying degrees of quality and that *some* HDL cholesterol is actually bad news.

"For many years, HDL has been viewed as good cholesterol and has generated a false perception that the more HDL in the blood, the better," said the lead researcher, Angelo Scanu, M.D., of the University of Chicago.[3] "It is now apparent that subjects with high HDL levels are not necessarily protected from heart

Knowing you have a "high" LDL level is pretty much a useless piece of information unless you know *how much* of that LDL is the small, dense kind (harmful) and how much is the big, fluffy kind (not harmful in the least).

THE GOOD, THE BAD, AND THE REALLY, REALLY UGLY!

This just in: As of this writing, new research funded by the British Heart Foundation has uncovered still another subtype of LDL cholesterol that is particularly bad. It's called the *MGmin-low-density lipoprotein*, and it's more common in people with type 2 diabetes and in the elderly. It's "stickier" than normal LDL, which makes it much more likely to attach to the walls of the arteries.

This new "ultra-bad" boy is actually created by a process called glycation, which sharp-eyed readers will recall is one of the Four Horsemen of Aging. Glycation happens when there's too much sugar hanging around in the bloodstream. The excess sugar starts gumming up the works, inserting itself in places where it doesn't belong—in this case, the LDL molecule. (We'll have a lot more to say about sugar and its role in heart disease later on in chapter 4. Preview: Sugar is way more of a threat to your heart than fat ever was!)

problems and should ask their doctors to find out whether their HDL is good or bad." Scanu's study found that the HDL of people with chronic diseases such as rheumatoid arthritis and diabetes is very different than the HDL of healthy individuals, even when their blood levels of HDL are similar. Normal, "good" HDL cholesterol reduces inflammation; dysfunctional, "bad" HDL does not.

"This is yet one more line of research that explains why some people can have perfect cholesterol levels, but still develop cardiovascular disease," said Gerald Weissmann, M.D., editor-in-chief of the *FASEB Journal*. "Just as the discovery of good and bad cholesterol rewrote the book on cholesterol management, the realization that some of the 'good cholesterol' is actually *bad* will do the same."[4]

The point is that there is, indeed, "bad" cholesterol— even "*ultra*-bad" cholesterol—but simply using a shotgun pharmaceutical approach to lowering all cholesterol doesn't accomplish anything and has significant unwanted side effects, as we will see in chapter 6.

Now that the four main characters in our drama have been introduced—oxidation, inflammation, cholesterol, and the arterial walls—let's see how they interact in real life, and how they work together to create a dangerous situation for your heart.

WHEN LDL *REALLY* IS BAD FOR YOU: THE SMOKER'S PARADOX

Here's a riddle for you: Why is it that smokers with *normal* LDL (the so-called "bad" cholesterol) levels have a much higher risk of heart disease than nonsmokers with elevated LDL levels?

Sure, we all know how cigarette smoke damages the lungs, and that cigarette smoking significantly increases the odds of getting lung cancer. But, really, what's the connection between smoking and heart disease, or, more specifically, between smoking and LDL cholesterol?

Glad you asked.

Besides the harsh smoke, cigarettes also graciously provide your body with myriad toxic chemicals, all at no extra charge, thank you very much. These chemicals and toxins both constrict the blood vessels and harm the arterial walls. Specifically, they cause your LDL to become oxidized—damaged by the free radicals that are found in abundance in cigarette smoke! (And, by the way, it's not just cigarette smoke that can oxidize LDL. Heavy metals like mercury can do it, as can insecticides, radiation, and all manner of toxins in the environment, the air, and the food supply.)

And listen carefully now: LDL is *never* a problem in the body *until* it becomes oxidized. Only oxidized LDL sticks to the arterial walls, contributing to plaque and causing further inflammation and injury. Non-oxidized LDL is pretty much harmless. It's oxidation that actually initiates the process that culminates in atherosclerosis.

So a smoker with a low amount of LDL, *most* of which has been damaged by oxidation, is at far greater risk for heart disease than a nonsmoker with a much *higher* level of LDL, only a tiny percentage of which has been damaged. It's not the LDL that causes the problem—it's *damaged* (oxidized) LDL.

So LDL floats around in the bloodstream, delivering cholesterol to the cells that need it, and *some* of this LDL, the LDL that's damaged by oxidation, infiltrates the endothelium. Once the endothelium becomes infiltrated with this damaged LDL, the process of inflammation begins in earnest.

Remember our earlier discussion about harmless "bad" cholesterol (LDL pattern A) and dangerous "bad" cholesterol (LDL pattern B)? Well, one of the reasons why pattern B molecules (those BB gun-pellet types) are so bad is that they are the ones most likely to be damaged and most likely to be oxidized. On top of that, they're small enough to penetrate the arterial walls in the first place. The smaller the particles (and pattern B particles are small indeed), the more inflammatory they are. Oxidized LDL is like "angry" LDL, and the smaller the particle, the angrier it is. So these nasty little damaged LDL particles stick to the endothelium and begin the process of inflammation. In the presence of oxidative damage—or in the presence of high blood sugar, which is such an important initiator of damage that we'll examine it separately in chapter 4—this LDL experiences chemical changes that the immune system perceives as dangerous.

Once the immune system notices this damaged (oxidized) LDL, it sends in the heavy artillery. First, cells known as *monocytes* rush to the scene of the action, releasing chemicals called *cytokines*. Cytokines are essentially chemical messengers that help regulate the immune system response, but many of these cytokines are themselves highly inflammatory. In the presence of some of these cytokines, the lining of the blood vessels (the endothelium) secrete sticky little molecules called *adhesion molecules* that act like molecular glue, grabbing on to the monocytes that have rushed to the scene of the crime to help put out the fire. Heart surgeon Dwight Lundell, M.D., cleverly refers to this as the "Velcro effect."

Monocytes now convert into a type of cell we like to call "Little Ms. Pac-Man." They're technically called *macrophages*, and their job, much like Ms. Pac-Man in the video game, is to eat up the enemy, in this case the damaged LDL particles and other molecular junk that have caused the problem in the first place. (The word *macrophage* literally means "big eater.")

The macrophages are like sugar addicts at a pie-eating contest. They have no off button; they'll keep eating, consuming oxidized LDL until they literally choke to death, leaving something called the *lipid core* of plaque. Once they reach a certain size they start to look like foam and actually become what pathologists call "foam cells," living cells that will continue the work of the macrophages, fighting and consuming until the "invader" is gone.

But it isn't an invader that sets them off. It's just plain old LDL experiencing chemical changes from sugar, starches, or oxidation and thus initiating an inflammatory process that can easily become an out-of-control "fire" within your arterial walls. As we've said, without inflammation, it's pretty irrelevant what your cholesterol levels are.

If inflammation isn't halted and if macrophages continue to feast away until they bust, they'll release a whole new set of toxins into the walls of the artery.

"We can see this in surgery as a yellow streak inside the artery wall," said Lundell, who has performed more than five thousand heart surgeries. "It is called the 'fatty streak,' and it is the beginning of significant heart disease."[5]

The body tries to contain this fatty streak by building a wall to hold it in—scarring is an example. But the immune system is now on full alert; it sends more soldiers to the front, and they try valiantly to break down the wall (the scar tissue), and the cycle continues—more scarring, more soldiers. Over time, if the body's immune system defenses are good enough, they will weaken the wall of the artery and literally "chew through" the scar tissue. A rupture will occur, resulting in more inflammation, and the potentially deadly cycle continues.

Not good news.

If the cycle is not stopped, the fatty streak grows into what's known as plaque. (Plaque is basically a big old collection of foam cells.) Some foam cells will die, and they will release a whole bunch of the accumulated fats (lipids), which in turn develop into the aforementioned lipid core, a soft, yellowy substance that resembles melted butter (but isn't nearly as good for you).

Now if you stop the inflammation at this point in time, the artery heals itself with what's called a *fibrous cap*. The fibrous cap is composed of fibrous scar tissue and will stay nice and stable. (Cardiologists like Steve call this "stable plaque.") Of course, if there's new inflammation, the cycle begins all over again.

So the more inflammation continues, the more foam cells accumulate. This means more macrophages (Ms. Pac-Man), which in turn means more oozy, slimy *lipid core*. This lipid core gets into the bloodstream, where the blood immediately puts out a signal saying, "What the heck is this? Foreign object! Foreign object!" And a blood clot is formed in an attempt to keep this foreign, gooey substance from spreading.

So the blood clot is actually a protective mechanism. It's the blood's—or the body's, if you prefer—way of saying, "Let's contain this threat and keep it from spreading!" But though this strategy makes sense, it has a big downside. That blood clot may block access to the heart muscle, preventing oxygen from getting through. Anytime you deprive cells of oxygen, the tissue they make begins to die.

And when that tissue is the muscle of the heart, you're looking at—you guessed it—a heart attack.

So overall, LDL can be likened to trees in a forest. A forest that has tons of trees but gets plenty of rain isn't likely to be the site of a wildfire, but a forest with far fewer trees can be a tinder box just waiting to ignite if all those trees are dried up (damaged) and there's very little rainfall! Getting rid of the trees is surely *one* crude way to prevent forest fires, just as lowering cholesterol indiscriminately *might* theoretically decrease the risk of a "fire" in your artery walls, but at what cost? Those trees serve a lot of ecological purposes, and removing them is not without consequences, both to the environment and to the landscape.

Wouldn't it be better to reduce the conditions under which a fire is likely to break out? That way we could have all the wonderful benefits of trees with none of the side effects of a compromised ecology.

We hope we've convinced you that inflammation is at the core of heart disease, and that it's inflammation—and its main initiator, oxidation—we need to be concerned about, not cholesterol.

But oxidation is only one of the conditions—albeit a very important one—that causes inflammation.

Another cause of inflammation is so important we're giving it its own chapter. It's something you eat every day and something you already know is bad for you, but only because of its well-documented role in diabetes and obesity. What you're about to learn is the connection between this common food and heart disease.

By the time you finish the next chapter, you'll be convinced—as we are—that this food is a far, far greater danger to your overall health, and specifically to your heart, than fat ever was.

We're talking about sugar.

CHAPTER 4

SUGAR: THE REAL DEMON IN THE DIET

FOR THOSE OF YOU WHO LIKE TO CUT RIGHT TO THE CHASE, here's this chapter's take-home point: Sugar is a far greater danger to your heart than fat ever was.

The full story of sugar, and of its often ignored influence on heart disease, requires that we venture into a topic we like to call Endocrinology 101. We understand this sounds like something an evil high school biology teacher designed for the express purpose of making your life miserable, but we promise not to make your eyes glaze over. In fact, by the time you finish this chapter, you will know more than many doctors do about the common link among heart disease, diabetes, obesity, and hypertension—conditions that are not exactly of casual interest to most readers.

Once you understand the link that joins all of these modern degenerative diseases and its connection to heart disease, we believe you'll come to the same conclusion we have: Our health gurus have tried and convicted the wrong man, your honor. Fat was innocent all the time.

It's *sugar* that's the true culprit in the American diet.

ENDOCRINOLOGY 101:
THE HORMONAL EFFECT OF FOOD

Our journey starts with one simple premise: Hormones control almost every metabolic event that goes on in your body, and *you* control some of the most critical hormones through your lifestyle. Food—along with several key lifestyle factors such as stress—is the drug that stimulates hormones, and those hormones direct the body to store or burn fat, just as they direct the body to perform a gazillion other metabolic operations.

"Food may be the most powerful drug you will ever encounter because it causes dramatic changes in your hormones that are hundreds of times more powerful than any pharmaceutical," said Barry Sears, Ph.D. Hormones are the air traffic controllers that determine the fate of whatever flies in (or in our case, "slides" in through the gullet!).

This fact has been conveniently ignored by many mainstream dietitians and doctors whose standard message to overweight people at increased risk for heart disease is to simply reduce calories and saturated fat. But all calories are not created equal. Some foods significantly boost levels of a hormone that *stores* fat, while other foods do not—even when the calories are the same. Not coincidentally, that fat-storing hormone also has some serious consequences for the heart.

The name of that fat-storing hormone? Insulin.

Insulin, a hormone first discovered in 1921, is the star actor in our little hormonal play. It is an anabolic hormone, which means it is responsible for building things up—putting compounds like glucose (sugar and amino acids) inside storage units (such as cells).

Its sister hormone, glucagon, is responsible for breaking things down—opening those storage units and releasing their contents as needed. Insulin is responsible for *saving*; glucagon is responsible for *spending*. Together their main job is to maintain blood sugar levels within the tightly regulated range it needs to be to keep your metabolic machinery running smoothly.

Insulin is at the hub of a significant number of diseases of civilization. When you control insulin, you reduce the risk for not only heart disease but also hypertension, diabetes, polycystic ovary syndrome, inflammatory diseases, and even, possibly, cancer.

Both insulin and glucagon are essential to health. Without insulin, blood sugar would skyrocket, and the result would be coma and death, the fate of virtually every type 1 diabetic in the early part of the twentieth century prior to the discovery of insulin. However, without glucagon, blood sugar would plummet, and the result would be brain dysfunction, coma, and death.

So the body knows what it's doing. This little dance between the force that keeps blood sugar from soaring too *high* (insulin) and the forces that prevent it from going too *low* (glucagon, for one) is essential for survival. It's interesting to note that although insulin is the only hormone responsible for preventing blood sugar from rising too high, there are several other hormones besides glucagon—cortisol, adrenaline, noradrenaline, and human growth hormone—that prevent it from going too low. You could say that insulin is such a powerful hormone that it needs five other hormones just to counterbalance its effects!

To see how insulin is *supposed* to work in the

body, let's take a look at a metabolism that hasn't been "screwed up" yet by years of bad diet and sedentary living. Let's look at the metabolism of a mythical five-year-old child who's been living on an organic ranch, eating nothing but whole foods, breathing clean air, and getting a vigorous amount of exercise on a daily basis. (We know, we know—we haven't seen too many of these kids, either, but let's just postulate one for the sake of our discussion.)

The kid comes home from school and eats an apple. His blood sugar goes up slightly, as it always does when you eat food. The pancreas responds to this slight elevation in blood sugar by secreting a little shot of insulin, and insulin promptly goes to work rounding up the excess sugar in the kid's bloodstream and escorting it over to the muscle cells. Which is just dandy, because this boy is now going to go out and play, or ride a bike, or work on the ranch, or do some other physical activity for which those muscle cells of his require fuel.

So far, so good.

The muscle cells welcome the extra sugar, which they use for fuel, and eventually blood sugar drops back down to normal and even goes down a bit further because the muscles are eating it right up. Now the boy gets hungry again, comes home, and eats supper. All is right with the world.

However, this ideal metabolism is not *your* metabolism.

Your metabolism looks like this: You wake up late, stress hormones coursing through your body. (These stress hormones are an important factor in heart disease, and we'll discuss them at greater length later.) One of the things stress hormones do is send a primitive signal to the brain that it's time to fuel up for an emergency. So you run out the door and stop at Starbucks for a sweetened latte and a "low-fat" bran muffin that contains a gazillion calories. Your blood sugar takes off like the *Challenger*. The pancreas says, "Uh-oh, better send in the big guns this time, the guy's gone mad, there's sugar all over the place!" And it produces a bucketful of insulin to try to start bailing all that sugar out of your bloodstream and get it to the muscle cells pronto!

Except the muscle cells aren't having it.

"What do we need all this sugar for?" they ask. "This guy's just going to sit around all day pushing a computer mouse, and when he goes home, he's going to sit on the couch and play with the clicker."

So the muscle cells begin to *resist* the effects of insulin. "We're good," they say, "go somewhere else." Insulin now has no choice but to take its sugar payload to another location, and guess where it winds up?

Your fat cells, which happily welcome it in.

At first.

For a while, your pancreas can manage to keep up with the added demand for more and more insulin, and your muscle cells may still absorb enough sugar to keep you from becoming officially diabetic. But those elevated levels of insulin produced by excess sugar (in the diet and in the bloodstream) are not without serious consequences, including ones that directly affect the heart.

For a stunning example of this phenomenon, all we need do is look at the effect of insulin on blood pressure.

- The number one dietary contributor to heart disease is sugar, which is a far greater danger to your heart than fat.
- Sugar contributes to inflammation in the artery walls.
- Sugar is the missing link among diabetes, obesity, and heart disease.
- High sugar intakes drive up the hormone insulin, which raises blood pressure *and* increases cholesterol.
- Sugar and processed carbs raise triglycerides, which are an important and independent risk factor for heart disease.
- When sugar in the bloodstream sticks to proteins, it creates damaging and toxic molecules called *advanced glycation end products*, or AGEs.
- This same process also damages LDL, contributing to inflammation and ultimately to heart disease.

INSULIN RESISTANCE AND HIGH BLOOD PRESSURE

High levels of insulin will increase your blood pressure in a couple of ways. For one thing, insulin can narrow the artery walls. Narrower walls translate into higher blood pressure because a harder pumping action is required to get the blood through the narrower passageways.

But there's an even more insidious way in which insulin raises blood pressure.

It talks to the kidneys.

Insulin's message to the kidneys is this: *Hold on to salt*. Insulin makes the kidneys do this even if the kidneys would much prefer not to. Because the body controls sodium within a tight range, as it does sugar, the kidneys figure, "Listen, if we have to hold on to all this salt, we'd better bring on more water to dilute it so that it stays in the safe range." And that's exactly what they do. Increased sodium retention results in increased water retention. More water means more blood volume, and more blood volume means higher blood pressure. Fully 70 percent of people with hypertension (high blood pressure) have insulin resistance.[1]

And this is not just theoretical. Research from Wake Forest Baptist Medical Center[2] demonstrates that insulin resistance is *directly* related to high blood pressure. "We found you can predict who's at higher risk for developing high blood pressure based on their insulin resistance," said lead researcher David Goff Jr., Ph.D., M.D. "The one-third of participants [in our study] with the highest levels of insulin resistance had rates of hypertension that were 35 percent higher than the one-third with the least resistance. These findings point out that reducing the body's resistance to insulin may help prevent hypertension and cardiovascular disease."[3]

Back to our story.

After a while, under the constant assault of more and more sugar and more and more insulin—all produced, mind you, by a sugar-heavy, high-carb diet—the fat cells start to say, "Enough, already!" They become somewhat resistant to the effects of insulin (a condition known, not surprisingly, as *insulin resistance*). Now your blood sugar is high (as it's got nowhere left to go!), your insulin is high, and you're on the way to full-blown diabetes.

A side note to those of you who are concerned about weight: Not only does insulin load up your cells with sugar, making you fatter, it also locks the doors to the fat cells, making it fiendishly difficult to lose

THE INSULIN-CHOLESTEROL CONNECTION

Interesting factoid: Insulin has a profound effect on cholesterol as well. It turns up the cholesterol-making machinery by turbocharging the activity of the enzyme that actually controls the cholesterol-manufacturing machinery in your body. This enzyme—with the unwieldy name of HMG-CoA reductase—is the very same enzyme that's shut down by cholesterol-lowering drugs! You could probably lower your cholesterol—if you still care about that—by simply lowering your insulin levels. And doing so would have none of the side effects of cholesterol-lowering medication, unless you call a longer life span and better health side effects!

By the way, we're not kidding about the "longer life span and better health" part. A 1992 study examined the blood work of healthy centenarians in an effort to find out whether there were any commonalities among the members of this unusually long-lived demographic. It found three: low triglycerides, high HDL cholesterol, and—wait for it—low fasting insulin.[4] Your diet affects two of these blood measures—triglycerides and fasting insulin—and both measures will fall like a rock when you reduce or eliminate sugar and processed carbs in your diet. Lowering triglycerides is one of the major health benefits of a diet lower in sugar, as high triglycerides are far more of a danger sign for heart disease than high cholesterol is.

weight. And one reason being overweight significantly increases the risk of heart disease is that all those fat cells are loaded with chemicals that contribute mightily to inflammation!

Beginning to connect the dots?

"Normally, insulin has some fairly positive effects on the body, such as being anti-inflammatory," says Jeff Volek, Ph.D., R.D., one of the top researchers in the field of diet and health.[5] "But if you're insulin resistant, chronically high insulin levels have the opposite effect. They actually promote inflammation and cardiovascular problems. That's not generally appreciated yet; what is well accepted is that high glucose (blood sugar) will cause problems over time."[6]

So insulin is *anti*-inflammatory in people with normal insulin sensitivity, but it is *highly* inflammatory in those with insulin resistance. Having insulin resistance is a double whammy when it comes to developing heart disease. Insulin resistance makes it more likely you'll have hypertension and puts you at significantly greater risk for diabetes and obesity—all major risk factors for cardiovascular disease. But to add insult to injury, that excess insulin has an inflammatory effect on your system as well. As we've seen, inflammation is a major player in the development of plaque, and a far more important risk factor for heart disease than cholesterol is.

The collection of diseases strongly influenced by insulin resistance has been given the acronym CHAOS: coronary disease, hypertension, adult onset diabetes, obesity, and stroke. They're all related, and what they have in common is insulin resistance. If you have any degree of insulin resistance, controlling your insulin by dietary means may be one of the most effective strategies for reducing the risk of coronary disease. It certainly beats the fairly irrelevant strategy of lowering cholesterol!

"[H]aving chronically elevated insulin levels has harmful effects of its own—heart disease for one," Gary Taubes wrote in the *New York Times*.[7] Elevated insulin increases triglycerides, raises blood pressure, and lowers HDL cholesterol—all making insulin resistance even worse and substantially upping the risk for heart disease.

At this point you may be wondering, "How do I know if I have insulin resistance?" Good question. Though there are blood measures to determine this, there's also a nice, simple, low-tech way to do it. Stand in front of a wall and walk toward it. If your belly touches the wall before the rest of your body, there's an excellent chance that you're insulin resistant. Men with waist sizes of 40 inches or more are almost certainly insulin resistant, as are women with waist sizes

Not only does insulin load up your cells with sugar, making you fatter, it also locks the doors to the fat cells, making it fiendishly difficult to lose weight.

Stand in front of a wall and walk toward it. If your belly touches the wall before the rest of your body, there's an excellent chance that you're insulin resistant.

of 35 inches or more. (Although there are, indeed, people with insulin resistance who are rail thin, the vast majority of people with insulin resistance are not.)

Insulin resistance *is* reversible. And it's hardly a rare phenomenon. The prevalence of insulin resistance has skyrocketed 61 percent in the past decade alone, according to Daniel Einhorn, M.D., cochair of the AACE Insulin Resistance Syndrome Task Force and medical director of the Scripps Whittier Diabetes Institute in California.[8] The prevalence of insulin resistance has probably been underestimated from the beginning. Gerald Reaven of Stanford University did the original work on insulin resistance in the 1980s. Here's how he approximated the number of people who were insulin resistant. He divided his test population—nondiabetic, healthy adults—into quartiles and tested their ability to metabolize sugar and carbohydrates. He found that while the top 25 percent of the population could handle sugar just fine, the bottom 25 percent could not—they had insulin resistance (or, in the parlance of researchers, impaired glucose metabolism). So for a long time, it was thought that the number of people with insulin resistance was one in four (25 percent).

But there's a problem.

What happened to the 50 percent of people *between* those two extremes? It turns out they had neither the terrific glucose metabolism of the top 25 percent nor the full-blown insulin resistance of the bottom 25 percent; instead, they fell somewhere in between. One could easily argue that because only 25 percent of the population had flawless glucose metabolism, the rest of us—up to 75 percent of the population—had *some* degree of insulin resistance! Also, Reaven used young, healthy adults as subjects, and their numbers were definitely not representative of the population as a whole—the fact is, sensitivity to insulin actually *decreases* (and insulin resistance *increases*) as you get older. The take-home point: Insulin resistance isn't just something that happens to other people. The American Association of Clinical Endocrinologists has estimated that one in three Americans is insulin resistant,[9] and we suspect that the number is a bit higher.

Back in chapter 3 we mentioned that calculating your ratio of triglycerides to HDL cholesterol is a much better way to predict heart disease than by assessing cholesterol levels. (Just so you don't have to go back and look it up, you calculate your ratio by simply looking at two line items on your blood test—triglycerides and HDL cholesterol. If, for example, your triglycerides are 150 mg/dL and your HDL cholesterol is 30 mg/dL, your ratio is 150:30, or five.) As it turns out, this same ratio is an excellent predictor of insulin resistance. In one study, a ratio of three or greater was a reliable predictor of insulin resistance.[10]

That same triglyceride-to-HDL ratio gives us other important information as well. As noted previously, only the small, dense, BB gun pellet-type LDL molecules are the ones that cause damage (the "bad" bad cholesterol). There are several blood tests your doctor can order that will tell you just how much of your LDL cholesterol is "bad" bad cholesterol (the BB gun pellets) and how much of your LDL cholesterol is "good" bad cholesterol (the cotton ball molecules). (Tests for particle size include the widely used NMR test; the Lipoprotein Particle Profile test, or LPP; the Berkeley cholesterol test from Berkeley HeartLab; and the Vertical Auto Profile test, or VAP.)

But the triglyceride-to-HDL ratio is also a great indicator of the kind of LDL you're packing. Those with high ratios have more of the BB gun pellet-type LDL (which is atherogenic), while those with low ratios have more of the cotton ball molecules (harmless). Triglyceride levels higher than 120 mg/dL and HDL levels below normal (less than 40 mg/dL in men and less than 50 mg/dL in women) are usually associated with the small, dense, atherogenic LDL particles you don't want![11]

In fact, if you prefer not to do any math, one single number on your blood test will tell you whether your LDL cholesterol is primarily the big, fluffy, harmless kind (pattern A) or the mean, angry, small, dense kind (pattern B). Just look at your triglyceride levels.

High triglycerides in general correlate strongly with high levels of those dangerous LDL-B particles. *Low* levels of triglycerides correlate with *higher* levels of the harmless LDL-A particles. In other words, the higher your triglycerides, the greater the chance that your LDL cholesterol is made up of the kind of particles that are way more likely to lead to heart disease. And the higher your triglycerides, the greater the chance that you're insulin resistant, which in turn means that insulin is contributing mightily to the very inflammation that damages LDL cholesterol in the first place and starts the whole cycle of plaque formation. The take-home point: Reduce your triglycerides (and raise your HDL), and you reduce your risk of heart disease.

Lowering your sugar intake probably won't affect your HDL level, but it will dramatically affect two of the other three indicators of a long and healthy life: triglycerides and fasting insulin, both of which will certainly drop when you lower the amount of sugar and processed carbs you're eating (or drinking).

SUGAR: CAUGHT AT THE SCENE OF THE CRIME

We're pretty sure that if you asked a random sampling of ordinary people what part of their diet is most dangerous to their heart, the majority of them would say "fat."

They'd be wrong.

The number one dietary contributor to heart disease is sugar.

Diets that are lower in sugar and processed carbs will reduce inflammation, blood sugar, insulin, insulin resistance, *and* triglycerides. And lowering triglycerides automatically improves that all-important ratio of triglycerides to HDL. (If your triglycerides were 150 mg/dL and your HDL was 50 mg/dL, you'd have a ratio of three, but if you brought your triglycerides down to 100 mg/dL, the ratio would automatically drop to two, or 100:50. Neat, huh?)

You may remember from chapter 3 a concept called the "Four Horsemen of Aging." We've already covered two of those horsemen—oxidation and inflammation—and seen how oxidation initiates the inflammation that ultimately leads to plaque formation and heart disease. Now it's time to tie up some loose ends and introduce the third horseman of aging: sugar.

Sugar is directly responsible for one of the most damaging processes in the body, something called *glycation*. (Previously, Dr. Jonny had named glycation as one of the Four Horsemen of Aging, but because glycation is impossible without sugar, and because sugar affects heart disease in other ways as well, in this book we're going to be talking about the heart-damaging effects of sugar in general.)

Here's how it works.

Glycation is what happens when sticky sugar molecules glom onto structures and get stuck where they don't belong, essentially gumming up the works.

You see, sugar is sticky (think cotton candy and maple syrup). Proteins, on the other hand, are smooth and slippery (think oysters, which are pure protein). The slippery nature of proteins lets them slide around easily in the cells and do their jobs effectively. But when you've got a lot of excess sugar in your system,

it keeps bumping into proteins, ultimately getting stuck onto the protein molecules. Such proteins are now said to have become *glycated*. The glycated proteins are too big and sticky to get through small blood vessels and capillaries, including the small vessels in the kidneys, eyes, and feet, which is why so many diabetics are at risk for kidney disease, vision problems, and amputations of toes, feet, and even legs. The sugar-coated proteins become toxic and make the cell machinery run less efficiently. They damage the body and exhaust the immune system. Scientists have given these sticky proteins the acronym AGEs—which stands for *advanced glycation end products*—partially because these proteins are so involved in aging the body.

What does this have to do with cholesterol and heart disease? Actually, everything. You may recall our earlier discussion about LDL cholesterol in which we pointed out that LDL cholesterol is never a problem until it becomes damaged. (Remember, damaged LDL cholesterol of the BB gun pellet variety [pattern B] gets stuck to the artery walls, ultimately triggering the immune system reaction that causes inflammation.) We discussed one primary way in which LDL cholesterol gets damaged—through oxidative stress generated by free radicals.

Can you guess the other way it gets damaged? Glycation.

So now you have sugar at the scene of several crimes, all related to heart disease. "High blood sugar causes the lining cells of the arteries to be inflamed, changes LDL cholesterol, and causes sugar to be attached to a variety of proteins, which changes their normal function," says Dwight Lundell, M.D., author of *The Cure for Heart Disease*. High blood sugar, as we've seen, also sends insulin levels skyrocketing, and in most people that will lead to insulin resistance, the central player in every condition we've examined that is intimately connected to heart disease: diabetes, obesity, high blood pressure, and metabolic syndrome.

Is it any surprise that we think reducing sugar is far more important than reducing fat or cholesterol?

And by the way, we're hardly the first people to say so.

The Voice of Dissent: Introducing John Yudkin

By 1970, Ancel Keys's research had been published and was being picked up by the media; the low- or no-cholesterol brigade was gearing up for an assault on the consciousness of the American public. Then in 1972, Robert Atkins published *Diet Revolution*, which became the de facto poster child for the low-carb movement two decades later. Atkins advocated an approach completely opposite to the one promoted by Keys: He said that insulin and carbohydrates, not fat and cholesterol, were the problem in the American diet.

Because his high-fat, high-protein, low-carb diet went so dramatically against the conventional wisdom of the times, Atkins was attacked mercilessly in the press and vilified by the medical mainstream, which turned him into a pariah in the medical community. But in the same year that Atkins published his book, an English doctor named John Yudkin was making waves by politely and reasonably suggesting to the medical establishment that perhaps its emperor, while indeed cholesterol-free and low-fat, was nonethe-less naked as a jaybird.

A professor of nutrition at Queen Elizabeth College, University of London, Yudkin was a highly respected scientist and nutritionist who had dozens of published papers in such renowned peer-reviewed journals as *The Lancet,* the *British Medical Journal,* the *Archives of Internal Medicine,* the *American Journal of Clinical Nutrition*, and *Nature*.

Yudkin was typically portrayed by his detractors as a wild-eyed fanatic who blamed sugar as the cause of heart disease, but in fact he was nothing of the sort. In his 1972 book, *Sweet and Dangerous*, he was the embodiment of reason when he called for a reexamination of the data—which he considered highly flawed—that led to the hypothesis that fat causes heart disease.

In the 1960s, Yudkin did a series of animal experiments in which he fed sugar and starch to a variety of critters, including chickens, rabbits, pigs, and college students. Invariably he found that the levels of triglycerides in all these subjects were raised. (Remember, high triglycerides are a major risk factor for heart disease.) In Yudkin's experi-ments, sugar also raised insulin, linking sugar to type 2 diabetes, which, as you now know, is intimately related to heart disease as well.[12]

Yudkin was one of the many who pointed out that statistics for heart disease and fat consumption existed for many more countries than those referred to by Keys, and that these other figures didn't fit into the "more fat, more heart disease" relationship that was evident when only the seven selected countries were considered. He pointed out that there was a better

In the same year that Atkins published the first edition of his book, an English doctor named John Yudkin was making waves by politely and reasonably suggesting to the medical establishment that perhaps its emperor, while indeed cholesterol-free and low-fat, was nonetheless naked as a jaybird.

and truer relationship between *sugar consumption* and heart disease, and he said that "there is a sizable minority—of which I am one—that believes that coronary disease is *not* largely due to fat in the diet." (Three decades later, Dr. George Mann, an associate director of the Framingham Heart Study, arrived at the same conclusion and assembled a distinguished group of scientists and doctors to study the evidence that fat and cholesterol cause heart disease, a concept he later called "the greatest health scam of the century."[13])

Around the same time, the brilliant Danish scholar Uffe Ravnskov, M.D., Ph.D., reanalyzed the original Keys data and came to an identical conclusion. His exemplary scholarship is supported by hundreds of referenced citations and studies from prestigious peer-reviewed medical journals and can be found in his book, *The Cholesterol Myths*, or on his website (www.ravnskov.nu/cholesterol.htm).

Though Yudkin did not write a low-carb diet book per se, he was one of the most influential voices of the time to put forth the position that sugar was responsible for far more health problems than fat was. His book called attention to countries in which the correlation between heart disease and sugar intake was far more striking than the correlation between heart disease and *fat*. And he pointed to a number of studies—most dramatically of the Masai in Kenya and Tanzania—in which people consumed copious amounts of milk and fat and yet had virtually no heart disease. Interestingly, these people also consumed almost no sugar.[14]

The Sweetening of America

To be clear, Yudkin never said that sugar *causes* the diseases of modern civilization, just that a case could easily be made that it deserved attention and study, certainly as much as, if not more than, fat consumption. Heart disease is associated with a number of indicators, including fat consumption, being overweight, cigarette smoking, a sedentary lifestyle, television viewing, and a high intake of sugar. (Yudkin himself did several interesting studies on sugar consumption and coronary heart disease. In one he found that the median sugar intake of a group of coronary patients was 147 g, twice as much as it was in two different groups of control subjects that didn't have coronary disease; these groups consumed only 67 g and 74 g, respectively.[15])

"Many of the key observations cited to argue that dietary fat caused heart disease actually support the sugar theory as well," Taubes wrote. "During the Korean War, pathologists doing autopsies on American soldiers killed in battle noticed that many had significant plaques in their arteries, even those who were still teenagers, while the Koreans killed in battle did not. The atherosclerotic plaques in the Americans were attributed to the fact that they ate high-fat diets and the Koreans ate low-fat. But the Americans were also eating high-sugar diets, while the Koreans, like the Japanese, were not."

As Yudkin put it, "It may turn out that [many factors, including sugar] ultimately have the same effect on metabolism and so produce coronary disease by the same mechanism." What is that mechanism? Fingers are beginning to point suspiciously to an *overload of insulin* as a common culprit at the root of at least some of these metabolic and negative health effects, such as heart disease; controlling insulin was the main purpose of the original Atkins diet and has become the raison d'être of the low-carb approach to living. Though the Atkins diet is certainly not the only way to control insulin, Atkins—

who was after all a cardiologist—is to be commended for being prescient when it comes to identifying carbohydrates and insulin resistance as causative factors in diabetes, obesity, hypertension, and, you guessed it, heart disease.

CHOLESTEROL INSANITY

Yudkin's warnings against sugar and Atkins's early low-carb approach to weight loss were mere whispers lost in the roar of anti-fat mania. By the mid-1980s, fat had been utterly and completely demonized, and fat phobia was in full bloom, with hundreds of cholesterol-free foods being foisted on a gullible public.[16] In November 1985, the National Heart, Lung, and Blood Institute launched the National Cholesterol Education Program with the stated goal of "reducing illness and death from coronary heart disease in the United States by *reducing the percent of Americans with high blood cholesterol* [italics ours]."[17]

In 1976, Nathan Pritikin opened his Pritikin Longevity Center in Santa Barbara, California, and for the next decade preached the super-low-fat dogma to all who would listen, which included most of the country. Pritikin died in 1985, but his mantle was quickly taken up by Dr. Dean Ornish. Ornish's reputation—and much of the public's faith in the low-fat diet approach—was fueled by his famous five-year intervention study, the Lifestyle Heart Trial, which demonstrated that intensive lifestyle changes may lead to regression of coronary heart disease. Ornish took forty-eight middle-aged white men with moderate to severe coronary heart disease and assigned them to two groups. One group received "usual care," and the other group received a special, intensive, five-part lifestyle intervention consisting of (1) aerobic exercise, (2) stress-management training, (3) smoking cessation, (4) group psychological support, and (5) a strict vegetarian, high-fiber diet with 10 percent of the calories coming from fat.

When Ornish's study showed some reversal of atherosclerosis and fewer cardiac events in the twenty men who completed the five-year study, the public perception—reinforced by Ornish himself—was that the results largely stemmed from the low-fat diet. This conclusion is an incredible leap that is in no way supported by his research. The fact is that *there's no way to know* whether the results were because of the low-fat diet portion of the experiment (highly unlikely in our view), the high fiber, the whole foods, the lack of sugar, or some combination of the interventions. It is entirely possible that Ornish would have gotten the same or better results with a program of exercise, stress management, smoking cessation, and group therapy plus a whole foods diet high in protein and fiber and low in sugar.

Yet low-fat eating managed to remain the dietary prescription of every major mainstream health organization. This recommendation was built on a foundation of two basic beliefs: that low-fat diets will reduce cholesterol, and that reducing cholesterol will actually reduce heart disease and extend life.

Although some studies have shown that low-fat diets do reduce overall cholesterol, many have shown nothing of the sort. When you replace fat in the diet with carbohydrates, which is exactly what low-fat diets do, you wind up with *higher* triglycerides and *lower* HDL cholesterol.

Bad news indeed. Higher triglycerides are an independent risk factor for heart disease—and raising them while lowering HDL cholesterol at the same time is a double whammy, a really bad "side effect" of the supposedly heart-healthy low-fat diet. Not only do you raise one important independent risk factor for heart disease (triglycerides) while at the same time lowering one *protective* measure (HDL cholesterol), but you *also* change the all-important ratio of triglycerides to HDL cholesterol in the worst way possible. A higher triglycerides number and a lower HDL cholesterol number mean a much *higher* ratio of triglycerides to HDL. As we've seen, you want your ratio to be *low*, not high; low-fat, high-carbohydrate diets make the ratio *higher*.

The Sugar Lobby in Action

So how did fat get demonized while sugar got a "get out of jail free" card?

Well, there's no political lobby for "fat," but there's a powerful one for sugar.

In 2003, the World Health Organization (WHO)—not exactly a bunch of wide-eyed radicals—published a conservative, reasonable report called *Diet, Nutrition and the Prevention of Chronic Diseases*.[18] In it, the WHO made the unexceptional statement that it would be a good idea for people to derive no more than 10 percent of their daily calories from added sugars. The report suggested that people could lower their risk of obesity, diabetes, and heart disease simply by curbing some of the sugar they were consuming. A completely mainstream, noncontroversial, "vanilla"

- Hypertension, high levels of triglycerides, and a high ratio of triglycerides to HDL are all better predictors of heart disease than cholesterol. Sugar, or more specifically fructose, raises every single one of these measures.
- Fat raises LDL cholesterol, but it raises the big, fluffy, harmless particles (producing the desirable pattern A profile) and lowers the nasty little BB gun–pellet LDLs that actually do cause heart disease. Sugar, in contrast, has the opposite effect, increasing the number of really bad LDL molecules (producing the harmful pattern B profile) and decreasing the number of harmless ones. On top of that, high levels of sugar and insulin damage those nasty little LDL particles, making them far more likely to start the process of inflammation.
- If you accept our theory that inflammation, not cholesterol, is at the "heart" of heart disease, it's worth pointing out that the metabolic effects of sugar are highly inflammatory to your artery walls.

recommendation if ever there was one. Who could possibly object, you might think?

Well, the U.S. sugar industry, for one.

"Hoping to block the report . . . the Sugar Association threatened to lobby Congress to cut off the $406 million the United States gives annually to the WHO," reported Juliet Eilperin in the *Washington Post*.[19] The *Post* quoted an April 14, 2003, letter from the Sugar Association's president, Andrew Briscoe, to the general director of WHO in which he stated, "We will exercise every avenue available to expose the dubious nature of the *Diet, Nutrition and the Prevention of Chronic Diseases* report."

Two senators wrote a letter to then Health and Human Services Secretary Tommy G. Thompson, urging him to squelch the report. Soon afterward, the U.S. Department of Health and Human Services submitted comments on the report, stating that "evidence that soft drinks are associated with obesity is not compelling."

Oh, really? Shades of the tobacco industry's defense of cigarettes.

In a 2005 report by the Institute of Medicine,

the authors acknowledged that there was a ton of evidence suggesting that sugar consumption could increase the risk of heart disease and diabetes—and that it could even raise LDL ("bad") cholesterol. The problem was they couldn't say that the research was definitive. "There was enough ambiguity, they concluded, that they couldn't even set an upper limit on how much sugar constitutes too much," Taubes wrote.

This dovetailed nicely with the last assessment of sugar by the Food and Drug Administration (FDA) back in 1986 that basically said "no conclusive evidence on sugars demonstrates a hazard to the general public when sugars are consumed at the levels that are now current."

"This is another way of saying that the evidence by no means refuted the [charges against sugar], just that it wasn't definitive or unambiguous," Taubes said. It's also worth noting that at the time, we were consuming approximately 40 pounds per year of "added sugars," meaning sugar beyond what we might naturally obtain from fruits and vegetables. (That comes to about two hundred extra sugar calories a day, about a can and a half of Coke.)

That doesn't sound so bad, really, and if that were all the sugar we were consuming, most nutritionists in America would be pretty happy. The problem was it wasn't 40 pounds a year. Even back then the Department of Agriculture said we were consuming 75 pounds a year, and by the early 2000s it was up to 90 pounds. As of late 2011, we're up to 156 pounds a year. That's the equivalent of thirty-one 5-pound bags for every man, woman, and child in America.[20]

What's So Bad about a Little Sugar?

The way in which sugar damages the heart can be directly related to insulin resistance.

Ordinary table sugar, known technically as *sucrose*, is actually composed of equal parts glucose and fructose, two simple sugars that are anything but metabolically equal. Glucose can be used by any cell in the body. Fructose, on the other hand, is metabolic poison. It's the fructose in our sweetened foods that we should fear the most.

Before you point the finger of blame exclusively at high-fructose corn syrup (HFCS), an additive that's made it into virtually every processed food on the market, consider the following:

- Regular sugar (sucrose) is 50 percent glucose and 50 percent fructose.
- High-fructose corn syrup is 55 percent fructose and 45 percent glucose, a difference that just doesn't matter very much.
- So sugar and high-fructose corn syrup are *essentially* the same thing.

Because high-fructose corn syrup has gotten so much heat in the press, some food manufacturers now proudly advertise that their products contain none of it and are instead sweetened with "natural" sugar (meaning ordinary sucrose). Meanwhile, the Corn Refiners Association has claimed that high-fructose corn syrup is being unjustly targeted and is no worse than "regular" sugar.

Sadly, the association is technically right. Fructose is the damaging part of sugar, and whether you get that fructose from regular sugar or from

HFCS doesn't make a whit of difference. That doesn't absolve HFCS at all; it just means that "regular" sugar is *just as bad* as HFCS. It's the fructose in each of them that's causing the damage, and here's why.

Fructose and glucose are metabolized in the body in completely different ways. They are *not* identical. Glucose goes right into the bloodstream and then into the cells, but fructose goes right to the liver. Research has shown that fructose is seven times more likely to form the previously mentioned artery-damaging AGEs (advanced glycation end products). Fructose is metabolized by the body like fat, and it turns into fat (triglycerides) almost immediately. "When you consume fructose, you're not consuming carbs," says Robert Lustig, M.D., professor of pediatrics at the University of California, San Francisco. "You're consuming fat."

Fructose is the major cause of fat accumulation in the liver, a condition known technically as *hepatic steatosis* but which most of us know as fatty liver. And there is a direct link between fatty liver and our old friend, insulin resistance.

A top researcher in the field of insulin resistance, Varman Samuel of the Yale School of Medicine, told the *New York Times* that the correlation between fat in the liver (fatty liver) and insulin resistance is remarkably strong. "When you deposit fat in the liver, that's when you become insulin resistant," he said.[21]

And all together now, class: What causes fat to accumulate in the liver? Fructose.

If you want to watch a bunch of lab animals become insulin resistant, all you have to do is feed them fructose. Feed them enough fructose and, sure enough, the liver converts it to fat, which then accumulates in the liver—with insulin resistance right behind it. This can take place in as little as a week if the animals are fed enough fructose, whereas it might take a few months at the levels we humans normally consume. Studies conducted by Luc Tappy, M.D., in Switzerland revealed that feeding human subjects a daily dose of fructose equal to the amount found in eight to ten cans of soda produced insulin resistance and elevated triglycerides within a few days.[22]

Fructose found in whole foods such as fruits, however, is a different story. There's not all that much fructose in, for example, an apple, and the apple comes with a hefty dose of fiber, which slows the rate of carbohydrate absorption and reduces insulin response. But fructose extracted from fruit, concentrated into a syrup, and then inserted into practically every food we buy at the supermarket—from bread and hamburger buns to pretzels and cereals—well, that's a whole different animal.

High-fructose corn syrup was first invented in Japan in the 1960s and made it into the American food supply around the mid-1970s. It had two advantages over regular sugar, from the point of view of food manufacturers. Number one, it was sweeter, so theoretically you could use less of it. Number two, it was much cheaper than sugar. Low-fat products could be made "palatable" by the addition of HFCS, and before long, manufacturers were adding the stuff to everything. (Doubt us? Take a field trip to your local supermarket and start reading labels. See if you can find any processed foods that don't contain it.)

The result is that our fructose consumption has skyrocketed. Twenty-five percent of adolescents today consume 15 percent of their calories from fructose alone! As Lustig points out in a brilliant lecture, "Sugar: The Bitter Truth" (available on YouTube), the percentage of calories from fat in the American diet has gone down at the same time that fructose consumption has sky-rocketed, along with heart disease, diabetes, obesity, and hypertension. Coincidence? Lustig doesn't think so, and neither do we.

Remember our mention of metabolic syndrome? It's a collection of symptoms—high triglycerides, abdominal fat, hypertension, and insulin resistance—that seriously increases the risk for heart disease. Well, rodents consuming large amounts of fructose rapidly develop it.[23] In humans, a high-fructose diet raises triglycerides almost instantly; the rest of the symptoms associated with metabolic syndrome take a little longer to develop in humans than they do in rats, but develop they do.[24] Fructose also raises uric acid levels in the bloodstream. Excess uric acid is well known as the defining feature of gout, but did you know that it also predicts future obesity and high blood pressure?

Fructose and glucose behave very differently in the brain as well, as research from Johns Hopkins has suggested. Glucose decreases food intake while fructose increases it. If your appetite increases, you eat more, thus making obesity, and an increased risk for heart disease, far more likely. "Take a kid to McDonald's and give him a Coke," Lustig said. "Does he eat less? Or does he eat more?"

M. Daniel Lane, Ph.D., of the Johns Hopkins University School of Medicine stated, "We feel that [the findings on fructose and appetite] may have particular relevance to the massive increase in the use of high-fructose sweeteners (both high-fructose corn syrup and table sugar) in virtually all sweetened foods, most notably soft drinks. The per capita consumption of these sweeteners in the USA is about 145 lbs/year and is probably much higher in teenagers/youth that have a high level of consumption of soft drinks."[25]

All told, the case against fructose consumption as a key factor in the development of heart disease seems to us to be far more cogent than the case against fat. It's also worth pointing out that every single bad thing that fructose does to increase our risk for heart disease—and it does a lot—has virtually nothing to do with elevated cholesterol.

The fact is that sugar is far more damaging to the heart than either fat or cholesterol are, but that has never stopped the diet establishment from continuing to stick to its story that fat and cholesterol are what we ought to be worried about.

As the old journalistic maxim goes, "Never let the facts get in the way of a good story."

Unfortunately, this story is long past its expiration date. Sticking to it in the face of all evidence continues to make many people very sick indeed.

CHAPTER 5

THE TRUTH ABOUT FAT: IT'S NOT WHAT YOU THINK

YOU CAN'T TALK ABOUT CHOLESTEROL WITHOUT ALSO TALKING ABOUT FAT, which is convenient, because it's exactly what we're going to discuss in this chapter.

When you're done reading it, you may have an entirely different perspective on fat and a much more accurate notion of what the terms "good fat" and "bad fat" mean. And no, we're not just going to tell you the stuff you've heard a million times, such as "fat from fish is good" (completely true) and "saturated fat is bad" (very far from always true).

But let's not get ahead of ourselves.

According to conventional wisdom, fat and cholesterol are the twin demons of heart disease, linked together in our minds as firmly as Hell and Damnation or Bonnie and Clyde. We've been admonished to lower our cholesterol and stop eating saturated fat. These two mandates are the basis of the diet-heart hypothesis, which has guided national health policy on healthy eating for decades and basically holds that fat and cholesterol in the diet are a direct and significant cause of heart disease.

Okay, so fat and cholesterol (whether they show up in your diet or in your bloodstream) are pretty much kissing cousins.

We've discussed cholesterol in the previous chapters, so let's clear up some misconceptions about fat—what it is, what it does, what it doesn't do—and why all this matters in the first place. Once we've done that, we'll be able to look at the relationship among heart disease, fat in the diet, and cholesterol in the blood with completely new eyes.

Let's get to work!

WHAT EXACTLY IS FAT, ANYWAY?

Fat is the collective shorthand name given to any big collection of smaller units called fatty acids. You can think of "fat" and "fatty acids" as analogous to paper money and a bunch of coins. The dollar bill is the "fat" and the coins are the "fatty acids." Just as a dollar can comprise different combinations of coins—one hundred pennies, four quarters, ten dimes, twenty nickels, and so forth—a "fat" comprises different combinations of fatty acids.

There are more fatty acids in a big fat blob of butter than there are in a spoonful of butter, just as there are more coins in $5 than there are in $1, but whether you're dealing with a spoonful of butter, a tub of lard, or a tablespoon of fish oil, all fat on earth is composed of fatty acids. The only difference between the fat in olive oil and the fat in lard is that if you looked at them under a microscope, you'd see that each is made up of a different mix of fatty acids (i.e., nickels, dimes, quarters, etc.).

There are three families of fatty acids: saturated fatty acids, monounsaturated fatty acids, and polyunsaturated fatty acids. (There's actually a fourth class of fatty acids called trans fats, a kind of "Franken-fat,"

but we'll address that later.) In this section we'll concentrate primarily on saturated fat, but keep a place on your dance card for two members of the polyunsaturated family called *omega-3 fatty acids* and *omega-6 fatty acids*. They're of special importance, and we'll be talking about them in depth later on.

Now a word of complete candor from your authors. We wrote this book for our families. We wanted the average intelligent person who didn't have a background in science to be able to follow the basic arguments and have a clear sense of the takeaway messages. We wanted the discussions within the book to be simple enough that they could be easily grasped by nonmedical people. And, frankly, fat is complicated.

So this is the part of the book where we could easily slip into a short course on the biochemistry of fats. It's interesting to write about, it fills a lot of pages—and it's deadly dull for readers. Don't worry, we're not going to write about the chemical structure of fat, and here's why. What makes one fatty acid "saturated" and another "unsaturated" has to do with fairly intricate details of fat architecture and composition that, frankly, most folks couldn't care less about. (If you're really dying to know, it has to do with the number of chemical double bonds that exist in the fatty acid's molecular chain. Mono-unsaturated fats have one double bond. Polyunsaturated fats have more than one. There. Now you know.)

And as much as we enjoy talking about this stuff and would be happy to chat about it if you met us at a cocktail party, the truth is it causes many people's eyes to glaze over pretty quickly. So if you're interested in reading about double bonds, saturation, chain length, and other cool biochemical stuff, please, by all means, be our guest! That information is widely available. It's not controversial, it's not debated, and it's not really germane to our story. So, mercifully, we've decided to forgo it here and instead give you the big picture—what you really need to know about saturated, poly-unsaturated, and monounsaturated fats.

SATURATED FAT 101: EVERYTHING WE LEARNED WAS WRONG!

Saturated fats are primarily found in animal foods (meat, cheese, butter, eggs) and, less often, in certain plant foods, such as coconut, coconut oil, and palm oil. They tend to be solid at room temperature (think butter) and soften when warm.

◀ **WHAT YOU NEED TO KNOW**

- Saturated fat has been wrongfully demonized.
- Saturated fat raises "good" (HDL) cholesterol.
- Saturated fat tends to change the pattern of your "bad" (LDL) cholesterol to the more favorable pattern A (big, fluffy particles).
- Several recent studies have shown that saturated fat is not associated with a greater risk of heart disease. One study from Harvard concluded that "greater saturated fat intake is associated with less progression of coronary atherosclerosis, whereas carbohydrate intake is associated with a greater progression."[7]
- In the Nurses' Health Study, refined carbohydrates were independently shown to be associated with an increased risk for coronary heart disease.
- Omega-6 fats—e.g., vegetable oils—are pro-inflammatory.
- The balance between omega-6 and omega-3 is far more important than saturated fat intake is.
- Low-fat diets work because they reduce omega-6 fats, not because they reduce saturated fat.

FAT 101: THE DIFFERENT TYPES OF FATTY ACIDS

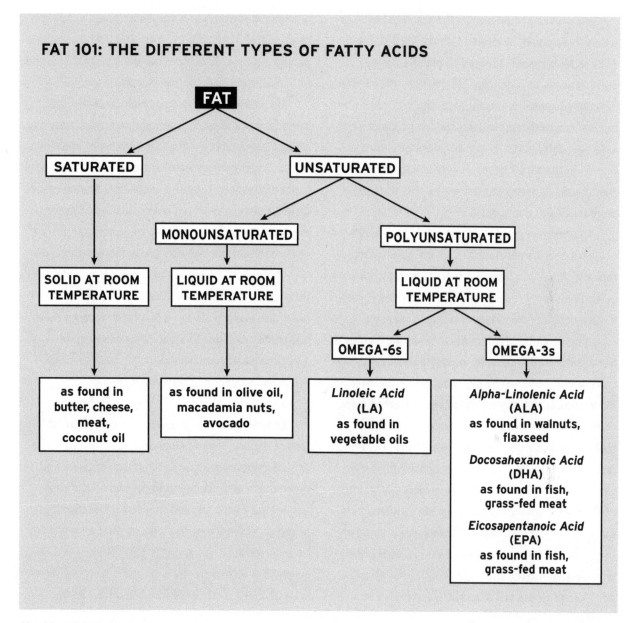

Chart by Michelle Mosher.

They also have a few other characteristics worth mentioning. Saturated fats are very stable. They're tough—when exposed to high heat they don't "mutate" or "damage" as easily as their more delicate cousins, the unsaturated fats do. That's one reason why lard (with its high concentration of saturated fatty acids) is actually a better choice for frying than the cheap, processed vegetable oils that gradually replaced it as restaurants tried to be more health conscious.

The problem with vegetable oils is that they're nowhere near as resistant to damage as saturated fats are. When you heat and reheat them for frying, as virtually every restaurant in America does, it causes the formation of all sorts of noxious compounds, including carcinogens. Compared to saturated fat, the unsaturated fatty acids in vegetable oils are much more easily damaged by high heat and more susceptible to oxidation and the production of free radicals. Those vegetable oils transform into all sorts of mutant molecules under the stress of high heat and reheating, but when high heat is applied to saturated fat, it behaves like the strong, silent uncle at the family gathering; everyone else is going nuts, but he's calm and serene! (We'll talk about some of the other problems with the overuse of vegetable oils in our diet later on.)

Now let us ask you a question, and please answer honestly: Did you just shudder in horror when we implied a few sentences ago that using lard for cooking might actually be a good idea? You probably thought to yourself, "Now they've gone too far. Did they really say lard is better to fry with than canola oil? That's nuts!"

We'd be surprised if you didn't recoil in horror. Most people would do just that—and it's because most people have totally bought into the idea that saturated fat is the worst thing on the planet.

The idea that lard—with its high content of saturated fat—could ever be a better choice than those high-omega-6 vegetable oils that are continually pushed on us is in direct opposition to fat theology, the deeply held belief that saturated fat and cholesterol are the root of all heart disease evil. That notion has been the prevailing dogma about saturated fat, cholesterol, and heart disease for decades. By now you're more than familiar with this notion, known as the diet-heart hypothesis—it's the mantra that has guided public policy on diet and heart disease for virtually every major governmental and mainstream health organization, such as the American Heart Association.

There's only one problem.

It isn't true.

Despite its horrible reputation, saturated fat is far from a dietary demon. More and more health professionals, researchers, scientists, doctors, and nutritionists are beginning to reexamine the case against saturated fat, and they're finding that it's based on very little solid evidence (and a lot of guilt by association).

Saturated Fat and Heart Disease: Where's the Evidence?

Look, there is no shortage of studies pointing to an association between increased saturated fat intake and cardiovascular risk, but there are a few things to know about those studies.

📄 Dr. Jonny:

When I was in fifth grade back in Queens, New York, there was a kid named A.J. who was always, and I mean *always*, getting in trouble. But it was for the most minor stuff: coming in a couple of minutes late from recess, whispering in class, or, worst case scenario, throwing a spitball. There could be five other kids doing the same thing, but A.J. would always be the one to get caught. Singled out, reprimanded, parents called in to school, the whole humiliating deal.

But there were a couple of other kids in the class who were real pieces of work. One kid, Gilbert, compulsively lit firecrackers, scaring everyone to death, and then disappeared before he could be caught at the scene of the crime. Another kid named Howie took delight in breaking people's windows with rocks. A third one, Corky, was a bully. And yet none of them ever managed to get caught. Rarely did any of these kids even get a stern talking-to. The role of the "bad kid" in the class was played by A.J., who would have to serve detention, sit in the corner, and be yelled at in front of the class, all for fairly meaningless infractions, while the kids who were doing all the really bad stuff got off scot-free.

Now it's not that old A.J. didn't do anything wrong. But unlike the other kids, he never beat anyone up, he never did anything mean, he never destroyed anyone's property—and yet whenever there was trouble, he was always the scapegoat.

I think saturated fat is like that kid A.J. It's not that it's perfect. It's just that it's far less important than the stuff we ignore—such as high intakes of omega-6 fatty acids, low intakes of omega-3s, and obscene intakes of sugar and processed carbs.

Is saturated fat so wonderful that we should all resolve to melt a ton of butter and add it to our smoothies right this minute? No, of course not. Saturated fat has some negatives. It is mildly inflammatory. It may contribute to insulin resistance.

If the dietary dictocrats are going to warn us against inflammatory food components, why choose saturated fat, a relatively minor factor in inflammation compared to the omega-6 to omega-3 ratio? If they're going to warn us about saturated fat because of its purported connection to insulin resistance, why do they continue to promote ridiculously high carbohydrate intakes, which are demonstrably worse?

Saturated fat is a lot like A.J. Not perfect, but it doesn't deserve to get beat up. And the irony is that while everyone's pushing him around and blaming him for everything bad that happens, the real culprits are getting away.

A WORD ABOUT META-ANALYSES AND WHY THEY'RE IMPORTANT

A little backstory about meta-analyses and why people do them. Say you want to learn about the sex habits of college students. There are probably a couple dozen relevant studies you could look at, but as with any other area of research, there's no guarantee that all the studies will reach the same conclusions. In fact, it's almost certain that they won't. One study might find, for example, that college kids are having more sex, while another study might find that they're actually having less. (A critical look at these two studies might uncover the fact that researchers in the two studies used slightly different definitions of the term "sex" when they surveyed the students, something that might account for the difference in results.)

Sometimes researchers overlook an obvious variable that could skew the results. Although researchers always try to control for these variables (such as age, sex, and smoking) and generally "match" subjects by the most important criteria, they don't–they can't–always control for every variable that might make a difference (and this is particularly true in diet research). The point is, if you look at anything worth studying you're going to find a whole bunch of research on it, and among those research studies you're almost guaranteed to encounter conflicting findings and areas of disagreement about how to interpret those findings.

Even something that now seems as clearly connected as the link between smoking and cancer started out as a hypothesis and had to be tested in all sorts of populations under all sorts of conditions. Studies can and do reach different conclusions depending on the statistical measures used, the populations studied, and even the definition of terms. (Is a "smoker" defined as anyone who has even one cigarette a week? Or is a "smoker" defined as someone who smokes at least half a pack a day?)

Which brings us, finally, back to meta-analysis.

Sometimes researchers gather up a whole bunch of these individual studies whose results are clustered all over the place like pins on CNN's election maps. Then they'll ask, "What do these studies, taken together as a whole, really tell us about what's going on?" They'll gather up all the studies on, say, smoking and cancer, college students and sex, or saturated fat and heart disease. They'll examine them scrupulously, tossing out any studies whose methods, designs, or data don't meet the highest standards of research excellence. (Meta-analyses typically exclude small pilot studies, unblinded studies, studies with too few participants, or studies that do not collect data on something the researchers consider important.)

Once the "best-of-the-best" studies are selected for inclusion (and lesser studies are eliminated), the researchers go to work and apply every statistical manipulation you can imagine to tease out the real relationships from the mass of accumulated data. They look at the findings of the individual studies and compare them. They pool the subjects from all the studies. They look for trends, directions, statistical significance, and hidden relationships. And though meta-analyses themselves are not infallible, they're a great way to look at the big picture to gauge what's really going on.

Number one, the associations are far weaker than one might suspect, given how entrenched the belief is that saturated fat clogs your arteries. In many of these studies, the major "risk" examined was cholesterol, so we wind up with a circular argument in which higher saturated fat intake increases the risk for heart disease, but *only* if you accept the use of cholesterol levels as a stand-in for heart disease. Studies that measure the effect of saturated fat on heart disease and mortality *directly*—rather than indirectly by measuring its effect on cholesterol—are few and far between. But there are some important ones, which we'll discuss in a moment.

Number two, as scientists have looked more carefully at the association between saturated fat in the diet and levels of cholesterol in the blood, they are beginning to see that even here the relationship is murky. Saturated fat, as we've pointed out, does in fact raise overall cholesterol levels, but its effect is still more positive than negative, because it causes HDL levels to go up more than LDL levels. Even more important, saturated fat has a positive effect on the particle sizes of both LDL and HDL, making *more* of the big, fluffy, benevolent particles and much *less* of the small, dense, inflammatory particles (such as LDL pattern B and HDL-3). (It's called *shifting the distribution* of LDL particles.) And, as we've been saying, the particle size of cholesterol molecules is far more important than their sheer numbers. Later, when we examine the twin principles of fat theology, you'll learn exactly why this is so and exactly why *particle size* is what we should be looking at.

One of the basic tenets of fat theology is that saturated fat increases the risk of heart disease. In the scientific literature, this issue is as far from being settled as you might think from listening to CNN. Recently, Patty Siri-Tarino, Ph.D., and Ronald Krauss, M.D., of the Children's Hospital Oakland Research Institute together with Frank B. Hu, M.D., Ph.D., of Harvard, decided to do a meta-analysis–a study of studies. In this case, they looked at all previously published studies whose purpose was to investigate the relationship of saturated fat to coronary heart disease (CHD), stroke, or cardiovascular disease (CVD). Note that this is one of those hard-to-find studies we mentioned earlier: a study of the *direct effect* of saturated fat on health. The researchers weren't just interested in the effect saturated fat had on *cholesterol*–they wanted to know the effect saturated fat had on *heart disease*. (Remember, they are *not* the same thing!)

Twenty-one studies qualified for inclusion in their meta-analysis, meaning these studies met the criteria for being well designed and reliable. All in all, the twenty-one studies included 347,747 subjects who were followed for between five and twenty-three years. Over this period of time, 11,006 of the subjects developed coronary heart disease (CHD) or stroke.

Ready for the findings?

How much saturated fat people ate predicted absolutely nothing about their risk for cardiovascular disease. In the researchers' own words, "Intake of saturated fat was not associated with an increased risk of coronary heart disease (CHD) or stroke, nor was it associated with an increased risk of cardiovascular disease (CVD)." Those folks consuming the highest amount of saturated fat were statistically identical to those consuming the least amount when it came to the probability of CHD, stroke, or CVD. Even when the researchers factored in age, sex, and study quality, it didn't change the results. Saturated fat did bupkis– it didn't increase or decrease risk in any meaningful way. Period.

"There is no significant evidence for concluding that dietary saturated fat is associated with an increased risk of CHD or CVD," the researchers concluded.[1]

Now–and this is a very important point–it's not that there's no evidence that saturated fat doesn't raise cholesterol. There is, and we'll examine that more in a moment. But the above meta-analysis didn't just look at cholesterol levels; it looked at what we really care about–heart disease and dying. So never mind whether saturated fat raises my cholesterol level. What I really want to know is, what does eating saturated fat do to my chances of getting a heart attack? The meta-analysis looked at exactly that real-life endpoint we truly care about, and on that all-important metric, it found that saturated fat in the diet has virtually no effect.

That meta-analysis is hardly the only study that has found saturated fat innocent of any direct involvement in cardiovascular disease. In the fall of 2011, a new study came out in the *Netherlands Journal of Medicine* titled "Saturated Fat, Carbohydrates, and Cardiovascular Disease." Like the above-discussed meta-analysis, its purpose was to examine the current scientific data on the effects of saturated fat, looking at all the controversies as well as the potential mechanisms for the role of saturated fat in cardiovascular disease.

Here's what the researchers wrote:

"The dietary intake of saturated fattty acids is associated with a modest increase in serum total cholesterol, but *not* associated with cardiovascular disease [italics ours]."[2]

As we've been saying throughout this book, cholesterol is only used as a marker. (In other words, it's a stand-in answer for what we *really* want to know—namely, what is the likelihood of developing heart disease?) But if you're looking for a metric to predict who is and isn't going to get heart disease, cholesterol—as we've seen in this book—is a lousy choice for a marker. If cholesterol really predicted heart disease (wrong belief number one), and if saturated fat really did terrible things to your cholesterol (wrong belief number two), then that might be reason to eliminate saturated fat from your diet.

But it turns out neither of those two things is true.

Let's take those two notions one by one, because they are the bedrock beliefs of fat theology.

FAT THEOLOGY: TWO MAIN TENETS DEBUNKED

Researchers in Japan examined the first of those beliefs—that cholesterol is a good predictor of heart disease—with another meta-analysis. They searched for all studies that had examined the relationship of cholesterol to mortality, excluding any done before 1995 and any that had fewer than five thousand subjects. Nine studies met the criteria, but four had incomplete data and so were excluded. The researchers then performed a meta-analysis on the remaining five studies, which together involved more than 150,000 people followed for approximately five years.

The researchers placed everyone into one of four groups depending on their cholesterol levels: less than 160 mg/dL, 160 to 199 mg/dL, 200 to 239 mg/dL, and higher than 240 mg/dL. (These categories mirror the American Heart Association guidelines, which state that 200 mg/dL or lower is "desirable," 200 to 239 mg/dL is "borderline high," and higher than 240 mg/dL is bad news indeed.)

Which group do you think would have the worst possible outcomes?

According to everything we've heard from the cholesterol zealots, the answer is simple: Those whose cholesterol readings were the highest (240 mg/dL and over), and even those with cholesterol readings in the "borderline" category (200 to 239 mg/dL), should be expected to die at a higher rate than those with a cholesterol level of 160 to 199 mg/dL. And those in the under 160 mg/dL category should live longest of all!

That is precisely and exactly what did *not* happen.

In fact, the group with the *lowest* cholesterol levels died at the *highest* rate.

In scientific terms, the risk for dying from any cause whatsoever (called "all-cause mortality") was highest in the group with low cholesterol. Compared with the reference group (160 to 199 mg/dL), the risk of dying from any cause whatsoever was significantly decreased in the group having "borderline high" cholesterol of 200 to 239 mg/dL and even further

Total cholesterol is so irrelevant as a metric that in 2007 the Japan Atherosclerosis Society stopped using it in any tables related to the diagnosis or treatment criteria in its guidelines.

decreased in the group having "high" (greater than 240 mg/dL) cholesterol. In contrast, your risk of dying from any cause was the highest of all if your cholesterol was under 160 mg/dL![3]

So *high ch*olesterol is associated with a *reduced* risk of death? Not exactly what you might expect but exactly what the study found.

Total cholesterol is so irrelevant as a metric that in 2007 the Japan Atherosclerosis Society stopped using it in any tables related to the diagnosis or treatment criteria in its guidelines.[4] It's not that the society abandoned the cholesterol theory, mind you. It just now relies entirely on LDL levels to determine who should be classified as having "high cholesterol," reasoning that if total cholesterol is high simply because you've got a terrifically high HDL level, that shouldn't be counted as a bad thing. Many American doctors—even the most conservative ones—would probably agree that the LDL number is the important one, even if they

don't fully embrace the notion that it is the *type* of LDL–not the LDL number–that matters the most.

But is the LDL level a better predicator of heart disease or mortality than the total cholesterol level?

Once again, let's go to the videotape.

Researchers in Japan set out to answer this question in something called the Isehara Study.[5] The Isehara Study was based on data collected from annual checkups of residents in Isehara, a smallish city (population: 100,000) located in the central Kanagawa Prefecture in Japan. A database of 8,340 men (average age sixty-four) and 13,591 women (average age sixty-one) was mined for cholesterol readings, and the 21,931 people were divided into seven groups ranked from lowest to highest LDL cholesterol levels (in mg/dL): <80, 80 to 99, 100 to 119, 120 to 139 (reference group), 140 to 159, 160 to 179, and >180.

In both men and women, overall mortality was significantly higher in the group with the lowest LDL cholesterol levels (under 80 mg/dL).

Although it's true that in this study mortality from heart disease was greater in the group with the highest LDL levels (over 180 mg/dL, which is, admittedly, pretty darn high), this was only true in men. In women the opposite was so—fewer women died of heart disease in the group with the highest LDL levels. In any case, this increase in heart disease in the high LDL group of men was apparently more than off-set by the increase in deaths from other causes.

Okay, hopefully this information will get you, and your doctor, to at least question the notion that cho-lesterol is an important marker or predictor of heart disease. But let's say for the sake of argument that you, or your doctor, is not quite willing to throw out the cholesterol theory. Fine, no problem. After all, you, like most of us, have been indoctrinated with the idea that anything that raises your cholesterol is bad news, and that's a hard thing to let go of, especially when you've been hearing it for your entire adult life.

But before you go back to demonizing saturated fat, let's examine the second belief that constitutes the bedrock of fat theology, the idea that saturated fat does really bad things to your cholesterol.

When cholesterol was assessed in the old-fashioned way—"total," "good," and "bad"—this idea might have made sense, because a number of studies show that saturated fat does raise total cholesterol and LDL cho-lesterol. And if you bought into the theory that choles-terol is a big cause of heart disease, this would be a good enough reason to give up the butter. But satu-rated fat actually raises HDL ("good") cholesterol more than it does LDL cholesterol, leaving the ratio between total cholesterol and HDL cholesterol—a ratio that's accepted as a measure of heart disease risk by just about everyone—unchanged or even improved.

If you eat less saturated fat and your cholesterol goes down as a result, your doc may think that's a good thing and stop looking any further. But that's the point: You can't just look at your LDL number and stop there. The reduction in LDLs that you may get from cutting out saturated fat, and the reduction in LDLs that makes everyone jump for joy and celebrate your newfound "health," comes with a hefty price: a big decrease in precisely the LDL molecules that you want more of—the "good citizen" LDLs, those big, fluffy LDL particles that, when they're predominant, make up a pattern A cholesterol profile.[6] When the number of big, fluffy particles goes down, the proportion of your LDL population shifts in favor of the nasty, angry, athero-genic, BB gun pellet-type particles, giving them a kind of "majority rule." Sure, your LDL number will go down and your doctor will be happy, but meanwhile, because of the shift in makeup of your LDL population, your risk for heart disease goes *up*.

Conversely, when saturated fat intake goes up—and carbohydrate intake goes down—the opposite happens. Now you'll see a significant shift to more of those big, fluffy, harmless LDL particles and less of those small, dense, angry LDL particles. Your LDL pop-ulation has just shifted, and the big, fluffy, harmless particles are now in the majority, leaving you in a sig-nificantly better place in terms of your heart disease risk. Sure, your overall LDL level may go up a bit, but what's actually happened is that there are now many more "good citizens" among your LDL population and far fewer "bad" ones. In other words, you're much better off.

The Carbohydrate Swap

For decades, most health professionals have told us that we'd be doing ourselves a huge favor if we just cut out saturated fat and replaced it with carbohydrates. And that's exactly what most people did. After all, this idea fit nicely with the prevailing ethos: Saturated fat is bad, and "complex" carbohydrates are good. If we just swap 'em, everyone will go home happy, and all will be right with the world.

So, as our old friend Dr. Phil might say, "How's that working for you?"

The answer is, "Not so well."

One important study shed light on the whole "carbs for saturated fat" swap but raised a lot of eyebrows because of its unexpected results. The study, titled "Dietary Fats, Carbohydrate, and the Progression of Coronary Atherosclerosis in Post-menopausal Women," was conducted by the distinguished researcher Dariush Mozaffarian and his associates from Harvard Medical School.[7]

As the study title suggests, Mozaffarian set out to investigate how various fats—saturated, polyunsaturated, and monounsaturated—influenced the progression of heart disease in postmenopausal women who ate a relatively low-fat diet. Noting that standard dietary advice has always been to eat less saturated fat, the researchers wondered exactly what terrific things would happen if you replaced terrible saturated fat

with other food substances. According to the standard advice, replacing saturated fat with good stuff (e.g., carbs or "good fats" such as vegetable oils) should substantially reduce your risk for heart disease.

Except that it didn't.

"Greater saturated fat intake is associated with *less* progression of coronary atherosclerosis, whereas carbohydrate intake is associated with a *greater* progression [italics ours]," the authors concluded. "Women with higher saturated fat intakes had less progression of coronary atherosclerosis."

Greater saturated fat intake was also associated with higher HDL levels, higher HDL-2 cholesterol levels, lower triglycerides, and an improved total-cholesterol-to-HDL ratio. Saturated fat, at least in this study, was hardly the dietary demon it's been made out to be.

And if this were not a knockout punch by itself, consider what was associated with a greater progression of coronary atherosclerosis.

Are you sitting down?

Carbohydrates.

Especially the high-glycemic, processed variety of carbohydrates, which is exactly what we tend to eat when we replace saturated fat in the diet with so-called "complex" carbs such as breads, pasta, rice, and cereal.

"The findings also suggest," wrote the researchers, "that carbohydrate intake may increase atherosclerotic progression, especially when refined carbohydrates replace saturated or monounsaturated fats."

"Wait a minute," you might well say. "When I take the saturated fat out of my diet and replace it with

Dr. Sinatra: The Case Against Canola Oil

Back in 1997, I wrote an article for *Connecticut Medicine* about oxidized LDL and free radicals. I was very gung ho about canola oil at the time—as were most of my colleagues—and I was emphatic in my recommendation of it.

But the paper was rejected.

A Yale professor of medicine who was on the peer review board—a biochemist, in fact—reviewed the paper and nixed it for publication. But he was kind enough to suggest some review articles on canola oil in the literature.

I read them.

My reaction: "What have I been smoking all these years?"

The success of canola oil and its reputation as the healthiest of oils is a triumph of marketing over science. It's a terrible oil. It's typically extracted and refined using very high heat and petroleum solvents (such as hexane). Then it undergoes a process of refining, degumming, bleaching, and—because it stinks—deodorization using even more chemicals. The only kind of canola oil that could possibly be okay is organic, cold-pressed, unrefined canola oil, and hardly anyone is using that.

Our friend Fred Pescatore, M.D., bestselling author of *The Hamptons Diet* and former medical director of the Atkins Center, is something of a cooking oil expert. Here's what he had to say about canola oil: "I would never use this stuff!"

If you'd like to read more about the dark side of canola oil, check out the definitive paper by lipid biochemist Mary Enig and Weston A. Price Foundation president Sally Fallon. Widely available online, it's called, tellingly, "The Great Con-Ola."

As for my 1997 paper, I revised it, removing the recommendation to use canola oil. The paper was accepted and published.

Dr. Jonny: Good Carbs, Bad Carbs

Whenever I give a talk about healthy eating and I mention that a diet very high in carbohydrates is problematic for most people, I'm very careful to add the caveat: "I'm not talking about fruits and vegetables!" So here's a quick cheat sheet on "good" versus "bad" carbs.

Good carbs include the following foods:

• Fruits
• Vegetables
• Beans and legumes

Bad carbs, which cover almost all carbs that come in a box with a bar code*, include:

• Cereals
• White rice
• Pasta
• Breads
• Cookies
• Pastries
• Snack foods
• Sodas
• Juice drinks
• Crackers

*There are exceptions in the categories of cereal and bread, but they are few and far between. Oatmeal is one example (but not the instant kind). Ezekiel 4:9 bread is another. But by and large if you stay away from most of the foods on the above list—or keep them to an absolute minimum—you'll be much better off healthwise.

high-glycemic carbohydrates I'm actually *increasing* my risk for heart disease?"

Um, yes.

By the way, Mozaffarian and his research team didn't just look at cholesterol. They looked at actual clinical events, such as heart attacks and deaths, from any type of cardiovascular disease. They also looked at lesser known metrics that only your doctor will appreciate (such as coronary revascularization and unstable angina).

Bottom line: Greater saturated fat intake didn't increase the risk for any of them.

Vegetable Oils:
Myths and Myth-Conceptions

The researchers also tested what happens when you replace saturated fat with polyunsaturated fat (such as vegetable oils), the conventional dietary advice given by just about every major health organization. Maybe high-sugar carbs aren't so good for us after all, but what about the much-touted vegetable oils, which contain the "healthy fat" our doctors keep telling us about? Swapping saturated fat for a nice helping of healthy vegetable fat has got to be just the ticket to heart health, right?

So the researchers looked at the effect of replacing saturated fat with polyunsaturated fat. Just for fun, they also took a look at what happens when you swap carbs for polyunsaturated fat.

When carbs were replaced with polyunsaturated fat there was no change in atherosclerotic progression—in terms of heart disease risk, it was a wash. But when saturated fat was replaced with polyunsaturated fat, there was a big change—but not in the expected direction. Replacing saturated fat with polyunsaturated fat actually led to an *increase* in the progression of coronary atherosclerosis![8] (This seemingly crazy finding will make a lot more sense when we discuss those special classes of polyunsaturated fat mentioned earlier in the chapter, omega-3s and omega-6s. Stay tuned.)

If you're confused by these findings, you're hardly alone. The *American Journal of Clinical Nutrition* devoted an entire editorial to the findings titled "Saturated Fat Prevents Coronary Artery Disease? An American Paradox."[9] But it's only a paradox if we refuse to question the bedrock belief of fat theology that saturated fat consumption increases the risk for heart disease. The research is showing that it does not.

We worry deeply about the wholesale, unqualified recommendation to reduce saturated fat at all costs, because it invariably means that people will replace it with processed carbohydrates. That switcheroo is just about guaranteed to both reduce HDLs and increase triglycerides, and if you're trying to prevent heart disease, those are very bad outcomes indeed.[10] In the Nurses' Health Study, for example, refined carbohydrates and their high glycemic load were independently shown to be associated with an increased risk for coronary heart disease.[11]

We worry deeply about the wholesale, unqualified recommendation to reduce saturated fat at all costs, because it invariably means that people will replace it with processed carbohydrates.

GLYCEMIC INDEX AND GLYCEMIC LOAD

Glycemic index is a measure of how quickly a given amount of food raises your blood sugar (and keeps it elevated). Glycemic load is a related (and more accurate) measure of the same thing. High-glycemic foods—such as most white breads, white rice, and cereals—are simply those that send your blood sugar on a roller-coaster ride. Low-glycemic foods include most fruits and vegetables as well as beans and legumes.

Now don't misunderstand us. If you wanted to swap some saturated fat out of your diet and trade it for some low-sugar, high-fiber, nutrient-rich carbohydrates, such as Brussels sprouts or kale, no one would complain. Substituting saturated fat with low-glycemic carbs such as vegetables doesn't increase the risk of heart attacks at all, but substitution of saturated fat with high-glycemic carbs does—by a fair amount, actually. A study in the *American Journal of Clinical Nutrition* found that replacing saturated fats with high-glycemic index carbs was associated with a 33 percent increase in heart attack risk.[12] Because most people replace saturated fat with exactly these kinds of processed, high-glycemic (high-sugar) carbs (e.g., breads, cereals, and pasta), the conventional wisdom to cut out saturated fat and consume lots of carbs instead is starting to look like an increasingly boneheaded notion. Although it's not perfect, saturated fat does a number of good things in the body. Its wholesale replacement by the worst kind of carbohydrates is turning out to be a cure worse than the disease.[13]

A recent Dutch study added to the list of accumulating research showing that when you substitute high-glycemic carbohydrates for saturated fat you actually increase cardiovascular risk.[14] But the Dutch researchers had an interesting take on this, one that appreciates that an accumulation of saturated fat in the body is not necessarily the best thing in the world.

They pointed out that eating a high amount of carbs causes your body to hold on to the saturated fatty acids that you're also consuming—and those saturated fats get preserved, stored in your body rather than burned for energy. Meanwhile, all those extra carbs you're eating get converted into more saturated fatty acids in the liver. Now you've got a serious excess of saturated fatty acids—you're holding on to the ones you're eating, and your liver is creating even more of them, fueled by the carbs you're consuming. Because large amounts of saturated fat can lessen the anti-inflammatory actions of HDL cholesterol,[15] this isn't a good situation.

However, the Dutch researchers correctly noted that cutting saturated fat out of the diet is not the most effective way to combat the accumulation of saturated fatty acids in the body. It's far better, they suggested, to reduce dietary carbohydrates. This way, your body makes fewer saturated fatty acids, and its tendency to hold on to those you do eat is reduced. "Attention should be shifted from the harmful effects of dietary saturated fat per se to the prevention of the accumulation of saturated fatty acids (in the body)," the authors wrote. "This shift would emphasize the importance of reducing dietary carbs, especially carbs with a high glycemic index, rather than reducing dietary saturated fat."[16]

Carbohydrates have a nasty effect on cholesterol particle size, which, as you've seen, is of significantly greater importance than total cholesterol, LDL, or even HDL. Two researchers from the Department of Atherosclerosis Research, part of the Children's Hospital Oakland Research Institute in California, decided to test the effect of dietary carbohydrates on the size and density of both LDL and HDL. They found that people who ate more carbohydrates—particularly simple sugars and starches with a high glycemic index—had significantly greater levels of those angry, dense, atherogenic particles of LDL (pattern B). They also had the greatest number of small, dense HDL particles.[17]

Fat in the Diet: Our Perspective

We want to propose a different way of looking at fat intake. We think what we are about to suggest goes a long way toward explaining the contradictory findings, or apparently contradictory findings, on saturated fat, diet, fat reduction, and cardiovascular disease.

To do this, we have to briefly introduce the other two categories of fats besides saturated: monounsaturated fats and polyunsaturated fats. (Remember, all fatty acids fall into one of these three broad categories.)*

Monounsaturated fat is the fat that's predominant in olive oil (as well as in nuts and nut oils, such as macadamia nut oil). Its health benefits have been well documented and are noncontroversial. Monounsaturated fat is the primary fat consumed in the highly touted Mediterranean diet, and it's generally accepted that this kind of fat is perfectly healthy. For that reason, we won't spend much time on it, because it is pretty irrelevant at this point to the case we're about to make.

The real action is with polyunsaturated fats.

Remember, polyunsaturated fats, which are primarily found in vegetable oils, are the very ones we've been admonished to include more of in our diets. When lard was slammed back in the early part of the twentieth century, the health dictocrats started their cheerleading effort for vegetable fats. (The first major beneficiary of this all-out campaign to make vegetable fats synonymous with "healthy" fat was actually the trans fat-laden Crisco, the most popular vegetable shortening of its time.) Even now, most people believe that substituting vegetable oil for animal fats is universally a good thing.

But is it always?

Let's, as they say, go to the videotape.

*Trans fats are a special category.

Polyunsaturated fats as a whole are divided into two subcategories: omega-3 fatty acids and omega-6 fatty acids. (For those who've always wondered what the heck an "omega" is anyway, you can think of the terms *omega-6* and *omega-3* as real estate terms; they're simply descriptions of the location of certain chemical structures—called double bonds—within the fatty acid. An omega-3 has its first double bond at the third carbon atom in the chain, while omega-6 has its first double bond at the sixth carbon atom in the chain. Now, for our purposes, you can promptly forget all that and just concentrate on what these two types of fatty acids— omega-3s and omega-6s—actually do in the body.)

Omega-6s, as mentioned, are found primarily in vegetable oils and some plant foods. Omega-3s are found primarily in fish, such as salmon, and certain animal foods, such as grass-fed beef, as well as in some plant foods, such as flax and flaxseed oil. So far, so good.

Here's where it gets tricky.

Both inflammatory and anti-inflammatory hormones, known as *eicosanoids*, are made in the body from polyunsaturated fats. (And to answer the inevitable question, yes, we actually need both. Inflammatory compounds are a necessary part of the immune system and play a big part in the healing process when you have a wound or other type of injury.)

Omega-6s are the precursors to the inflammatory compounds in our body—they're the building blocks the body uses to make these inflammatory hormones (specifically *series 2 prostaglandins*). And omega-3s have the opposite function: The body uses omega-3s as building blocks for the anti-inflammatory compounds (known as *series 1 prostaglandins* and *series 3 prostaglandins*).

A ton of research has established that the ideal ratio of omega-6s to omega-3s in the human diet is somewhere between 1:1 and 4:1. This seems to be the best balance to keep inflammation in check and everything running smoothly. It's the ratio found in the diets of both hunter-gatherers and healthy indigenous societies where heart disease is rare.[18]

But the ratio of omega-6s to omega-3s in Western diets is anywhere from an astonishing 15:1 to an even more astonishing 20:1 in favor of omega-6s.[19] If you think of the inflammatory and anti-inflammatory hormones as two armies that work together to create balance in the body, that means we're overfunding the inflammation army by 1,500 to 2,000 percent!

The Law of Unintended Consequences

Our extraordinarily high intake of vegetable oil has another unintended consequence, and one that may have a profound effect on cardiovascular health. To understand it, though, you have to take a short excursion into the world of omega-3 fatty acids. (Trust us, it's a short and easy trip.)

You see, there are actually three omega-3 fatty acids—ALA (*alpha-linolenic acid*), EPA (*eicosapentaenoic acid*), and DHA (*docosahexaenoic acid*). The only one that is "essential" in the diet is ALA, which is found in green, leafy vegetables and in flaxseeds, chia seeds, perilla seeds, and walnuts. That doesn't mean the other two aren't important. In terms of their overall effects on human health, the other two are probably *more* important than ALA. The reason the other two—EPA and DHA—aren't considered "essential" is that scientists use the word *essential* in a different way than regular people use it in ordinary conversation. In this context, *essential* simply means that it's something the body can't make, so you have to get it from your diet. Your body can make EPA and DHA, so technically they're not classed as "essential." Because the body can't make ALA, however, it's considered an "essential" omega-3.

But the fact that the body can make EPA and DHA from ALA doesn't mean it does a particularly good job of it. It converts the ALA from the diet into EPA and DHA using enzymes and a complicated series of operations known as *elongation* and *desaturation*, the success of which is influenced by many different factors, including the amount of inflammatory omega-6's

in the diet. Even under the best of circumstances, only a small amount of ALA successfully gets converted into the very critical EPA and DHA.

Omega-6s and omega-3s compete for the same enzymes, and when omega-6 intake is very high, it wins the competition by default. A high intake of omega-6 reduces the conversion of ALA into EPA and DHA, which might be another reason why high omega-6 diets contribute to heart disease.[19] So not only are those omega-6 fatty acids pro-inflammatory on their own, but they also reduce the body's ability to produce two of the most anti-inflammatory substances on the planet: the omega-3s EPA and DHA. It's a double whammy, and your heart is the loser.

No, the omega-6s that have been the darling of the high-carb, low-fat movement, the vegetable oils we've been told to use instead of animal fats—the very vegetable oils that "saturate" (no pun intended) our diet through their incorporation into virtually every baked, fried, and processed food available in the supermarket, the very vegetable oils that restaurants proudly boast of

The vegetable oils we've been told to use instead of animal fats are actually turning out to be as bad as, or worse than, the original saturated fats (such as lard) that they replaced, just as margarine turned out to be far worse than butter.

using because they're so "healthy"—are actually turning out to be as bad as, or worse than, the original saturated fats (such as lard) that they replaced, just as margarine turned out to be far worse than butter.

For example, the primary omega-6 fatty acid—linoleic acid—has been shown to increase the oxidation of LDL cholesterol, thus increasing the severity of coronary atherosclerosis.[21] One research study showed that a diet enriched with linoleic acid increased the oxidation of the small, nasty LDL particles, precisely the cholesterol particles that are most dangerous and most involved in the formation of arterial plaque.[22] Omega-6s even inhibit your body's ability to fully incorporate the EPA you get from fish or fish oil supplements into the cell membranes, which is meaningful because EPA is the omega-3 that has the most profound effect on the heart.[23]

Published values for omega-6 intake closely track observed coronary heart disease death rates for all sorts of populations worldwide.[24] And in the famous MRFIT study, subjects with the lowest ratio of omega-6 to omega-3 (i.e., those with the lowest intakes of omega-6 relative to their omega-3 intakes) had the lowest death rate.[25]

The Paradox of the Ultra-Low-Fat Diet

At this point you may well be wondering why low-fat, high-carb diets work at all when they do work. If saturated fat is not the bad guy we thought it was, and if carbohydrates aren't always the good guys, why is it that some of these high-carb, super-low-fat programs seem to work sometimes?

Glad you asked, because we have a theory about that.

Although many people may believe that extremely low-fat diets work because they cut out saturated fat, we suspect the real benefit comes from reducing omega-6s. Omega-6 is the predominant fat we consume, and as we've seen, we consume way too much of it. When we follow a very low-fat diet we consume less of it, which automatically lowers the pro-inflammatory to anti-inflammatory ratio. The fact that saturated fat is lowered is actually incidental.

In addition, those famous low-fat, high-carb diets, such as those promoted by McDougall, Ornish, and Esselstyn, are remarkably low in sugar. The carb content may be high, but they're not the carbs most people are gorging on. The carbs in these high-carb diets tend to be vegetables, fruits, and a smattering of starches, such as beans and brown rice. And although some of the starches may be high-glycemic (such as potatoes), they don't contain a ton of fructose (as do most processed carbs and virtually all packaged goods). Fructose is the most metabolically dangerous of the sugars, and it is a very minor player in any of the low-fat, high-carb diets that are successful. We suspect that when very low-fat, high-carb diets work at all—and they frequently don't—they work because of these three dietary factors: fewer inflammatory omega-6s, fewer high-glycemic carbs, and much less fructose or sugar. We believe that whatever benefits might sometimes accrue from extremely low-fat, high-carb diets could be easily achieved by simply reducing sugar and processed carbs, eliminating trans fats, *in*creasing omega-3s, and *de*creasing omega-6s. Reducing saturated fat and dietary cholesterol intakes has virtually nothing to do with it.

Besides, what is the mechanism by which saturated fat could cause heart disease? In 2008, the distinguished biochemist Bill Lands attempted to answer this and other related questions about conventional dietary advice in a closely argued review (complete with 231 scientific references) that was published in the scientific journal *Progress in Lipid Research*.

Here's what Lands had to say about saturated fat and heart disease:

"Advice to replace saturated fat with unsaturated fat stimulated my early experiments in lipid research. It made me ask by what mechanisms could saturated fats be 'bad' and unsaturated fats 'good' ... Fifty years later, I still cannot cite a definite mechanism or mediator by which saturated fat is shown to kill people ... The current advice to the public needs to identify logical causal mechanisms and mediators so we can focus logically on what food choices to avoid."[26]

When it comes to the theory that saturated fat kills people, Lands was essentially challenging his researcher colleagues to "prove it."

And they haven't.

CHAPTER 6

THE STATIN SCAM

STEPHANIE SENEFF ALWAYS WANTED TO BE A BIOLOGIST.

For as long as she can remember, she has been fascinated by how things work, particularly how living things work. She wanted to know how frogs jump, how grasshoppers breathe, how cells communicate, how the heart talks to the brain, all of which scientists study in detail, frequently by spending hours a day peering into a microscope. She was interested in systems, and to her the human body was the most fascinating system of all. So she was more than a little delighted when, after high school, she was accepted into the biology program at MIT.

After completing her B.S. in biophysics, she entered the MIT Ph.D. program and spent a year working under Professor Harvey Lodish in the laboratory headed by future Nobel Prize winner David Baltimore.

But there was a problem.

After a year in Baltimore's lab, Seneff realized two things. One, she wasn't really cut out for the isolation required by a life in the lab, and two, she wanted to start a family. So she quit the Ph.D. program.

But she didn't quit MIT. "In those days," she told us, "you could get a job as a programmer with no prior experience. I got a job at MIT Lincoln Laboratory, where I lucked into a group of pioneers in the fledging field of computer speech processing."

Voilà. Seneff found a home, a perfect blend of her two great interests—biology and computer dialogue systems. She went on to earn a Ph.D. in electrical engineering from MIT, ultimately publishing more than 170 papers and becoming one of the world's leading experts in blending biological systems with computer intelligence. (It was her pioneering work in the field of voice recognition and computer systems that led to commercial applications such as SIRI, the virtual assistant built into the iPhone, which has an uncanny ability to recognize what you say to it and execute voice commands.

Then something happened: Seneff's husband was diagnosed with heart disease.

His doctor put him on a high-dose statin—four times the usual dose—and told him it was imperative that he stay on it. "If you go off this, or even reduce the dosage, I can no longer be your doctor," his physician told him.

Almost immediately, the side effects started. He developed debilitating shoulder problems; muscle aches and weakness (he could no longer open drawers or jars); cognitive and memory problems; and depression, something he had never experienced before.

We all know what we do when we first get a diagnosis, or are prescribed a medication we're not familiar with, or begin having a bunch of unexplained symptoms or side effects: We go on the Internet, which is exactly what Seneff did.

Except Seneff, as you can probably imagine, is no ordinary Googler. She applied her not inconsiderable, methodologically precise skills as a researcher to the task at hand and proceeded to try to learn everything

there was to learn about cholesterol, heart disease, and statin drugs. She had no agenda, other than to help her husband get well. She had not spent four years in medical school being subtly influenced by the drug companies, had not been a consultant to the pharmaceutical industry, had not been visited daily by a charming crew of pharmaceutical company reps spinning studies—paid for by those same pharmaceutical companies—that tout the unabashed benefits of their products. And she had not been paid hefty fees by those same pharmaceutical companies (like Dr. Sinatra had) to give "educational" lectures on behalf of their products (lectures that are little more than marketing tools disguised as scholarship).

Basically, she wasn't bought or influenced by or beholden to anyone in the heart disease-cholesterol-statin drug establishment. She had no preconceived ideas, either positive or negative, about what she'd find. Her research for the next few years was motivated primarily by two things: one, helping her husband get well, and two, her lifelong interest in biology and nutrition.

And let's remember that we're talking about someone whose ability to understand systems, theory, statistics, interpretation, experimental bias, confounding variables, and all the rest of the esoterica associated with evaluating studies is nothing short of world-class.

Here's what Seneff told us about statin drugs when we contacted her for this book: "Statin drugs are toxic. I liken them to arsenic, which will slowly poison you over time." (P.S.: Seneff's husband terminated his statin therapy, and all of his symptoms disappeared. Needless to say, he switched to a different doctor.)

THE NEXT MEDICAL TRAGEDY?

Seneff has become one of the most respected and outspoken critics of the cholesterol hypothesis, and she is quite vocal about her opposition to statin drugs, which she believes are the next medical tragedy waiting to happen.

Let's be clear: Although Seneff and other independent researchers are pretty unequivocal in their negative appraisal of statin drugs, we are a little more moderate. (Just a little.) Neither of us, especially Steve, believes that statin drugs are all bad. As mentioned earlier, Steve still prescribes them very occasionally, in certain limited circumstances (to middle-aged men who have already had a heart attack and are at very high risk for another). Even Duane Graveline, M.D., perhaps the most outspoken critic of statins on the planet and author of *Lipitor: Thief of Memory*, lists low-dose statin therapy as one possible option for "high-risk" people.

Statin drugs do some good in some circumstances, but their benefits, and the circumstances in which they are appropriate, are much more limited than the pharmaceutical companies would have us believe. Furthermore, any good they may accomplish has little to do with cholesterol lowering, as you will soon see.

Statin drugs are anti-inflammatory. They lower C-reactive protein (a protein in the blood that's an excellent measure of systemic inflammation), and they decrease blood viscosity (meaning they make the blood flow more easily). Any of the benefits, however mild they are in reality and however overstated they

are in promotional materials, are almost definitely related to these other two effects, not to the drugs' fairly meaningless ability to lower cholesterol.

(In fact, when you finish reading this section, you may find that you agree with a growing number of health professionals who think that statin drugs would be even *more* effective if they *didn't* lower cholesterol. But we digress.)

If you still doubt that the cholesterol-lowering effect of statins is the least important thing they do, put on your detective hat for a moment, and consider the following:

Prior to the introduction of statin drugs in the 1990s,* there were a number of studies done in which cholesterol was successfully lowered by other drugs, notably the class of drugs known as *fibrates*, the go-to treatment for high cholesterol prior to the near-universal switch to statins in the last decade of the twentieth century. These drugs actually lowered cholesterol quite well, thank you very much. If lowering cholesterol does in fact prevent heart attacks or strokes, then we should see a significant reduction in heart attacks and strokes anytime we successfully lower it, regardless of the particular drug (or diet) used to accomplish this.

But investigations of the cholesterol-lowering studies prior to the mainstream use of statin drugs showed quite the opposite. And there's proof, all cataloged, collected, and assembled in one place, thanks to a man named Russell Smith.

---

*Mevacor, a statin drug, was actually introduced in 1987, but statins didn't become popular until the 1990s.

"DYING WITH CORRECTED CHOLESTEROL IS NOT A SUCCESSFUL OUTCOME"

Back in the late 1980s, Russell Smith, Ph.D., an American experimental psychologist with a strong background in physiology, math, and engineering, decided to write the most comprehensive and critical review of the diet-heart disease literature yet seen. Published in two volumes that spanned more than six hundred pages and contained three thousand references, it was titled *Diet, Blood Cholesterol, and Coronary Heart Disease: A Critical Review of the Literature*.

◀ WHAT YOU NEED TO KNOW

- The benefits of statin drugs have been widely exaggerated, and any benefit of these drugs has nothing to do with their ability to lower cholesterol.
- Statin drugs deplete coenzyme Q_{10}, one of the most important nutrients for the heart. Depletion of CoQ_{10} can cause muscle pain, weakness, and fatigue.
- The brain depends on cholesterol to function optimally. Cholesterol helps stimulate thinking and memory.
- Statin drugs lead to a reduction in sex hormones, as shown by several studies. Sexual dysfunction is a common (but underreported) side effect of statin drugs.
- Statins interfere with serotonin receptors in the brain.
- There are troubling indicators that statin drugs may be associated with a higher risk for cancer and diabetes.
- A comprehensive study by a University of California, San Diego, School of Medicine researcher showed that a majority of doctors *dismiss* complaints of side effects from statins and do *not* report them to MedWatch, the FDA's system for reporting any undesirable experiences associated with the use of medical products or drugs (experiences collectively known as "adverse events"). In other words, side effects are grossly underreported.
- Statins should not be prescribed for the elderly or for the vast majority of women, and they should *never* be prescribed for children.
- Research shows that (with rare exceptions) any benefit from statin drugs is seen only in middle-aged men wth documented coronary artery disease.

In the vast majority of studies reviewed, there was no difference in the number of deaths between the group that lowered its cholesterol and the group that didn't.

Then in 1991, together with Edward Pinckney, M.D., an editor of four medical journals and former coeditor of the *Journal of the American Medical Association*, Smith published a summary of this massive work in a book called *The Cholesterol Conspiracy*.

Among many other things, Smith and Pinckney reviewed all of the cholesterol-lowering trials that had been done prior to 1991. The studies found that using drugs to lower cholesterol was quite effective—at lowering cholesterol. The problem was that they weren't much good for anything else. If cholesterol lowering was in fact the holy grail of preventing heart disease and death, then we would expect the research to show a reduction in heart attacks, strokes, and deaths when cholesterol was effectively lowered, wouldn't we?

Let's see what Smith and Pinckney had to say about that:

"Drugs were used to lower blood cholesterol levels in twelve trials (i.e., studies). Eight of these trials were both randomized and blinded.* Of the eight that met this standard, total deaths in six trials were the same or greater in the treatment group than in the control group. For the remaining four trials (either nonrandomized or unblinded), there were no differences between the treatment group and the control group."

Translated into clear English: In the vast majority of the studies reviewed, there was no difference in the number of deaths between the group that lowered its cholesterol and the group that didn't. In fact, in a few cases, more people died in the group that lowered its cholesterol.

Okay, so much for ten out of those twelve trials— pretty dismal results. But what about the remaining two trials?

In these two trials, there were fewer deaths in the group treated with cholesterol-lowering drugs than in the control group. These two studies, accounting for only a sixth of the total number of drug studies conducted, the rest of which showed no benefit, were

* Randomized, double-blind studies are the "gold standard" of these kinds of trials and considered much more reliable than those that are either nonrandomized, nonblinded, or both.

exactly the ones the cholesterol establishment seized on as "proof" of the link between cholesterol and heart disease. "However," reported Smith and Pinckney, "one of these trials was conducted by a pharmaceutical company, which evaluated its own cholesterol-lowering drug.[1] The second trial involved an estrogen drug that produced more harm than good in three other trials.[2] Therefore, both of these trials are suspect."

Scorecard: Out of twelve studies, ten showed no benefit; the two that did were both questionable.

Choosing one or two studies that show a positive result and burying the ones that don't is a well-documented tactic of the pharmaceutical industry. It's akin to finding two white checkers in a bucket of black ones and then holding up the white ones and claiming they're proof that all checkers are white.

Back to the scorecard.

Smith and Pinckney now turned their attention to sixteen randomized and blinded studies that looked at the combined effect of drugs and diet on lowering cholesterol. "The total numbers of all-cause deaths in the treatment groups were the same as or greater, statistically speaking, than those in the control groups for fourteen of those trials," they wrote. "The total numbers of coronary heart disease deaths in the treatment groups were the same as or greater than those in the control groups for fifteen of these trials. And the total number of nonfatal coronary heart disease events in the treatment groups were the same as those in the control groups for fifteen trials."

Did your eyes just glaze over? No problem. Allow us to translate. If you define "benefit" as a lower amount of fatal or non-fatal heart attacks, a whopping fifteen out of sixteen studies showed exactly zero benefits from lowering cholesterol. Whoops.

The authors of this exhaustive review of the literature summed up their findings thusly:

"In effect, the clinical trial data overwhelmingly demonstrated no benefits of cholesterol-lowering for either coronary heart disease deaths, nonfatal coronary heart disease events, or all-cause deaths."

So prior to the introduction of statin drugs, it was overwhelmingly clear that lowering cholesterol by itself did virtually nothing to prevent a single death or even to affect coronary heart disease in any meaningful way. Therefore, if any positive effects were to be seen in the studies using the new statin drugs (as opposed to the old cholesterol-lowering drugs), these beneficial effects couldn't possibly be due to lowered cholesterol.

As Smith and Pinckney conclusively demonstrate, all thirty or so studies completed prior to 1990 showed that you could lower cholesterol to your heart's content without adding a single day to your life. John Abramson, M.D., a professor of medicine at Harvard Medical School and the author of *Overdosed America*, recently summed up the problem perfectly in the medical journal *The Lancet*: "You can lower cholesterol with a drug, yet provide no health benefits whatsoever. And dying with corrected cholesterol is not a successful outcome."

Statin Drugs: Risks versus Benefits

Let's review: Lowering cholesterol, as the thirty-some odd studies prior to 1990 showed, accomplishes nothing (except, of course, lowering cholesterol). If there's a benefit to statin drugs at all, that benefit has to be coming from something *other* than their ability to lower cholesterol.

Now, one might reasonably argue, *so what*? Suppose you're right that the ability of statin drugs to lower cholesterol is irrelevant, but suppose they do a lot of good anyway? Why not just use them for their other benefits?

Good question. But to answer it, we need to know two things: One, just how great a benefit do we actually *see* with statin drugs? And two, what are the side effects?

In simple terms, we'd want to know: What are we risking, and what are we getting?

Only when we know the answers to these two questions can we make a smart decision about whether to go on a statin drug (or any drug, for that matter). We want to know what the risks are so we can calculate whether those risks are worth taking, which means we have to know exactly what we're likely to gain. For example, if your risk in taking a drug was a one in one hundred chance of getting a mild tummy ache, but the potential benefit was lowering your risk of cancer by 25 percent, you would probably take that drug in a heartbeat. Why? Because the potential benefit is so great and the potential downside

is so small. On the other hand, if the risk of taking a drug was a 40 percent chance of hair loss, and the potential benefit was shortening the length of a cold by a few hours, you might decide that the benefit is way too insignificant to justify even the possibility of going bald!

With that in mind, let's take a look at the side effects of statin drugs you probably don't know about. (No surprise—this is not exactly data that manufacturers of these drugs are dying to publicize.)

THE DARK SIDE OF STATIN DRUGS

Besides being far less effective than you've been led to believe, statins have myriad unpleasant, and in some cases acute—or even fatal—side effects, such as many of those Seneff's husband experienced. These include muscle pain, weakness, fatigue, memory and cognition problems, and—as you will soon see—very serious problems with sexual functioning.

The executive summary of what statin drugs do is this: They cut off cholesterol production in the body. That's pretty obvious, right? But to understand why the side effects of this seemingly "innocent" action are so severe and troubling, you have to understand how statin drugs cut down on the body's production of cholesterol. When you do, you'll see that cutting off

Besides being far less effective than you've been led to believe, statins have myriad unpleasant, and in some cases acute—or even fatal—side effects.

cholesterol production in the way that statin drugs do is like trying to stop the growth of a branch at the top of a tree by starving the roots at the trunk. The "side effect" of starving the roots is that you destroy the rest of the tree. The irony is that there was no need to remove the branch in the first place.

Let us explain.

Statin Drugs and Your Brain: Memory, Thinking, and Alzheimer's

Cholesterol is synthesized in the liver through a pathway called the *mevalonate pathway*, also known as the *HMG-CoA reductase pathway*. Don't worry about those long names, but do pay attention to what this pathway does. The HMG-CoA reductase enzyme is the one directly responsible for initiating the manufacture of cholesterol, and it is this enzyme with which the statin drugs interfere. (Statin drugs are technically known as HMG-CoA reductase inhibitors.)

But HMG-CoA reductase is at the base of the mevalonate pathway, much as the trunk of the tree is the base from which all branches grow. In the case of the mevalonate pathway, a lot more branches "grow" than just the cholesterol "branch." The mevalonate pathway produces cholesterol, but it is also responsible for the production of coenzyme Q_{10}, one of the most vital nutrients for the heart. Cutting off the mevalonate pathway at the root also blocks or lowers the production of nuclear factor kappa B (NF-kB)—more on this in a moment—and disrupts the activities of pathways that regulate the production of tau proteins, dolichols, and selenoprotein.

Now don't worry. We're not going to go into all these branches and what they do. Suffice it to say that these are all-important pathways producing all-important compounds for the body, and the long-term effect of messing with such a complicated system is unpredictable at best. But we are going to go into a bit of detail when it comes to four of the actions of cholesterol drugs that may account for the lion's share of their effects, including, unfortunately, their significant and numerous side effects.

The first of these actions is the most obvious one: Statin drugs lower cholesterol, and they do a great job of it. So good, in fact, that they lower cholesterol in the brain, and that is very far from a good thing.

The brain absolutely depends on cholesterol for optimal functioning. Although the brain makes up only about 2 percent of the total weight of the body, it contains 25 percent of the body's cholesterol. Cholesterol is a vital part of cell membranes in the brain, and it plays a critical role in the transmission of neurotransmitters. Without cholesterol, brain cells can't effectively "talk" to each other, cellular communication is impaired, and cognition and memory are significantly affected, usually not in a good way! (See the sidebar, "SpaceDoc: The Strange Case of the Missing Memory.")

Cognitive and memory problems are one of the most dramatic and frequent side effects of statin drugs, and a 2009 study from Iowa State University demonstrates why. Yeon-Kyun Shin, Ph.D., a biophysics professor in the department of biochemistry, biophysics, and molecular biology at Iowa State, tested the whole neurotransmitter machinery of brain cells in a novel

THE MEVALONATE PATHWAY: THE CHOLESTEROL CORRIDOR

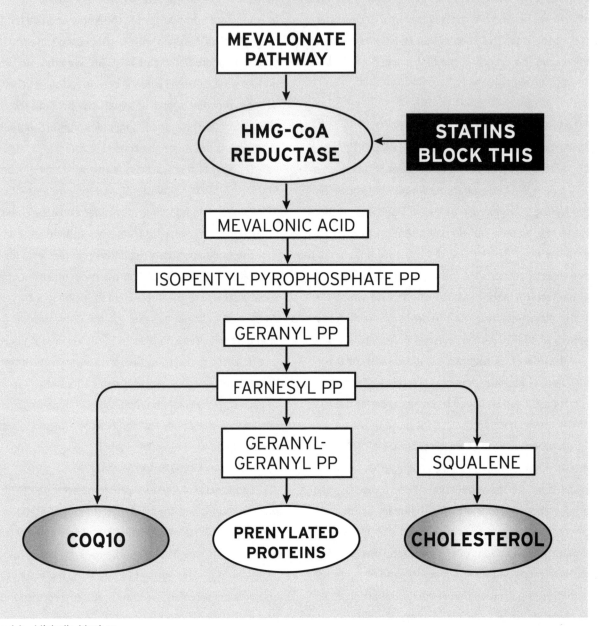

Chart by Michelle Mosher.

experiment. (Neurotransmitters affect data-processing and memory functions.) He measured how the system released neurotransmitters when cholesterol was removed from the cells and compared that with how the system functioned when cholesterol was put back in.

Cholesterol increased protein function fivefold.

"Our study shows there is a direct link between cholesterol and neurotransmitter release," said Shin. "Cholesterol changes the shape of the protein to stimulate thinking and memory."[4] In other words—how smart you are and how well you remember things.[5]

Note to parents: Now that you understand this, the fact that some groups are currently advocating statin drugs for children, whose brains aren't even fully developed until they're twenty-five, should be as utterly frightening to you as it is to us.

Adults should be no less sanguine. Speaking at a 2008 luncheon discussion put on by Project A.L.S.—a nonprofit dedicated to raising money for brain research and the understanding of Lou Gehrig's disease—the vice chairman of medicine at New York Presbyterian Hospital, Orli Eingin, M.D., had this to say regarding the number-one-selling statin drug in the world, Lipitor: "This drug makes women stupid."[6]

Statin Drugs and Your Energy

Here is one noncontroversial and incontrovertible fact: Statin drugs significantly deplete your body's stores of coenzyme Q_{10} (CoQ_{10}).

If you don't already know what CoQ_{10} is, this would be a great time to become familiar with it. Once you understand the importance of CoQ_{10} to human health, you'll immediately appreciate why the depletion of CoQ_{10} by statin drugs is such a big deal. The depletion of CoQ_{10} is one of the most important negative effects of statins, and the one that is pretty much responsible for a host of common side effects involving muscle pain, weakness, and loss of energy.

CoQ_{10} is a vitamin-like compound found in virtually every cell in the human body, and when your CoQ_{10} levels fall, so does your general health. CoQ_{10} is used in the energy-producing metabolic pathways of every cell. It's a powerful antioxidant, combating oxidative damage from free radicals and protecting your cell membranes, proteins, and DNA. In a previous book, Dr. Sinatra has referred to CoQ_{10} as "the spark of life," and Dr. Jonny has written about it at length in *The Most Effective Natural Cures on Earth*.

Without CoQ_{10}, our bodies simply can't survive.

The production of CoQ_{10} happens in one of the branches of the mevalonate pathway tree that is blocked by the action of statin drugs. When cholesterol production is interfered with in this way, so is the production of CoQ_{10}. Interestingly, the most important muscle in the body—the heart—contains the greatest concentration of CoQ_{10}. The severe reduction in CoQ_{10} caused by statin drugs damages not only the heart but also the skeletal muscles that rely on CoQ_{10} for energy production. How ironic that a drug given to prevent heart disease—which it barely does, and then only in extremely limited circumstances—substantially weakens the very organ it's meant to protect!

The fact that statin drugs cause depletion of CoQ_{10} levels has been known for decades. Merck, the manufacturer of Zocor (one of the best-selling statin drugs), has had a patent on a combination statin-CoQ_{10} drug since around 1990 but never

SPACEDOC: THE STRANGE CASE OF THE MISSING MEMORY

In 2006, magician and performance artist David Blaine decided to do a stunt in which he was immersed in water for seven days. To prepare for this grueling event, he decided to train with a man named Duane Graveline.

Graveline has a particularly interesting resume: He's both an M.D. and an astronaut, one of six scientists selected by NASA for the Apollo program. He's also a renowned expert in the field of zero gravity deconditioning research. The reason Blaine chose him as a consultant was because Graveline himself had once spent seven days immersed in water as part of his own zero gravity conditioning program.

Ask Graveline how terrifying it was to be immersed in water for seven days, and he'd probably tell you it was a walk in the park compared to what he went through when he suddenly lost his memory.

Graveline's story began in 1999, when he took his annual astronaut physical. The doctors said his cholesterol was too high and prescribed Lipitor, the biggest selling drug in the history of medicine.

But shortly after starting the medication, Graveline experienced a six-hour episode of transient global amnesia (TGA). TGA is the medical term for a rare phenomenon that can last anywhere from fifteen minutes to twelve hours. TGA sufferers suddenly lose the ability to retain new memory and often fail to recognize familiar surroundings. Often they can't even identify members of their own family, and they frequently become confused and disoriented. People experiencing TGA will literally regress in time—hours, days, weeks, or even years—and not have any memory of their life after the time they've regressed to.

Following the episode, Graveline discontinued the statin. But during his next physical a year later, he was persuaded to restart the statin at half the previous dose. Two months after doing so, he experienced another episode of TGA. This time it lasted for twelve hours. His awareness was tossed back fifty-six years to when he was thirteen years old—he knew the names of every teacher and kid in his classes, but he had no memory of his subsequent life. He didn't even recognize his wife, who was with him when the incident occurred. Decades had been erased from his mind as if they had never happened.

Fortunately, the amnesia lifted, and his memory reverted back to normal. He stopped taking the statin again, too—this time for good.

Graveline began his own personal search for the facts about statins, and what he found was more than a little disturbing.

He learned that TGA had befallen hundreds of other patients taking statin drugs. He also discovered that the side effects of statin drugs in general were both potentially serious and vastly underreported—they included elevated liver enzymes, muscle wasting, sexual dysfunction, and fatigue. He began digging a little deeper into the whole issue of statin drugs and heart disease. He started questioning some of the accepted notions about cholesterol, ideas he himself had once embraced wholeheartedly: for example, the idea that cholesterol causes heart disease and the idea that lowering cholesterol is one of the most important things you can do to protect your heart.

"I came to realize that cholesterol was in no way the heinous foe we had been led to believe it was," he wrote. "Instead, I realized that cholesterol was the most important substance within our bodies, a substance without which life as we know it would simply cease to exist. That billions of dollars have been spent in an all-out war on a substance that is so fundamentally important to our health is undoubtedly one of the great scientific travesties of our era."[3]

manufactured it. Although no one knows for sure why, it's widely believed that Merck never produced this drug because there was no real economic incentive to alerting the public to the CoQ_{10} problem and then "solving" it with a combo drug. No one else was doing it, so why should Merck bother?

As we age, we make less CoQ_{10}, so keeping what we have is even more important during our middle-age and older years, when statin drugs are prescribed the most. Lower CoQ_{10} means less energy production for the heart and muscles. Stephanie Seneff and her associates at MIT collected a large number of subjective reports by patients on various drugs. They gathered more than 8,400 online reviews by patients on statin drugs and compared them for mentions of side effects with the same number of age-matched reviews randomly sampled from a broad spectrum of other drugs.

You can see the comparison of side effects from statin and non-statin drugs in the chart on the next page.

To this day, many doctors are completely clueless about the CoQ_{10} connection and are unaware of its

PATIENT REPORTS ON STATIN AND OTHER DRUG SIDE EFFECTS

Side effects	Number statin reviews that mention side effects	Number nonstatin reviews that mention side effects	Associated p-value* (how likely the difference is because of chance)
Muscle cramps	678	193	0.00005
General weakness	687	210	0.00006
Muscle weakness	302	45	0.00023
Difficulty walking	419	128	0.00044
Loss of muscle mass	54	5	0.01323
Numbness	293	166	0.01552
Muscle spasms	136	57	0.01849

Source: Stephanie Seneff. "How Statins Really Work Explains Why They Don't Work," http://people.csail.mit.edu/seneff/why_statins_dont_really_work.html.

*P-value (probability value) is a measure of the likelihood that such results could be found by chance. In statistics, a probability of 0.05 or less means the result would be obtained by chance five (or fewer) times in a hundred. When this happens, statisticians consider the results not to be due to chance. All of the above findings meet this criteria (some of them by a long shot), meaning they are considered statistically significant.

significance. One of us, Dr. Jonny, played tennis for years with a terrific eighty-year-old named Marty. Although in great shape, Marty was always winded, had trouble catching his breath, and frequently experienced muscle pain and fatigue, which he (and his doc) attributed to "getting older." It turns out that Marty's doctor had put him on a statin drug for his cholesterol; his symptoms marked a classic case of CoQ_{10} depletion. When Dr. Jonny pointed this out to him and suggested he immediately start supplementing with CoQ_{10}, Marty said, "I'll ask my doctor about that!"

The doctor barely knew what CoQ_{10} was, was utterly clueless about its importance, and was completely unaware of this critically important side effect of the drug he had prescribed—a drug that is especially unnecessary in this case, because high cholesterol is actually *protective* for older people.

This, folks, is just one example of what we like to call "cholesterol madness."

If you are on a statin drug and need to remain on one for whatever reason, don't spend one more day without supplementing with CoQ_{10}. Run, don't walk, to your nearest pharmacy or health food store and pick some up. We recommend a minimum of 100 mg twice a day, preferably of the ubiquinol form or a highly bioavailable ubiquinone.

Statin Drugs and Immunity (NF-kB)

One of the good things about statin drugs is that they are anti-inflammatory. This is important and probably one of the main reasons statins show any of the benefit they sometimes do. Inflammation, as you learned in chapter 3, is one of four major contributors to heart disease.

We want our anti-inflammatory arsenal to be as powerful as possible, because inflammation is a major component of every degenerative disease known to humankind. Anti-inflammatory foods, supplements, drugs? Bring 'em on!

So the fact that statins are anti-inflammatory is a good thing. But the way they accomplish this anti-inflammatory action may not be without problems.

One of the compounds made in the mevalonate pathway is something called nuclear factor kappa B, also known as NF-kB. NF-kB is an important part of the immune system, but it is highly inflammatory. (Remember, inflammation is an important part of the healing process, so you need some inflammatory compounds in your body to help fight infectious microbes.) It's widely believed that the main reason statins are so anti-inflammatory is because they turn down the volume on NF-kB production (just as they turn down the volume on CoQ_{10} production, another "branch" in the mevalonate pathway that's short-circuited by statins).

You might well ask how this could be anything but a good thing, right? Statins lower NF-kB, which is an inflammatory chemical, and the less we have of those the better!

Well, maybe.

Although at first blush it might seem that lowering this powerful inflammatory chemical produces a wholly good effect, the problem is that NF-kB is neither "good" nor "bad." Some infectious organisms—*E. coli* and salmonella, for example—actually manage to infect the body by inhibiting NF-kB, just as statin drugs do. Other microbes, such as the bacterium that causes chlamydia, actually *enhance* NF-kB. The Epstein-Barr virus inhibits NF-kB at some points in the life of the virus and activates it at other points.

The point is, no one knows the long-range consequences of constantly suppressing NF-kB by cutting off the mevalonate pathway, as statin drugs do. Some of the results—for some people, with some conditions—are indeed positive. Some of the results—for *other* people, with *other* conditions—could be disastrous. There are far easier, safer, and more natural ways to reduce inflammation than by using a drug that has been shown to have a strong link to serious side effects and may—as in the case of long-term suppression of NF-kB—have consequences we don't even know about yet.

But the impact of cholesterol lowering on the immune system is not limited to the effect on NF-kB. Research has shown that human LDL (the so-called "bad" cholesterol) is itself able to inactivate more than 90 percent of the worst and most toxic bacterial products.[7]

A number of studies have linked low cholesterol to a greater risk for infections. A review of nineteen large, peer-reviewed studies of more than 68,000 deaths found that low cholesterol predicted an increased risk of dying from respiratory and gastrointestinal diseases, both of which frequently have an infectious origin.[8] Another study that followed more than 100,000 healthy individuals in San Francisco found that those who had low cholesterol at the beginning of the fifteen-year study were far more likely to be admitted to the hospital because of an infectious disease.[9] And an interesting finding from the MRFIT study found that sixteen years after their cholesterol was first checked, the group of men whose cholesterol level was 160 or under were four times more likely to die from AIDS than the group of men whose cholesterol was over 240![10]

STATINS FOR CHILDREN?

Dr. Sinatra will sometimes—not often, but sometimes—prescribe a statin drug for people in this specific population: middle-aged men who have already had a heart attack or have documented coronary artery disease. Both of us believe there is no other good use for statin drugs. They definitely should not be prescribed for most women, they do not need to be prescribed for people who have not had a heart attack, and they definitely—emphatically, positively—should not be prescribed for children.

We want to clarify this position once again, partly to help counteract the enormous lobbying efforts of the pharmaceutical companies, which, as of this writing, are working tirelessly to expand the market for statin drugs to include children, one of the worst ideas in history. In *The End of Illness*, author David Agus, M.D., recommends that everyone in the country be on a statin drug. Agus is well-meaning but completely wrong. His idea, if accepted, may be the next medical disaster just waiting to happen.

So a middle-aged man who has already had a first heart attack may indeed find that a statin drug, along with coenzyme Q_{10} and fish oil, fits into his overall treatment plan.

For anyone else, proceed with caution!

Statin Drugs and Your Sex Life

And now for the part that no one is talking about. The dirty little secret about statin drugs. Please don't shoot the messengers. Ready?

Statin drugs have a terrific ability to completely mess up your sex life.

No kidding.

Not only is this a common side effect of cholesterol lowering, but it's also vastly underreported. And worst of all, many people who experience sexual dysfunction, especially men, have no idea that it might very well be related to the drug they're taking to lower their cholesterol.

Erectile dysfunction affects more than half of all men between the ages of forty and seventy years.[11] We've already seen how lowering cholesterol can have serious consequences for memory, thinking, and mood. Just as the brain needs cholesterol for neurotransmitters to properly function, the gonads need it to produce the hormonal fuel to keep our sex lives humming. All the major sex hormones—testosterone, progesterone, and estrogen—come from cholesterol. It's utterly preposterous to assume that lowering cholesterol, which is tantamount to downsizing your body's own sex hormone factory, is not going to have a profound effect on sexual functioning.

Of course it is. And it does.

Several studies have shown beyond any doubt that statin drugs lead to a reduction in sex hormones, most notably testosterone.[12] And this is a very big deal indeed.

Remember, low testosterone is not just a male problem—women also make testosterone (albeit much less of it), and it's increasingly clear that even this small amount of testosterone strongly influences women's sexual desire. (Most anti-aging clinics now routinely prescribe small, physiologic doses of testosterone to postmenopausal women to treat sagging libido levels and improve general well-being. Testosterone is vitally important to both sexes!)

We know for sure that low cholesterol is linked to low testosterone in women from studies conducted on women with a condition known as polycystic ovary syndrome (PCOS). Women with PCOS suffer from an abnormal increase in their testosterone levels, but when you lower their cholesterol their testosterone plummets, leaving little doubt about the anti-hormone effect of statin drugs.[13] The effect on men is pretty easy to document, and many studies have done just that. One study showed that Crestor, one of the most popular statin drugs, increased the risk of erectile dysfunction at least two and up to seven times![14]

If libido and sexual health were the only things disturbed by diminishing levels of testosterone, that would be reason enough to be deeply concerned. But low testosterone has a much more global influence on overall health. Low testosterone is associated with decreased life expectancy, as well as increased risk of mortality from cardiovascular disease.[15] And for those who have testosterone levels below a certain threshold, the risk is doubled!

As important as it is, testosterone certainly isn't the only driver of sex and desire in either males or females. Another important hormone—known as the "hormone of love"—is oxytocin.

Oxytocin is produced in the brain, and levels are very high during childbirth and nursing because one of its functions is to help the mother bond with the child. When you cuddle after sex, you're flooded with oxytocin. (Males also make oxytocin, just a lot less of it than females do.) Researchers love to study male prairie voles because they are a rare exception to the male-female oxytocin dichotomy; male prairie voles, unlike males of most species, make a ton of the stuff. Male prairie voles are also a rare example of monogamy in the animal kingdom, and this has long been attributed to their oxytocin production, resulting in fairly permanent "pair-bondings." The bottom line is that oxytocin, which helps you feel good and bond with another

person (or another prairie vole!), is an important part of human sexual desire, expression, and satisfaction.

So what does oxytocin have to do with cholesterol?

Unlike testosterone, oxytocin is not made from cholesterol. But oxytocin gets into its target organs via cell receptors, and those cell receptors are highly dependent on cholesterol-rich membranes. Critically important parts of the membranes known as lipid rafts don't work well without cholesterol, meaning that lowering cholesterol interferes with the ability of hormones such as oxytocin to reach their destination and work their magic. (As we've seen, this also happens with neurotransmitters in the brain that depend on cholesterol-rich membranes for cellular communication.)

Finally, statins also interfere with serotonin receptors in the brain.

In case you're not familiar with serotonin, it's one of the critical neurotransmitters involved in mood. The most commonly used antidepressants, including the blockbuster drugs Prozac, Zoloft, Lexapro, and the like, are known as *selective serotonin reuptake inhibitors* (SSRIs) because they act mainly to keep serotonin hanging around the brain longer. Serotonin has a great deal to do with our feelings of relaxation, well-being, and satisfaction.

So how exactly do statins act on the physiology of serotonin?

Simple. Much like oxytocin (discussed above), serotonin depends on cell receptors to get into the cells. Serotonin receptors—just like oxytocin receptors—are anchored into the cholesterol-rich lipid rafts in the cell membrane. If you lower cholesterol you're going to interfere with serotonin getting into the cells. It's that simple. In fact, research has convincingly demonstrated that serotonin receptors can be rendered dysfunctional by statin drugs.[16]

The noted French researcher Michel de Lorgeril, M.D. (lead author on the Lyon Diet Heart Study), is so strongly convinced that statins are screwing up our sex lives that he devoted an entire book to the subject. His only book in English, it offers a brilliant argument supported by ninety-two references from peer-reviewed journals and textbooks. The name of the book—*A Near-Perfect Sexual Crime: Statins Against Cholesterol*—pretty much tells you what de Lorgeril thinks about statins and our sex lives.

Statins and All-Cause Mortality, Diabetes, and Cancer

Earlier, we discussed how the majority of cholesterol-lowering studies didn't show any difference in death rates between patients who took cholesterol-lowering meds and patients who didn't. In some of these cases, a slight reduction in heart disease deaths was clearly offset by a slight increase in deaths from other causes, so the overall net "gain" in terms of lives saved was a big fat zero.

But studies show even more troubling results. For example, a study in the *Journal of Cardiac Failure* showed that low cholesterol was actually associated with a marked increase in mortality in heart failure cases.[17] And the Italian Longitudinal Study on Aging, published in the *Journal of the American Geriatric Society*, found that those with cholesterol levels lower than 189 were far more likely to die than those with the highest cholesterol levels. The researchers concluded, "Subjects with low total cholesterol levels are at higher risk of dying even when many related factors have been taken into account," adding that ". . . physicians may want to regard very low levels of cholesterol as potential warning signs of occult disease or as signals of rapidly declining health."[18]

There are also troubling indications that statin drugs may be associated with a higher risk for cancer and diabetes, though the evidence is far from conclusive. Researchers from the Department of Medicine at Tufts Medical Center and Tufts University School of Medicine examined twenty-three statin trials looking for any connection between cholesterol levels and cancer. They concluded that "the risk of cancer is significantly associated with lower achieved LDL-cholesterol levels," adding that "the cardiovascular benefits of low achieved levels of LDL-cholesterol may in part be offset by an increased risk of cancer."[19] Further, a meta-review of five statin trials found that an increased risk of diabetes was associated with "high-dose" statin therapy.[20] This finding was also seen in the well-known JUPITER trial, about which we'll have a lot more to say in a bit.

Remember Duane Graveline? The astronaut medical doctor who came down with transient global amnesia as a result of statin drug use? Graveline has spent the past decade or so accumulating data on statin side effects. Hundreds if not thousands of people have written to Graveline detailing their side effects with statin drugs, and his website contains dozens of essays on these various syndromes, conditions, and side effects.[21] In addition, Teresa Graedon, Ph.D., and Joe Graedon, M.S., authors of the popular *The People's Pharmacy*, have published a number of letters from readers on their website regarding statin side effects. Three examples:

"I have been on cholesterol-lowering medication for some time. I had been telling my doctor that my medication was doing something to my muscles and he would not believe me. I changed doctors and the new one discovered that my muscles' enzymes were 800 (normal is 200). He took me off the medication and my enzymes came down. When I went on a different statin, they climbed back up again."[22]

"My doctor insists I must take statins to lower my cholesterol even though I experience pain with all of them. Sometimes the pain gets so bad that I struggle not to cry when I walk down the hall of my child's school. My doctor says I should accept 'a little discomfort.' He says this pain is rare but I know a lot of people who have had the same muscle pain."[23]

"I have taken Lipitor for several years. I now notice numbness in my feet and sporadic memory loss, difficulty balancing my checkbook and using the computer. I have a Ph.D., so this is alarming. My doctor says Lipitor is not to blame. My cholesterol is great and not to stop. Is there any evidence that Lipitor could be connected to these symptoms?"[24]

Okay, so it's pretty clear that statin drug side effects are hardly uncommon. But if so many people have so many symptoms as a result of taking statin drugs, why, you might well ask, have you not heard about them? Don't doctors know about this stuff?

Interesting question. And one that was exhaustively investigated in a groundbreaking study by Beatrice Golomb, M.D., Ph.D., who wanted to find out exactly how doctors routinely handled patient reports of statin side effects.[25] What she found was disturbing: A comfortable majority of doctors dismissed the complaints. Patients in the study described symptoms of muscle pain, tightness, cramping, or weakness to a total of 138 doctors, 62 percent of whom dismissed the possibility that the symptoms were related to statins. Patients presented symptoms of nerve injuries, known as neuropathies, to 49 physicians, 65 percent of whom dismissed the possibility that the symptoms were statin-related. And they presented symptoms of impaired thinking or memory to 56

doctors, a whopping 71 percent of whom dismissed any possibility of a relationship to the meds![26]

This research is important for many reasons, but there's one in particular that's worth mentioning: If docs aren't acknowledging these symptoms—known as *adverse effects*—that means they're also not reporting them to MedWatch, the Food and Drug Administration's reporting system for adverse events. Virtually every doctor we know who is knowledgeable about this believes that the side effects of statin drugs are deeply underreported, a fact that should concern all of us (though it certainly doesn't cause the drug companies to lose any sleep).

Okay, we've answered the first question—"What are the risks?"—in our two-question inquiry. Now it's time to take a look at the second question: "What are the benefits?" Only then can we make an intelligent decision about the risk-benefit ratio and decide whether it really makes sense to take (or stay) on a statin drug.

Let's go to the proverbial videotape.

THE "BENEFITS" OF STATIN DRUGS: NOT EXACTLY WHAT WE'VE BEEN LED TO BELIEVE

To understand how you may have been misled about the benefits of statin drugs, it'll be useful to first understand something about how it's possible to mislead with numbers.

Imagine, if you will, that you are on a game show and the host asks you, "Would you rather have 90 percent of the money behind door number one, or 10 percent of the money behind door number two?" All things being equal—that is, if there were the same amount of money behind both doors—you'd pick the

90 percent option. But that wouldn't be much of a game show, would it? The point is that unless you know how much money is behind the doors, it's impossible to know the real significance of the 90 percent and the 10 percent. Obviously, you'd choose 10 percent of $1 million over 90 percent of $100.

So we must know the real, *absolute* amount of anything if we're to evaluate its significance. The *percent alone* is a kind of meaningless number unless you know what it's a percentage *of*.

Suppose we choose 90 percent of the money behind door number one and find $100 there. You can refer to your take-home haul as "90 percent of the total," or you can refer to it as $90. Both are accurate, but the first (90 percent) is misleading. (It reminds us of what Jack, Dr. Jonny's wisecracking tennis partner, says when the score is 2 to 1: "I've got a 100 percent lead over you!")

When you refer to your take-home money as "90 percent" you are expressing the amount in relative terms. Relative to the whole, your $90 is, in fact, 90 percent. Sure sounds like a lot, doesn't it? But when you refer to your take-home money as $90, you are expressing the real amount in absolute terms. Ninety dollars is the actual, *real* amount of money we're talking about here. Who cares what percentage it was?

Absolute and *relative*. Hold that thought.

Now there's a parallel concept to absolute and relative amounts that's used in clinical studies all the time. It's called absolute versus relative risk. One—the absolute risk—is the real, true reduction in risk that you get when you take, for example, a drug that is reputed to help prevent heart disease. That's the number you really want to know. The other—the relative risk—is a big smokescreen that *obscures* what you really want to know, just like "90 percent of the money behind door number one" *sounds* like a lot but really isn't.

Here's an illustration of what we're talking about. Let's say you're a gambler, and you are offered the chance to buy a special magic wand that guarantees you a 100 percent increase in your chance of winning the lottery. This sounds like a really good deal, right? But remember, it's a relative number. To evaluate your real chances of winning the lottery, we have to look at the *absolute* numbers. Your normal chance of winning the lottery without that magic wand is 1 in 87,000,000, so the magic wand just upped your chances to 2 in 87,000,000. Whoop-de-doo. Sure, it's a *100 percent improvement*, which sounds impressive, but *so what*? You still have virtually *no chance* of winning the lottery, and you're out of pocket for the cost of the wand. It's like having 90 percent of a "fortune" that's only worth a dollar.

The above example may seem silly, but it illustrates exactly what researchers do to make their results seem more dramatic, particularly when those research results are being used to tout the benefit of a drug. (Remember, most drug companies fund their own studies. Many if not most of these studies wind up being little more than marketing materials for the drugs being studied, wrapped up in the guise of science.) The researchers use percentages, specifically percentages that make the results sound far more impressive than they actually are. Yes, what they say is technically true—just as it's true that the magic wand offers you a 100 percent increase in your lottery chances—but it's wholly misleading. A more accurate way to express what you've bought with the magic wand is to say your chances went from 1 in 87,000,000 to 2 in 87,000,000. Forget the "100 percent increase"—what really happened is you went from *one* chance in a zillion to *two* chances in a zillion. Not something you'd probably pay a lot of money for.

Fuzzy Math, Anyone?

Now let's see how the drug companies use the same misleading "relative" numbers to mislead you about the effects of their drugs.

The makers of Lipitor, for example, famously advertised a 33 percent reduction in heart attack risk in their magazine ads. But read the fine print. It's a relative number. Here's how it's computed. Let's say you have a hundred randomly chosen men who are not taking medication; and let's say that out of that hundred, it's statistically likely that three of them would be expected to experience a heart attack at some point over the course of five years—in other words, 3 percent of the total number of men (one hundred) would be expected to have a heart attack.

Now, if you had put those same men on Lipitor over the course of the same five years, only two would be expected to have a heart attack (2 percent of the total number of men). A reduction from three heart attacks to two heart attacks is in fact a 33⅓ percent reduction in relative risk, but the real, *absolute* number of heart attacks prevented is only *one*. One heart attack among a hundred men over the course of five years. The real *absolute reduction in risk* is 1 percent (the difference between the 3 percent in the no-drug group who would

have had a heart attack and the 2 percent in the Lipitor group). The "33 percent reduction" figure is, again, a relative number, and because it's way more impressive than the much more truthful "1 percent" (the absolute number), researchers frequently choose to use relative risk instead of absolute risk when they report results! (Doesn't it sound much better to say Lipitor reduces risk by 33 percent than to say Lipitor reduces heart attack risk from 3 percent to 2 percent?)

Keep this in mind when you read our review of some of the studies used to promote the idea that statins save lives.

There's a second concept that would be helpful to understand before we venture into the studies themselves, and that's the distinction between *primary prevention* and *secondary prevention*. Primary prevention refers to treating people who have not had a heart attack for the purpose of preventing one. Secondary prevention refers to treating people who've already had a heart attack for the purpose of preventing another. As you'll soon see, the effect of statins on these two populations is quite different.

Before we get to that, there's something else you should know about study interpretation in general that may help you make more sense of some of the statin propaganda. Studies usually produce a mass of data that can be spun in a number of ways. Let's take one common substance we're all familiar with: alcohol. There are no shortages of studies demonstrating that moderate alcohol consumption lowers the risk of heart disease. So far, so good. But those same studies have also teased out a troubling connection—alcohol consumption increases the risk for breast cancer! Both facts—that alcohol helps your heart and that alcohol increases the risk for breast cancer—are absolutely true, but if you're a manufacturer of alcoholic beverages you're going to be talking up the reduction in heart disease risk and not calling attention to the association with breast cancer.

In much the same way, a drug company-sponsored study might indeed find a beneficial effect on heart disease associated with a particular drug, a beneficial effect similar to that of alcohol. But if in addition to lowering the risk for heart disease the drug increased the risk for diabetes—a finding that's shown up in a couple of statin drug studies—that finding might easily be buried in the text where only the most determined investigators would be likely to uncover it.

Now that you understand these concepts—relative versus absolute percentage, primary versus secondary prevention, and burying inconvenient associations where they are less likely to be noticed—let's look at some representative studies on statin drugs and see what they *really* say, as opposed to what their manufacturers would like you to *think* they say.

The ALLHAT Study: Not a Single Life Was Saved

The Antihypertensive and Lipid-Lowering Treatment to Prevent Heart Attack Trial (ALLHAT), conducted between 1994 and 2002, was the largest North American cholesterol study ever undertaken, and as of 2002, it was the largest study ever done using the statin drug pravastatin (brand name Pravachol). Ten thousand participants with high LDL cholesterol levels were divided into two groups. One group was treated with pravastatin, and the other group was simply given the standard advice on "lifestyle changes."

Twenty-eight percent of the pravastatin takers did lower their cholesterol by a small but statistically significant amount (compared to 11 percent who did so in the "lifestyle change" group). This allowed the pravastatin folks to trumpet a significant reduction in cholesterol and declare the trial a success.

Not so fast.

When the death rates from heart attack were examined, there was no difference between the two groups. The statin drug lowered cholesterol in 28 percent of the people taking it, but not a single life was saved. Pravastatin neither significantly reduced "all-cause" mortality (death from any reason whatsoever), nor reduced fatal or nonfatal coronary heart disease in the patients who took it.[27]

The ASCOT-LLA Trial: Not Exactly a Slam Dunk for Lipitor

The Anglo-Scandinavian Cardiac Outcomes Trial-Lipid Lowering Arm (ASCOT-LLA) was a multicenter randomized controlled trial in which more than ten thousand patients with high blood pressure and at least three other cardiovascular risk factors were assigned to one of two groups. Half were given Lipitor, half were given a placebo (an inactive substance in a pill form). Remember, too, that all patients in this study were hypertensive. Most were overweight (average BMI 28.6), 81 percent were male, and about a third were smokers.

In this study, even after a year, those taking Lipitor saw clear benefits, though as we've pointed out, this may be because of the many other things statin drugs do besides lower cholesterol. And the folks in this study certainly had risk factors (e.g., being overweight, having high blood pressure, etc.), so any one of the positive effects of statin drugs (e.g., its antioxidant, blood-thinning, or anti-inflammatory qualities) could easily have made a difference. Sure enough, fatal and nonfatal strokes, total cardiovascular events, and total coronary events were all significantly lowered.

Sounds like a slam dunk for Lipitor, doesn't it?

Well, maybe.

After three years, there was no statistical difference in the number of deaths between the two groups. (In fact, there were actually a few more deaths among the women taking Lipitor than among the women taking the placebo.) So approximately $100 million was spent, and not a single life was saved.

Worth noting: Of the fourteen authors credited in the ASCOT-LLA study, all of them served as consultants to—and received travel expenses, speaking fees, or research funding from—pharmaceutical companies marketing cholesterol-lowering drugs, including Merck, Bristol-Myers Squibb, AstraZeneca, Sanofi, Schering-Plough, Servier, Pharmacia, Bayer, Novartis, and Pfizer. Pfizer (maker of Lipitor) was the principle funding source for the study. That fact alone certainly doesn't make the results invalid, but it's still worth mentioning.

The Heart Protection Study: Pretty Weak Protection

The Heart Protection Study (HPS) divided more than twenty thousand adults with either coronary artery disease or diabetes into two groups and gave one group 40 mg of the statin Zocor daily while the other group received a placebo.[28] It was claimed that "massive benefits" were obtained by lowering cholesterol with the statin drug, and indeed fewer people died in the Zocor group than in the placebo group.

But let's look at the absolute numbers. Those in the Zocor group had an 87.1 percent survival rate after five years, but those in the placebo group had an 85.4 percent survival rate, an absolute difference of 1.8 percent. Most important, the survival rates were independent of lowering cholesterol. In other words, lowering LDL levels made essentially no difference in the risk of death from heart disease. (This is not difficult to understand when you factor in the other things statins do besides lower cholesterol. If anything, it simply shows that statin drugs may be useful in certain populations, but if they are, it's independent of their ability to lower cholesterol. In fact, it increasingly looks like lowering cholesterol may be the least significant thing statins do.)

As Uffe Ravnskov, M.D., Ph.D., stated in a letter to the editor of the *British Medical Journal* regarding the Heart Protection Study results, "Tell a patient that his chance not to die in five years without statin treatment is 85.4 percent and that [statin] treatment can increase this to 87.1 percent. With these figures in hand I doubt that anyone should accept a treatment whose long-term effects are unknown."[29]

Japanese Lipid Intervention Trial: No Relationship between LDL and Dying

In this trial, more than forty-seven thousand patients received Zocor over the course of six years. There was quite a variety in their response to this treatment. Some folks saw dramatic lowering of their LDL levels, some saw a moderate fall in their levels, and some experienced essentially no reduction in their levels.

After five years, the researchers examined the death rate among the participants and cross-referenced these deaths with the patients' LDL levels. You'd think this would be the perfect study to demonstrate a correlation between lower LDL levels and a decreased risk for heart disease, right? Clearly, those whose LDL levels had dropped dramatically would have been far more likely to live, while those whose cholesterol levels had not dropped at all would have been far more likely to die, and those who had lowered their cholesterol only a modest amount would have fallen somewhere in between.

We're sure that's what the researchers expected to see.

But they didn't.

After five years there was exactly no correlation between LDL levels and death rate in the three groups. In other words, whether your cholesterol had been lowered or not had no correlation to whether or not you died. Patients with the highest levels of LDL died at pretty much the exact same rate as patients with the lowest LDL levels (and as patients with LDL levels in between the highest and the lowest). Bottom line: Lowering LDL levels didn't give you even a drop of protection against dying.

PROSPER: Some Benefits, but Only for Certain People

The Prospective Study of Pravastatin in the Elderly at Risk (PROSPER) was interesting for a number of reasons. In this study, older patients were divided into two groups. The first group consisted of patients with no history of heart disease (primary prevention group), and the second group consisted of patients with current or past cardiovascular disease (secondary prevention group). Half of each group received Pravachol (a statin drug), while the other half received a placebo.

There was some reduction in heart attacks or strokes, but only, in the secondary prevention group (those who had current heart disease or a history of heart disease). There was, however, no reduction in heart attacks or strokes in the primary prevention group, the group that had no history of heart disease to begin with. This is pretty much in keeping with the findings of the vast majority of other studies.

But there were two other interesting findings, one of them quite troubling.

When pharmaceutical reps spin the data from the PROSPER study, they concentrate on the single fact that Pravachol reduced heart attacks and strokes (while downplaying the fact that it did so only in the group that already had heart disease). Okay, that's good; the prevention of a few heart attacks and strokes, even in a limited population, is always nice. But what about other measures of health, disease, and well-being besides heart attacks and strokes?

To answer this question, researchers decided to look at other measures of total health impact. They looked at "total deaths" and "total serious adverse events" and found that both were completely unchanged by Pravachol. Once again, a statin drug had a beneficial effect on heart attacks and strokes in the secondary prevention population but not in the primary prevention population, and once again, not a single life was saved overall.

The second finding was more troubling. Both groups receiving Pravachol had an increased risk of cancer. Amazingly, the investigators simply dismissed this statistically significant finding as "the play of chance."

The JUPITER Trial: "Flawed"

We saved this one for last, because it's the juiciest, most perfect example of utter cholesterol madness, media hype, behind-the-scenes manipulation, and intellectual dishonesty.

If you read the papers or watched the news in 2009, you probably heard about this study, though you may not have known what it was called. Its name—JUPITER—stands for the Justification for the Use of Statins in Primary Prevention: An Intervention Trial Evaluating Rosuvastatin. (Even the title of the study should give you pause; you don't do a study to justify the use of a drug you've already decided to use. What if the results of the study indicated the opposite? An objective scientific study wouldn't know the results in advance.)

Anyway, on to the study, about which there's much to dislike and critique—for example, everything.

The JUPITER trial looked at nearly eighteen thousand people whose cholesterol was perfectly normal or even on the low side. What these folks did have, however, were elevated levels of C-reactive protein (CRP). As we've said, CRP is a general measure of inflammation, and for the record, it's a measure we consider important. (You'll read more about CRP testing in chapter 9.) Now it's abundantly clear that what the manufacturers of the drug were aiming for here was a demonstration that statin drugs help prevent deaths even in people with normal cholesterol!

So here's the party line on the JUPITER trial, the line that was robotically repeated in virtually every news outlet in America: The JUPITER trial was such a resounding success that they had to stop it early because it would be "unethical" to continue, given that the group being treated with the drug (Crestor) experienced half as many deaths, strokes, and heart attacks as the control (untreated) group.

The JUPITER trial was touted everywhere as proof that the cholesterol guidelines needed to be changed. Clearly, the drug manufacturers argued, people who met or exceeded the existing standards for cholesterol were demonstrably helped by lowering their "normal"

*When the results of JUPITER came out, the stock of AstraZeneca—the company that makes Crestor—shot up by double digits.

cholesterol even further, virtually cutting their risk for all kinds of terrible things in half! Obviously, they argued to anyone who would listen, we need to make the recommended "normal" levels even lower! (Can you imagine the cheers that would erupt at stockholders' meetings if your product just expanded its market by roughly eleven million people?[30] Why that's almost as good as expanding an adult market by targeting children! Oh, that's right. As of 2011, that's what the statin lobbyists were doing. Never mind.)*

Well that was then. This is now.

Nine respected authors, including a Harvard Medical School faculty member, teamed up to write a critical reappraisal of the JUPITER trial, a reappraisal that was published in 2010 in *Archives of Internal Medicine*, one of the most respected, and conservative, medical journals in the world.[31] "The trial was flawed," they wrote. "It was discontinued (according to pre-specified rules) after fewer than two years of follow-up, with no differences between the two groups on the most objective criteria." The authors also said, "The possibility that bias entered the trial is particularly concerning because of the strong commercial interest in the study." They concluded that "[t]he results of the trial do not support the use of statin treatment for primary prevention of cardiovascular diseases."

So how did this study manage to garner headlines like this one: "Heart Attack Risk Lowered More Than 50 Percent by Taking Crestor!"?

Let's take a look.

The JUPITER trial took 17,800 people—men over sixty, women over fifty—and put them into two groups.

One group received 20 mg of Crestor daily, while the other group received a placebo.

Now before we tell you the results, let's recall the distinction between relative versus absolute numbers, a distinction we talked about earlier.

The study went on for 1.9 years, and at the end of that time it was determined that the risk of having a heart attack in the placebo group was 1.8 percent, while the risk of having a heart attack in the Crestor group was 0.9 percent.

So, yes, there was a 50 percent reduction in risk! Relatively speaking. But let's do the math on the number that really matters, the absolute risk.

The placebo group had a 1.8 percent risk, and the Crestor group had a 0.9 percent risk, so the absolute, real reduction in risk was 1.8 minus 0.9, or 0.9 percent. In absolute numbers, this means that if you took a group of 100 untreated people, 1.8 of them would have a heart attack at some point over the course of almost two years. If you took that same group of 100 people and treated them all with Crestor for the same period, 0.9 of them would have a heart attack. Researchers calculate that this translates into 120 people needing treatment for 1.9 years in order to prevent one event. At a cost of well over a quarter of a million dollars for almost two years' worth of Crestor, that's an awful lot to spend to prevent one event. Especially when there's a significant chance of experiencing really bad side effects from the medicine that's costing you a fortune.

Commenting on the JUPITER study in the *New England Journal of Medicine* in November 2008, Mark A. Hlatky, M.D., wrote: "[A]bsolute differences in risk are

WHAT ABOUT PLAQUE?

Okay, so maybe statin drugs don't cut the risk of dying, except possibly in middle-aged men with previous histories of heart disease (and even then the effect is modest). But what about plaque? Doesn't aggressive lowering of LDL cholesterol at least reduce plaque? (This could, you might argue, have a positive long-term effect on quality of life, even if it doesn't actually save lives.)

Well, no.

A study published in the *American Journal of Cardiology* in 2003 used electron beam tomography to evaluate plaque in 182 patients after 1.2 years of treatment with either statins alone or statins in conjunction with niacin.[34] And yes, just like in many other studies, cholesterol did indeed go down in those patients treated with cholesterol-lowering medication. But plaque?

Sorry.

The authors wrote, "Despite the greater improvement in [cholesterol numbers] . . . there were no differences in calcified plaque progression." In fact, subjects in both groups had—on average—a 9.2 percent increase in plaque buildup. "[W]ith respect to LDL cholesterol lowering, 'lower is better' is not supported by changes in calcified plaque progression," concluded the authors.

more clinically important than relative reductions in risk in deciding whether to recommend drug therapy, since the absolute benefits of treatment must be large enough to justify the associated risks and costs." He added that "[l]ong-term safety is clearly important in considering committing low-risk subjects without clinical disease to twenty years or more of drug treatment."[32]

Did we mention that there was a significantly higher incidence of diabetes in the group treated with Crestor?[33] (In her studies on statin side effects,

Stephanie Seneff also observed a highly significant correlation—p = 0.006—between mentions of diabetes and statin drug side effect reports.)

THE DARKER SIDE OF CHOLESTEROL LOWERING

Now, if you're still on the cholesterol-lowering/statin bandwagon, you might be forgiven for trying to look on the bright side. "Look," we can almost hear you saying, "maybe you guys are right. Maybe lowering cholesterol

Statins are being prescribed left and right to people who have absolutely no business being on them, and to populations for which they have shown no real benefit.

doesn't matter all that much. But clearly there are some good things statins do besides lower cholesterol, as you yourselves have pointed out. They're anti-inflammatory, they're powerful antioxidants, and they thin the blood. So what's the harm if people take them?"

Fair enough. For some people, especially middle-aged men who've already had a first heart attack, the good statins do may indeed outweigh the risks. The problem is twofold: One, statins are being prescribed left and right to people who have absolutely no business being on them, and to populations for which they have shown no real benefit. Two, the risks are significant, serious, varied, and highly underpublicized.

Before we get to our evaluation of the risks and benefits of statin drugs, let's review exactly what it is that cholesterol does in the first place. Understanding the functions of this much maligned molecule will help you understand why so many things can go wrong when we pursue lower and lower cholesterol numbers.

Cholesterol is a hormone factory. Cholesterol is actually the parent molecule for the whole family of hormones known as *steroid hormones*. These hormones include cortisol (known as the fight-or-flight hormone)

and the entire family of sex steroids, including estrogens, progesterones, and testosterone. (No wonder statins produce such serious sexual side effects!)

Cholesterol is used by the body to synthesize bile acids. Bile acids are vitally important for the digestion of fat. The acids are synthesized from cholesterol and then secreted into the bile. Bile acids are so important to the body that the body holds on to most of them. It keeps them from being lost in the feces by causing them to be reabsorbed from the lower intestine, put into a kind of "metabolic recycling" container, and taken back to the liver. Still, even with its best efforts, the body loses some bile acids. To make up for this, the liver synthesizes approximately 1,500 to 2,000 mg of new cholesterol a day (that's about seven to ten times the amount in a large egg). Clearly, the body thinks you need that cholesterol.

Cholesterol is an essential component of all the cell membranes in the body. It's especially important in the membranes of the brain, the nervous system, the spinal cord, and the peripheral nerves. It's incorporated into the myelin sheath, a kind of insulation or "cover" for the nerve fibers that facilitates nerve impulse transmission. And, as we've already seen, cholesterol is an integral part of the lipid raft, essentially allowing for cellular communication. (That's why there are so many cognitive problems associated with aggressive cholesterol lowering.) Cholesterol is also important for stabilizing cells against temperature changes.

Cholesterol is important for the immune system. Cholesterol has an important connection to the immune system. Research has shown that human LDL (the so-called "bad" cholesterol) is able to inactivate more than 90 percent of the worst and most toxic bacterial products.[35]

A number of studies have linked low cholesterol to a greater risk of infections. One review of nineteen large, peer-reviewed studies of more than 68,000 deaths found that low cholesterol predicted an increased risk of dying from respiratory and gastrointestinal diseases, which frequently have an infectious origin.[36] Another study that followed more than 100,000 healthy individuals in San Francisco found that those who had low cholesterol at the beginning of the fifteen-year study were far more likely to be admitted to the hospital because of an infectious disease.[37] And an interesting finding from the MRFIT study showed that sixteen years after their cholesterol was first checked, the group of men whose cholesterol level was 160 mg/dL or lower was four times more likely to die from AIDS than the group of men whose cholesterol was higher than 240 mg/dL![38]

We make vitamin D from cholesterol. It's almost impossible to overstate how important the cholesterol-vitamin D connection is. Vitamin D, which is actually a hormone, not a vitamin, is made from cholesterol in the body. If you lower cholesterol indiscriminately, it stands to reason that you may negatively affect vitamin D levels. And that's hardly insignificant.

Virtually every health practitioner worth his or her salt will tell you that massive numbers of people in the United States (and probably the world) have less than optimal vitamin D levels. According to the Centers for Disease Control and Prevention, "only" 33 percent of the U.S. population is at risk for either vitamin D "inadequacy" or vitamin D "deficiency,"[39] but the levels considered "sufficient" are still being debated, and "sufficient" is hardly "optimal."

In 2010, the Life Extension Foundation conducted a survey of its members—a self-selected sample of people who really care about these things and pay particular attention to their health, blood tests, and supplementation—and found that even in this highly health-conscious population, a whopping 85 percent had blood tests with vitamin D levels below 50 ng/mL, considered the low end of "optimal" (50 to 80 ng/mL).[40]

Why does this matter? Because there is compelling research that links less than optimal levels of vitamin D with heart disease, poor physical performance, osteoporosis, depression, cancer, difficulty in losing weight, and even all-cause mortality. Vitamin D is so important that Dr. Gregory Plotnikoff, medical director of the Penny George Institute for Health and Healing, Abbott Northwestern Hospital in Minneapolis, recently commented, "Because vitamin D is so cheap and so clearly reduces all-cause mortality, I can say this with great certainty: Vitamin D represents the single most cost-effective medical intervention in the United States."[41]

Undoubtedly, there are multiple reasons why so many people are walking around with suboptimal levels of vitamin D, not the least of which is that we are so darn sun-phobic that we now slather SPF 90 on our skin just to go to the grocery store. But is it a coincidence that vitamin D deficiencies and insufficiencies are showing up all over the place at the same time that 11 million to 30 million Americans are on statin drugs, the purpose of which is to lower the very molecule that gives "birth" to this vitally important nutrient?

An Overall Health Benefit of Zero

So what to make of all this? Therapeutics Initiative—a group whose mission is to provide physicians and pharmacists with up-to-date, evidence-based, practical information on prescription drug therapy—wondered the same thing.

Therapeutics Initiative was established in 1994 by the Department of Pharmacology and Therapeutics in cooperation with the Department of Family Practice at the University of British Columbia. To reduce bias as much as humanly possible, it made Therapeutics Initiative wholly independent from the government, the pharmaceutical industry, and other vested interest groups. A telling statement on the website of Therapeutics Initiative sums up the group's mission: "We strongly believe in the need for independent assessments of evidence on drug therapy to balance the drug industry-sponsored information sources."[42]

So it would be interesting to see what Therapeutics Initiative has to say about these statin trials, wouldn't it?

In Therapeutics Letter #48, an issue of its bimonthly letter series, the group tackled the question: "What is the overall health impact when statins are prescribed for primary prevention?" (Remember, primary prevention refers to the use of statin drugs to prevent a first heart attack or coronary "incident," whereas secondary prevention refers to the use of statin drugs to prevent a second heart attack.)

Interesting question, indeed. The scientists at Therapeutics Initiative analyzed five of the major statin trials—the PROSPER, ALLHAT-LLT, and ASCOT-LLA trials mentioned above, plus two published earlier.[43] Taken together, these five trials involved an overall population that was 84 percent primary prevention and 16 percent secondary prevention. In the pooled data, the statins reduced cardiovascular measures—total myocardial infarction (heart attack) and total stroke—by 1.4 percent. Yes, you read that right. Less than a 1.5 percent reduction in the very thing the drugs are supposed to prevent (heart attacks and strokes). "This value indicates that 71 mostly primary prevention patients would have to be treated for three to five years to prevent one such event," wrote the authors. (We wonder how many patients would eagerly sign on for statin therapy if they were asked the following question: Would you be willing to take an expensive drug that has the possibility of serious side effects for three to five years in order to reduce your chances of a cardiovascular event by 1.4 percent?) Note that Therapeutics Initiative used the word "patients" in its analysis of the findings. Instead of the generic term "patients," it should have used the more specific term

Dietary factors and therapeutic lifestyle changes have no side effects. They should be considered the first line of defense in preventive cardiology.

"men." Commenting on the evidence of benefit for primary prevention in women, the researchers reported that in women—28 percent of the total population of the studies—when coronary events were pooled, they were not reduced by statin therapy. "The coronary benefit in primary prevention trials appears to be limited to men," they wrote.

And do we need to remind you that the stated benefit was a mere 1.4 percent reduction in heart attacks and strokes?

It gets worse.

"The other measure of overall impact—total mortality—is available in all five trials, and is not reduced by statin therapy."

In other words, there was a small reduction in cardiovascular deaths but a corresponding increase in deaths from other causes, resulting in an overall mortality benefit of, let's see, that would be . . . zero. And although the researchers clearly acknowledged that paltry less-than-2-percent reduction in heart attack and/or stroke, they also pointed out that this cardiovascular benefit was not reflected in two measures of overall health impact: total mortality (overall death rate) and total number of serious adverse events. "Statins have not been shown to provide an overall health benefit in primary prevention trials," the researchers concluded.[44]

A few years ago, John Abramson, M.D., author of *Overdosed America*, analyzed eight randomized trials that compared statin drugs with placebos. His findings and conclusions were published in a column in *The Lancet*, and they echo the findings and recommendations of the researchers at Therapeutics Initiative. Here's what he wrote:

"Our analysis suggests that . . . statins should not be prescribed for true primary prevention in women of any age or for men older than 69 years. High-risk men age 30 to 69 years should be advised that about 50 patients need to be treated for five years to prevent one event. In our experience, many men presented with this evidence do not choose to take a statin, especially when informed of the potential benefits of lifestyle modification on cardiovascular risk and overall health. This approach, based on the best available evidence in the appropriate population, would lead to statins being used by a much smaller proportion of the overall population than recommended by any of the guidelines."[45]

Statins: A Final Cautionary Note

Millions of Americans will be taking statin drugs for decades, as recommended by the National Cholesterol Education Program's (NCEP) guidelines, and long-term side effects will become apparent, creating a whole host of pathologic situations. What does all this confusion and controversy mean to practicing physicians and the patients for whom they care? Dietary factors and therapeutic lifestyle changes have no side effects. They should be considered the first line of defense in preventive cardiology.

Look, there's not much doubt that statin therapy can significantly reduce the incidence of coronary morbidity and mortality for those who are at great risk of developing coronary artery disease.[46] But as research continues to implicate inflammation as the major coronary risk factor, cholesterol recommendations by groups such as the NCEP may need to be modified. Ultimately, hopefully, the attention paid to cholesterol will be proportional to its importance as a causative factor in heart disease, which is to say, not much.

Rather than selecting treatment options as a technician or a computer would do and targeting cholesterol numbers alone, doctors owe it to their patients—and patients owe it to themselves!—to look further into these controversial issues before embracing potent drugs that might not truly serve the needs of the people for whom they're being prescribed.

Although the use of statins in high-risk coronary patients—especially those with inflammatory markers—might be good medicine right now, overuse of these potent pharmacologic agents (that have both known and unknown side effects) for long-term use in otherwise healthy people is simply not justifiable.

CHAPTER 7

HELP YOUR HEART WITH THESE SUPPLEMENTS

ASK YOUR TYPICAL MAINSTREAM DOCTOR ABOUT NUTRITIONAL SUPPLEMENTS and the first thing you're likely to hear is this: "There's no good research showing they work." Both of us have heard this refrain time and time again when we discuss nutritional medicine with our more conservative colleagues.

It's not true.

You or your doctor can go online to the National Institute of Medicine's library (www.pub-med.com), enter into the search box the name of virtually any vitamin or herb you can think of, and, depending on what you choose, hundreds to thousands of citations will pop up. So the problem isn't an absence of research.

The problem is twofold. One, the conventional training of medical doctors in this country is highly biased toward pharmaceuticals. From the time they enter med school, doctors are courted by the pharmaceutical companies in myriad ways, some subtle, some not so subtle. Free lunches, symposiums, honorariums, consulting and lecturing contracts, vacations, perky pharmaceutical reps showing up at offices with the latest studies that show their products in a favorable light, free samples, and pens and prescription pads bearing the company's name—all create a culture in which pharmaceuticals are the first choice in any treatment plan. (Most docs will tell you these practices have no influence on them or what they choose to prescribe, but the research tells a very different story.[1])

The second part of the problem is that much of the research on vitamins flies beneath the radar. Your overworked doctor barely has time to scan the abstracts of the *New England Journal of Medicine* every month, let alone dig deeply into the hundreds of studies that are published every year on vitamins and nutrients in journals like the *American Journal of Clinical Nutrition*. The vast majority of doctors in this country get no training whatsoever in nutrition, and those who do receive only the most rudimentary and superficial introduction to the subject. Put this together with the built-in medical school bias in favor of patent medicines, and it's easy to see why doctors often fail to think of natural substances as legitimate tools that can help keep people healthy.

Let's be clear. Conventional medicine is simply terrific at keeping people alive in emergencies. Both of us know that if we were to be in a car accident, we wouldn't want the ambulance rushing us to the nearest herbalist's office. We'd want to go to the emergency room of the best hospital we could find. But as good as conventional medicine is at treating people in acute situations, it's astonishingly bad at overall preventive care. It's great at keeping your heart beating if you've just had a heart attack. It's not nearly as good at keeping your heart healthy for the long run and keeping you, the heart's owner, out of the hospital in the first place.

The supplements listed in this chapter are some of the superstars for heart health that Dr. Sinatra uses in his practice (as he has for decades) and that Dr. Jonny has recommended to clients and written about extensively in his books and newsletters.

Neither of us is saying you should just throw out your prescriptions and start randomly taking vitamins. But we *are* saying that natural substances such as vitamins, antioxidants, omega-3 fats, and many of the thousands of compounds found in foods may affect the health of the heart in an even more profound way than many of the medicines routinely prescribed as the first order of business.

Even if you're already on medication, nutritional supplements can still improve your health. In the case of coenzyme Q_{10} (CoQ_{10}), for example, supplementation is an absolute must if you're on a statin drug (more on that in a moment). Magnesium is often used in conjunction with blood sugar drugs such as metformin (Glucophage) or blood pressure medications such as beta blockers. And virtually everyone needs a little help in reducing oxidation and inflammation, two of the most important drivers in the development of heart disease. Omega-3 fatty acids, for example, can be used by just about anyone, whether he or she is on medication or not (check with your doctor for any possible contraindications, such as right before going into surgery).

The following list is far from exhaustive, but it will give you a good idea of how you can use supplements to keep your heart healthy, either alone or, in some cases, as an adjunct to conventional therapy.

COENZYME Q_{10}: THE SPARK OF LIFE

Coenzyme Q_{10} is a vitamin-like substance found throughout the body and made in every cell. Among the many important things it does, CoQ_{10} helps

A CoQ$_{10}$ deficiency affects your heart as profoundly as a calcium deficiency would affect your bones. We create less of it as we age, making it all the more important to supplement with CoQ$_{10}$ as we grow older.

create energy from fuel (food) in the human body, just as a spark plug creates energy from fuel (gasoline) in a car.

Here's how it works: Your body uses a molecule called *adenosine triphosphate*, or ATP, as a source of energy (which is why ATP is nicknamed "the energy molecule"). Much like gasoline is the fuel that allows you to actually drive a car to any of a million destinations, ATP is the fuel that allows your body to perform any of a million activities, ranging from cellular metabolism to doing bench presses to dancing the tango. The body makes ATP by stripping electrons—tiny subatomic particles that carry a negative electrical charge—from food and then delivering those electrons to oxygen, which is an *electron receptor*. CoQ$_{10}$ is one of the carriers of these electrons, so it essentially helps the cells use oxygen and create more energy. Bottom line: CoQ$_{10}$ has the ability to increase the body's production of the energy molecule ATP, and this is a very good thing indeed.

Just as a gasoline engine can't work without spark plugs, the human body can't work without CoQ$_{10}$. It's an essential component of the *mitochondria*, which is command central for the production of cellular energy (ATP). Not coincidentally, the heart is one of the two organs where the most CoQ$_{10}$ is concentrated (the other being the liver). The heart never sleeps, and it never takes a vacation. It beats more than one hundred thousand times a day, making it one of the most metabolically active tissues in the body, so it's very dependent on the energy-generating power of CoQ$_{10}$. A CoQ$_{10}$ deficiency affects your heart as profoundly as a calcium deficiency would affect your bones. We create less of it as we age, making it all the more important to supplement with CoQ$_{10}$ as we grow older. (Although it's present in food, the only foods that have any CoQ$_{10}$ to speak of are organ meats such as heart and liver. It's also easily destroyed by too much heat or overcooking.)

As we've said, one of the biggest problems with statin drugs is that they significantly deplete CoQ$_{10}$ levels. You may recall from the previous chapter on statins that the same pathway that produces cholesterol (the mevalonate pathway) also produces CoQ$_{10}$, so when you block that pathway at its virtual starting gate (as statin drugs do), you not only reduce the body's ability to make cholesterol but you also interfere with its ability to make CoQ_{10}.

We've said this before, but in case you missed it the first time, it's important enough to repeat: If you are on a statin drug you must, repeat *must*, supplement with CoQ_{10}. We recommend at least 100 mg twice a day.

But CoQ_{10} isn't just essential for those on statin drugs. We believe it's essential for everyone else as well, and *especially* for anyone at risk for heart disease.

CoQ_{10} has been approved in Japan as a prescription drug for congestive heart failure since 1974. And even in the United States, the benefits of CoQ_{10} for the heart have been well known since at least the mid-1980s. A study published in the *Proceedings of the National Academy of Sciences of the United States of America* in 1985 gave either CoQ_{10} or a placebo to two groups of patients having class III or class IV cardiomyopathy according to the definitions put forth by the New York Heart Association (NYHA).[2] These are seriously ill folks. Class III patients have marked limitation in activity because of symptoms and can basically only be comfortable at rest or with minimal activity; class IV patients have severe limitations and experience symptoms even while resting. (Most class IV patients are bedbound.)

So what happened when these very sick patients were given CoQ_{10}? Here's how the researchers themselves summarized the results: "These patients, steadily worsening and expected to die within two years under conventional therapy, generally showed an extraordinary clinical improvement, indicating that

CoQ_{10} therapy might extend the lives of such patients. This improvement could be due to correction of a myocardial deficiency of CoQ_{10} and to enhanced synthesis of CoQ_{10}-requiring enzymes."[3]

Another study that lasted six years and was published in 1990 looked at 143 patients, 98 percent of whom were in the same two classes as the patients in the 1985 study.[4] The participants were given 100 mg of CoQ_{10} (orally), in addition to being treated in their conventional medical program. Eighty-five percent of the patients improved by one or two NYHA classes, and there was no positive evidence of toxicity or intolerance. "CoQ_{10} is safe and effective long-term therapy for cardiomyopathy," the study authors concluded.

CoQ_{10} also has the ability to reduce blood pressure. A recent meta-analysis of CoQ_{10} in the treatment of high blood pressure reviewed twelve different clinical trials and found that across the board, patients who received CoQ_{10} supplementation had significant reductions in blood pressure compared to control subjects who didn't receive supplemention.[5] It's no wonder that several studies have demonstrated a strong correlation between severity of heart disease and severity of CoQ_{10} deficiency.[6]

You might recall that oxidative damage (oxidation) is one of the four major culprits in heart disease, and you might also remember that cholesterol in the body is never a problem until it becomes oxidized. It's only this oxidized cholesterol—specifically, pattern B LDL cholesterol—that is a problem, because pattern B LDL molecules are the ones that adhere to the cell walls and initiate or accelerate the process of inflammation.

◀ WHAT YOU NEED TO KNOW

- Coenzyme Q_{10} (CoQ_{10}) is a kind of "energy fuel" for the heart.
- Statins deplete CoQ_{10}; supplementation is an absolute necessity if you're on a statin drug, and it is a very good idea even if you're not.
- D-ribose is one of the components of the energy molecule ATP, which the body uses to power all activity.
- L-carnitine supplementation after a heart attack increases survival rate and makes it less likely you'll suffer a second heart attack.
- Magnesium relaxes the artery walls, reduces blood pressure, and makes it easier for the heart to pump blood and for the blood to flow freely.
- Niacin will lower both triglycerides and the "bad" kind of LDL cholesterol. It also reduces a toxic substance called lipoprotein(a)—Lp(a) for short—and raises HDL. Don't use the time-release kind.
- Omega-3s—especially from fish—lower the death rate from heart disease. They also lower triglycerides, resting heart rate, and blood pressure.
- Omega-3s are highly anti-inflammatory.
- At least twenty-eight clinical trials in humans show that pantothenic acid (vitamin B_5) produces positive changes in triglycerides and LDL cholesterol. It also increases HDL.
- Nattokinase and lumbrokinase are natural "clot busters."
- Other supplements worth considering include vitamin C, curcumin, resveratrol, and cocoa flavanols.

Why do we mention that here? Simple. CoQ_{10} is a powerful antioxidant, inhibiting oxidative damage to LDL cholesterol and thus helping to prevent cholesterol from becoming a "problem" in the first place. It's far smarter to prevent LDL from getting damaged and sticky in the first place than to use a sledgehammer pharmaceutical to reduce LDL as much as possible!

Coenzyme Q_{10} and vitamin E have a strange, almost symbiotic relationship. In rats given supplemental vitamin E, increases in blood levels of CoQ_{10} were observed; in baboons given supplemental CoQ_{10}, the anti-inflammatory effects of vitamin E were increased; and in one study, CoQ_{10} plus vitamin E actually lowered C-reactive protein (CRP), a systemic measure of inflammation. We think it's wise to make sure you're getting about 200 IUs or so of vitamin E a day (from mixed tocopherols with a high gamma vitamin E formula) in addition to your CoQ_{10} supplement. (But read the section on vitamin E, "The Good, the Bad, and the Ugly," first!)

D-RIBOSE: THE MISSING LINK

D-ribose, a five-carbon sugar, is one of the components of ATP, the energy molecule the body uses to power all activities. Without D-ribose, there would be no ATP; without ATP, there would be no energy.

Both CoQ_{10} and the nutritional supplement L-carnitine help facilitate the process by which the body manufactures ATP. Metaphorically speaking, they act like little elves, shuttling the material needed to make ATP to the factories where it's made, resulting in more efficient production of this important energy molecule. CoQ_{10} and L-carnitine can be said to function like very efficient trucks transporting building materials to the factories where stuff actually gets built, but D-ribose is one of the actual building *materials*. A shortage of D-ribose means a shortage of ATP, and a shortage of ATP, especially in the heart, is bad news indeed.

D-ribose is synthesized in every cell in the body, but only slowly and to varying degrees depending on the tissue. Tissues such as the liver, adrenal cortex, and adipose tissue make plenty of D-ribose because

they produce chemical compounds used to synthesize fatty acids and steroids, which are in turn used to make hormones.

But molecules of D-ribose made by these tissues are the opposite of rollover minutes on your cell phone—they have to be used right then and there and can't be "transferred" to other tissues that might need them, such as the heart. The heart, as well as the skeletal muscles and brain, can only make enough ribose for their day-to-day needs. They have no D-ribose saving account. When the cells of the heart, for example, encounter a stressor such as oxygen deprivation, they lack the metabolic machinery needed to quickly whip up some badly needed D-ribose. Tissues that are stressed because they don't get enough blood flow or oxygen can't make enough D-ribose to replace lost energy quickly. And when oxygen or blood flow deficits are chronic—as in heart disease—tissues can never make enough D-ribose, and cellular energy levels are constantly depleted.

The D-ribose connection to cardiac function was first discovered by the physiologist Heinz-Gerd Zimmer at the University of Munich. In 1973, Zimmer reported that energy-starved hearts would recover much faster if D-ribose was given prior to or immediately following ischemia (an insufficient supply of blood to the heart, usually as a result of blockage). Five years later, Zimmer demonstrated that the energy-draining effects of certain drugs used to make the heart beat stronger (called *inotropic agents*) could be significantly lessened if D-ribose was given along with the drugs.

The most important finding from Zimmer's research was that D-ribose plays an enormous part in both energy restoration and the return of normal diastolic cardiac function. (Diastolic *dysfunction* is basically a kind of heart failure.) One 1992 clinical study from Zimmer's group showed that administering D-ribose to patients with severe but stable coronary artery disease increased their ability to do exercise and delayed the onset of moderate angina (chest pain). Since then, the benefits of D-ribose have been reported for heart failure, cardiac surgery recovery, restoration of energy to stressed skeletal muscles, and control of free radical formation in tissues that have been deprived of oxygen.

Here's one dramatic story from Dr. Sinatra's practice that illustrates the almost miraculous power of D-ribose supplementation to improve the quality of life of cardiac patients:

Dr. Sinatra:
The Case of Louis and D-Ribose

Louis came to my office suffering from severe coronary artery disease. He had been previously treated by having a stent placed in a major coronary artery, but he still had severe blockage in a small arterial branch that was difficult to dilate with a stent and next to impossible to bypass with surgery. He had what's called refractory angina, which means he experienced chest pain even with normal activities such as walking across a room. He'd also feel chest pain anytime he had even mild emotional stress. Louis had visited a number of cardiologists for his heart problem and had been placed on a number of common heart drugs, but his problems persisted.

When Louis came to my office I noticed high levels of uric acid in his blood, indicating faulty ATP metabolism. At the time, he was already taking L-carnitine and CoQ$_{10}$ at "maintenance doses." Realizing that it would help him enormously if he could build up his ATP stores, I immediately recommended D-ribose as well as increased doses of L-carnitine and CoQ$_{10}$. In just a few short days, Louis showed remarkable improvement. His son-in-law, a dentist, called me a few days later and reported, "You fixed Louis!"

An adequate dose of D-ribose usually results in symptom improvement very quickly, sometimes within days, as in Louis's case. If initial response is poor, the dose should be increased to 5 g (1 teaspoon) three times a day. Logically, those who are the sickest and the most energy depleted will notice the most improvement in the quickest time.

Despite accumulating scientific evidence of the benefit of D-ribose, very few physicians in the United States have even heard of it outside of their first-year med school biochemistry class. Fewer still recommend it to their patients. Those who are familiar with it have the wonderful gratification of seeing it help patients on a regular basis.

Although the optimal level of D-ribose supplementation will differ depending on the person and the particular condition, here are some good recommended starting points for supplementation:

- 5 g daily for cardiovascular prevention, for athletes on maintenance, and for healthy people who engage in strenuous activities or hard-core workouts
- 10 to 15 g daily for most patients with heart failure, ischemic cardiovascular disease, or peripheral vascular disease; for individuals recovering from heart attacks or heart surgery; for treatment of stable angina; and for athletes who engage in chronic bouts of high-intensity exercise
- 15 to 20 g daily for patients with advanced heart failure, dilated cardiomyopathy, or frequent angina; for individuals awaiting heart transplant; and for individuals with severe fibromyalgia, muscle cramps, or neuromuscular disease

Reported side effects are minimal and infrequent, and there are no known adverse drug or nutritional interactions associated with D-ribose use. The toxicology and safety of D-ribose have been exhaustively studied, and the supplement is 100 percent safe when taken as directed. (Thousands of patients have taken D-ribose at doses of up to 60 g a day with minimal, if any, side effects.)

However, even though there are no known contraindications for supplementation with D-ribose, we recommend that pregnant women, nursing mothers, and very young children refrain from taking D-ribose simply because there is not enough research on using it in these populations.

L-CARNITINE: THE SHUTTLE BUS FOR FATTY ACIDS

As previously stated, the best way to conceptualize L-carnitine is to think of it as a transportation system. It acts as a kind of shuttle bus, loading up fatty acids and transporting them into tiny structures within each cell called *mitochondria*, where they can be burned for energy. Because the heart gets 60 percent of its energy from fat, it's very important that the body has enough L-carnitine to shuttle the fatty acids into the heart's muscle cells.

Studies of patients being treated for various forms of cardiovascular disease provide the strongest evidence for the benefit of L-carnitine supplementation. One study showed that people who took L-carnitine supplements after suffering heart attacks had significantly lower mortality rates compared to those of a control group (1.2 percent of the L-carnitine takers died versus 12.5 percent of the subjects in the control group).[7] One randomized, placebo-controlled study divided eighty heart failure patients into two groups. One group received 2 g of L-carnitine a day, and the other group received a placebo. There was a significantly higher three-year survival rate in the group receiving L-carnitine.[8]

L-carnitine improves the ability of those with angina to exercise without chest pain.[9] In one study, the walking capacity of patients with intermittent claudication—a painful cramping sensation in the muscles of the legs because of a decreased oxygen supply—improved significantly when they were given oral L-carnitine. In another study, patients with peripheral arterial disease of the legs were able to increase their walking distance by 98 meters when they supplemented with L-carnitine; they were able to walk almost twice as far as those who were given a placebo. Further, congestive heart failure patients have experienced an increase in exercise endurance on only 900 mg of L-carnitine a day.

And if that were not enough to establish L-carnitine's bonafides, it has been shown to be a powerful cardioprotective antioxidant. One paper published in the *International Journal of Cardiology* found that L-carnitine had a direct stimulatory effect on two important oxidative stress-related compounds (HO-1 and ecNOS). Both of these markers have antioxidant, antiproliferative (meaning they have an inhibitory effect on tumor cells), and anti-inflammatory properties, so ratcheting up their activity a notch is a very good thing indeed. The researchers concluded that this action of L-carnitine "would be expected to protect from oxidative stress related to cardiovascular and myocardial damage."[10]

Dr. Sinatra: L-Carnitine and CoQ$_{10}$

Eighty-five percent of my patients with congestive heart failure have improved significantly on CoQ$_{10}$. But I was concerned about the 15 percent who, despite supplementation with CoQ$_{10}$, still had symptoms that severely compromised their quality of life.

These folks were supplementing with CoQ$_{10}$ and had excellent blood levels to show for it, typically 3.5 ug/mL or higher (the normal level of CoQ$_{10}$ is 0.5 to 1.5 ug/mL.) Nonetheless, these folks seemed to be unable to utilize what was in their own bodies.

As I read more about L-carnitine, I came to see that it might work in synergy with coenzyme Q$_{10}$, stoking the fire in the ATP production phase of the Krebs cycle (a sequence of reactions by which living cells generate energy). I finally got comfortable enough to recommend to some of my worrisome patients that they give it a try in combination with CoQ$_{10}$, and wow, what a difference!

These treatment-resistant folks came in with better color, breathed easier, and walked around the office with minimal difficulty. I was genuinely amazed. It was as if the L-carnitine provided a battery, working perfectly with the coenzyme Q$_{10}$.

The bottom line is that the heart is the most metabolically active tissue in the body, and thus it requires a huge and constant amount of energy molecules, or ATPs.

Remember, the heart has to pump sixty to one hundred times a minute, twenty-four hours a day, for years and years with no time off for good behavior! Cardiac muscle cells burn fats for fuel, so the heart is especially vulnerable to even subtle deficiencies in the factors contributing to ATP supply: coenzyme Q$_{10}$, D-ribose, and L-carnitine.

These nutrients make up three of what Dr. Sinatra calls the "Awesome Foursome" in metabolic cardiology. Now let's introduce the fourth.

MAGNESIUM: THE GREAT RELAXER

Dr. Robert Atkins once referred to magnesium as a "natural calcium channel blocker," and he was 100 percent correct. A few paragraphs from now, you'll understand just why magnesium's ability to block the channels by which calcium gets into the cells is so important for the health of your heart.

Recent research strongly suggests that calcium in the heart can be a huge problem. One meta-analysis examined fifteen eligible trials with the objective of investigating the relationship between calcium supplements and cardiovascular disease. The researchers concluded that calcium supplements (administered without vitamin D) were associated with a modest but significant *increase* in the risk of cardiovascular disease—an increase, they noted, that might well translate into "a large burden of disease in the population." The authors called for a reassessment of the role of calcium supplements in the management of osteoporosis.[11]

A second study had a different purpose, one particularly relevant to our story.[12] The researchers began with the premise that statins reduce cardiovascular risk and slow the progression of coronary artery calcium. The purpose of the study, then, was to determine whether lowering LDL cholesterol (as statins do) is in some way complementary to slowing the progression of coronary artery calcium. The researchers basically wanted to illuminate the relationship of these two phenomena as they relate to heart disease.

Here's what they did. They measured the change in coronary artery calcium in 495 patients who were basically symptom-free at the beginning of the study. They did this by using a method known as electron beam tomography scanning. Right after their first scan, the patients were started on statin drugs, and they were followed for an average of 3.2 years, during which time their cholesterol was checked and they were scanned on a regular basis. Over the course of the 3.2-year follow-up period, 41 of the patients had heart attacks.

On average, the 454 patients who did *not* suffer heart attacks saw their arterial calcium go up by approximately 17 percent every year. But the 41 patients who *did* experience heart attacks saw a whopping 42 percent increase per year in their arterial calcium. According to the researchers, having a faster progression of coronary artery calcium gives you an astonishing 17.2-fold increase in your heart attack risk.[13]

And get this: LDL cholesterol did *not* differ between the two groups. Ironically, the LDL levels of the folks who did *not* suffer heart attacks were slightly *higher* (though not significantly so) than the average LDL levels of the folks who *did* suffer heart attacks.

So let's summarize the results. Both groups—the 41 folks who *had* heart attacks and the 454 folks who didn't—essentially had the *same* LDL levels. (So if you were using patients' LDL levels to predict heart attacks, you'd get no better accuracy than you would by reading their horoscopes!) But if instead of LDL levels you looked at the levels of calcium in the arteries, it would be a whole different story. Those who suffered myocardial infarctions were the *most* likely to have higher calcium levels in their arteries, especially when the arteries became totally blocked.

Coronary artery calcification has long been recognized as a big risk factor for heart disease, but for some reason we continue to obsessively focus on cholesterol, while few people have heard much about the calcium connection.

Arthur Agatston, M.D., a Florida cardiologist best known as the author of *The South Beach Diet*, actually invented a scoring method to determine the severity of calcification in the arteries—it's known as the Agatston score. (Research shows that people with Agatston scores higher than 400 are at a significantly increased risk for coronary "events"— myocardial infarctions—as well as for most coronary artery procedures [bypasses, angioplasty, etc.].[14])

Calcium in the bones? Very good. Calcium in the arteries? Not so good.

Enter magnesium.

Magnesium and calcium have an interesting, symbiotic relationship. When magnesium is depleted, intracellular calcium rises. Magnesium also inhibits platelet aggregation, an important step in the development of clots. Calcium channel blockers widen and relax the blood vessels by affecting the muscle cells found in the arterial walls, which is exactly what magnesium does—splendidly, we might add. Magnesium dilates the arteries, thus reducing blood pressure and making it far easier for the heart to pump blood and for the blood to flow freely.

In most of the epidemiologic and clinical trials, a high dietary intake of magnesium (at least 500 to 1,000 mg a day) resulted in reduced blood pressure.[15] These studies showed an inverse relationship between magnesium intake and blood pressure; people who consumed *more* magnesium had *lower* blood pressure. One study of 60 hypertensive subjects who were given magnesium supplementation showed a significant reduction in blood pressure over an eight-week period.[16]

So basically, you can think of magnesium as a "relaxer." One of the most relaxing things you can do is to bathe in Epsom salts, which is basically a compound of magnesium with a little bit of sulfur and oxygen. If you've ever worked with an integrative medicine practitioner who happens to use vitamin drips, you might have found that the most amazing and restful sleep you've ever had occurred after getting a magnesium-heavy vitamin push.* Just as magnesium has a relaxing effect on your body, it also has a relaxing effect on your arteries. And that's a very good thing from the perspective of the heart, which instead of having to push blood through a narrow or constricted vessel (dangerously raising blood pressure) now has the much easier task of pumping it through a relaxed, widened vessel that doesn't put up so much resistance. Your heart doesn't have to work as hard, your blood pressure goes down, and all is well with the world.

There's another interesting connection between magnesium and the heart, and if you've followed our argument so far, you'll love the elegance of how it all comes full circle. The connection? Sugar.

You'll recall from chapter 4 that sugar is one of the worst things you can eat if you want to have a healthy heart. (To save you the trouble of looking it up, here's why: Sugar is highly inflammatory. It also

---

*A form of vitamin injection administered slowly over the course of ten to fifteen minutes.

creates dangerous compounds known as advanced glycation end products, or AGEs, which play a pivotal role in atherosclerosis.[17]) AGEs play a role of particular importance in type 2 diabetes, which, as you know, is a condition in which blood sugar and insulin are essentially at unhealthy levels and have to be brought under control. (And diabetes is one way to fast-track your path to heart disease.)

One of the very best things magnesium does is help manage blood sugar. In several studies of diabetic patients, magnesium supplements of 400 to 1,000 mg per day, given for anywhere from three weeks to three months, improved a number of measures of glycemic (blood sugar) control, including the requirement for insulin.[18] One study measured serum concentrations of magnesium in 192 people with insulin resistance and found that the prevalence of a low magnesium level was about 65 percent among those with insulin resistance, as opposed to only 5 percent of those in a control group.[19]

Clearly, there's a strong association between magnesium deficiency and insulin resistance. You'll recall that people with insulin resistance are at great risk for diabetes, which in turn puts them at great risk for heart disease. Helping to control blood sugar and insulin is just one more important way in which magnesium is critical for heart health.

Magnesium is necessary for more than three hundred biochemical reactions in the body, and many of these are enzymatic reactions, essential for heart health (or what scientists call *myocardial metabolism*).[20] Even borderline deficiencies of magnesium can nega-tively affect the heart, and not surprisingly, there is a considerable amount of evidence associating low levels of magnesium with cardiovascular disease.[21]

Bottom line: Magnesium supplements are a must for those who want to protect their hearts. Magnesium lowers blood pressure, helps control blood sugar, and relaxes the lining of the blood vessels. And almost all dietary surveys show that Americans aren't getting nearly enough.[22] We recommend supplementing with at least 400 mg per day.

NOTE: Magnesium supplementation is *not* recommended for anyone with renal insufficiency (kidney disease).

NIACIN AND ITS EFFECT ON CHOLESTEROL

Even if your doctor hasn't studied nutrition and is skeptical (or worse) when it comes to supplements, chances are he or she will be familiar with the benefits of niacin. It's been known since 1955 that cholesterol can be effectively lowered with doses of 1,000 to 4,000 mg of niacin daily.[23] Subsequent studies have shown that niacin will lower triglycerides by 20 to 50 percent and LDL cholesterol by 10 to 25 percent.[24]

Niacin is one of two major forms of vitamin B_3—the other is nicotinamide. Although both forms can be used for different things in the body, only the niacin form has an effect on your cholesterol, triglycerides, and related compounds. And the effect is not just on overall cholesterol. Studies have shown that when LDL cholesterol is reduced with niacin, there is a pref-erential reduction of the really nasty LDL molecules, the hard, small, BB gun pellet-type particles that stick to the artery walls, get oxidized, and cause damage.

Niacin also reduces lipoprotein(a), or Lp(a). Lipoprotein(a) is basically a special kind of LDL, and it's a really bad one. This, folks, is the *real* cholesterol story! Lp(a) is an independent risk factor for heart disease and for heart attacks, yet it doesn't get as much attention as cholesterol does because there aren't effective drug treatments for lowering it, and no one really knows what to do about it. Niacin lowers Lp(a) levels by a remarkable 10 to 30 percent.[25]

Equally terrific, if not more so, is the fact that niacin *raises* HDL cholesterol. That alone would be worth shouting from the rooftops, because we consider HDL cholesterol to be a much undervalued player in the heart disease story. (We'll delve into this topic later on in the book.) Niacin raises HDL levels by 10 to 30 percent.[26] But even better is the fact that it *preferentially* increases HDL-2, which is the most beneficial of the HDL subclasses.[27] (HDL-3 is actually pro-inflammatory, even though it's a member of the so-called "good" cholesterol family—HDL—once again demonstrating how obsolete and ridiculous the classification of cholesterol into just "good" and "bad" really is!)

The most clinically important side effect of too much niacin is that it can be very taxing on the liver (a condition known as hepatotoxicity), although as Dr. Alan Gaby points out in his exhaustive review of nutritional supplements and disease, this is almost never seen in patients taking 3 g or less per day.[28]

Abram Hoffer, M.D., the great pioneer of nutritional and integrative medicine, stated that his thirty years of experience with niacin therapy (usually 3 g a day or more) showed that one out of every two thousand patients will develop hepatitis from large doses of this vitamin. However, Hoffer also pointed out that in all of his patients who developed hepatotoxicity, liver function returned to normal after treatment was discontinued.[29]

Sustained-release niacin is actually more hepatotoxic than regular niacin, and liver problems may occur at lower doses.[30] Nausea may be an early warning sign of niacin-induced hepatotoxicity; if nausea occurs, the dose should be reduced, or treatment should be stopped.[31] For folks taking therapeutic doses of niacin, it's a good idea to have your doctor check your liver enzymes periodically using a standard liver function test.

Dr. Jonny: Niacin Flush

The first time I experienced the "niacin flush" I was working as a personal trainer. It was five o'clock in the morning, and I was getting ready for my six a.m. client. I remember drinking my protein shake, swallowing my vitamins, and then, a very short time later while getting dressed, having the distinct feeling that I was going to die. My skin was flushed, warm to the touch, and my cheeks (and arms) were pinkish red. It wasn't painful, but it was deeply unpleasant.

My six a.m. client happened to be the president of a high-end makeup company whose husband was an equally well-known Manhattan dermatologist (as well as the only doctor I knew who was likely to be awake at this ungodly hour). I called my client, and she immediately put her husband on the line. I described my symptoms, and he asked me if I'd taken or eaten anything unusual. "Just my vitamins," I said, to which he replied without hesitation, "Oh, it's just the niacin. Nothing to worry about, it'll pass in a few. I'm going back to bed now."

So that was my first encounter with the infamous "niacin flush." It's basically a temporary flushing of the skin, not at all dangerous (especially if you know it's coming!), and it's actually a result of the dilation of the blood vessels in the skin (which is why my skin turned pink). Some people experience itching as well or even a mild burning sensation. It typically goes away within a couple of weeks and can usually be counteracted with a baby aspirin taken beforehand.

NOTE: If you are diabetic or have a liver ailment, be sure to check with your doctor before supplementing with niacin.

Dr. Sinatra's Niacin Know-How

- Look for straight, non-time-release niacin (also known as nicotinic acid). Take after meals at dosages of 500 mg to 3 g daily (see below).
- Start slowly at 100 mg. Work your way up gradually to a higher level, in divided doses.
- If the flush is too uncomfortable, take a baby aspirin before the first meal of the day and then take the niacin after the meal. Use the aspirin only as long as you experience the flush and whenever you increase your niacin dosage, which will trigger a flush.
- You can also try taking an apple pectin supplement with the niacin to reduce a flush.
- Niacin may increase the enzyme levels in liver function tests. This does not necessarily mean

that niacin is causing a liver problem, but have your doctor keep an eye on it. He or she may suggest stopping the niacin for five days before your next liver test to avoid possible confusion. Be aware, though, that when you resume the niacin you will develop a flush.

VITAMIN E: THE GOOD, THE BAD, AND THE UGLY

For decades, the nutritional world revered vitamin E as something of a heart savior, a major antioxidant that defended against lipid peroxidation, which was thought to be the cause of cardiovascular disease. (*Lipid* simply means fat, and *peroxidation* is a fancy way of saying oxidative damage from free radicals.) During the 1990s the adulation for vitamin E even extended to mainstream medicine, going as far as the American Heart Association. In 1996, for instance, vitamin E was celebrated in a well-publicized study for significantly reducing cardiovascular events over the course of one year among some 2,000 patients with documented heart disease.

The successes and reputation of vitamin E prompted many to believe that if a little vitamin E was good, then more would be even better! Critical studies that followed, however, began demonstrating that daily doses of vitamin E at 400 IUs and above didn't necessarily generate beneficial results, and, in fact, might be detrimental to health. (As early as 2003, Dr. Sinatra wrote in his newsletter about his own reluctance to back high-dose vitamin E because the emerging research indicated possible pro-oxidant effects.)

That said, both of us found ourselves puzzled by the negative study results that have popped up since then. Sure, problems could come from using the synthetic form of vitamin E (designated *dl-alpha-tocopherol*) instead of the "natural" form (designated *d-alpha-tocopherol*). But a *pro*-oxidant effect from natural vitamin E, considered one of the powerhouses in the anti-oxidant armamentarium? How could that be?

Sharp-eyed readers may have noticed that we put quotation marks around the word *natural* when referring to natural vitamin E in the above paragraph. That's because d-alpha-tocopherol by itself is only one *part* of natural vitamin E. Vitamin E is actually a collection of eight related compounds that are divided into two classes: *tocopherols* and *tocotrienols*. The tocopherols come in four forms: *alpha, delta, beta,* and *gamma.* Of these four forms, the best known is alpha. When you purchase a "natural" vitamin E supplement, most of the time it is 100 percent *alpha*-tocopherol.

And therein lies the problem.

Gamma-tocopherol is turning out to be the most potent of the four tocopherols, and the one most responsible for vitamin E's positive effects as an anti-oxidant. Thus, people taking high-dose alpha-tocopherol alone and not getting enough gamma-tocopherol in their diets, or in their supplements, could run the risk of experiencing a pro-oxidant effect from vitamin E. Moreover, large doses of alpha-tocopherol could also deplete the body's existing gamma-tocopherol stores.

A 2011 study provided an even sharper image of the two faces of vitamin E. In laboratory experiments, researchers in Belfast found that vitamin E (alpha- and gamma-tocopherol) protects very low-density lipoprotein (VLDL) and LDL cholesterol against oxidation. That's a good thing! Yet they found a "surprising" pro-oxidant effect on HDL (high-density lipoprotein), the cholesterol particle that acts like a garbage truck, picking up harmful oxidized LDL and transporting it back to the liver for removal. Anything that can hinder HDL is of real concern.

Worth noting is that the researchers referenced a previous study in which taking a small amount of vitamin C along with your alpha-tocopherol helped *prevent* the negative, pro-oxidant effect of vitamin E on HDL. That wouldn't be the first time one nutrient helped another one out. We already know that CoQ_{10} helps protect vitamin E in the body and gives it a hand by recycling it back to an active form after it's been oxidized in biochemical reactions. (We are big fans of the synergistic effects of nutrients.)

The other half of the vitamin E story concerns the four components known as the *tocotrienols.* Tocotrienols are turning out to be the real heavy lifters in the vitamin E family, at least when it comes to benefits for the heart. They have more potent antioxidant activity than tocopherols do.[32] They also increase the number of LDL receptors, which helps with LDL removal.[33] Tocotrienols provide significant lipid-lowering effects in experimental animals, and most prospective studies have demonstrated the same thing in humans.[34]

If you take vitamin E, we recommend that you always get it from a supplement labeled "mixed tocopherols" in order to avoid the problems that can occur with pure alpha-tocopherol supplementation. A vitamin E supplement that is 100 percent alpha-tocopherol is less effective and may even be problematic in high doses. Virtually all the studies showing negative results used the alpha-tocopherol form or, worse, the synthetic dl-alpha-tocopherol form. (The dl-alpha-tocopherol form should be left on the shelf to rot!)

If you add 200 IUs of mixed tocopherols or high-gamma vitamin E to a regimen that also includes vitamin C and CoQ$_{10}$, you should be fine!

FISH OIL'S OMEGA-3: THE ULTIMATE WELLNESS MOLECULE

If you've read this book sequentially, you're already familiar with omega-3 fatty acids from our extensive discussion of them in chapter 5, so here we'll highlight just a few of the many studies demonstrating the value of omega-3 fats for the heart. (We should also point out that there is equally compelling research documenting the positive effect of omega-3s on the brain as well,[35] but because this is a book on cholesterol and cardiovascular disease, we'll focus on the heart.)

More than thirty years ago, scientists began to notice very low rates of cardiovascular disease among Greenland Eskimos compared to age- and sex-matched Danish control subjects. Shortly afterward, they were able to link these low rates of heart disease to high consumption of omega-3s in the Greenland diet.[36] This discovery triggered an enormous amount of research on the role of fish oil in preventing heart disease. (On the day of writing this—December 7, 2011—a National Library of Medicine search for the term "omega-3 fatty acids cardiovascular" produced 2,524 citations.)

One recent review of omega-3s and cardiovascular disease by Dariush Mozaffarian, M.D., of the Harvard School of Public Health, concluded that omega-3 consumption "lowers plasma triglycerides,

resting heart rate, and blood pressure and might also improve myocardial filling and efficiency, lower inflammation, and improve vascular function."[37] Mozaffarian also noted that the benefits of omega-3s seem most consistent for coronary heart disease mortality and sudden cardiac death.

In case your eyes were beginning to glaze over from all the medical journal speak, let's sum it up in plain English: *There is reliable and consistent research evidence demonstrating that omega-3 fats, mainly from fish, lower the death rate from heart disease and lower the risk of sudden cardiac death.* This is hardcore evidence that fish oil saves lives.

One of the landmark clinical studies of omega-3 supplementation in a high-risk population was published in 1999 and was known as the GISSI-Prevenzione trial.[38] More than 11,000 patients who had suffered a heart attack within the past three months were randomly assigned to receive either 1 g a day of omega-3s, 300 mg of vitamin E, both, or neither, in addition to whatever standard therapy they were receiving. Vitamin E had no effect, but omega-3s were associated with a 20 percent reduction in mortality and a whopping 45 percent reduction in the risk of sudden death. These effects were apparent within a mere three months of therapy.[39]

International guidelines recommend 1 g of omega-3 fats daily for all people who've already had a heart attack or for patients with elevated triglycerides.[40] Experts believe these guidelines will soon be extended to patients with heart failure as well.[41]

It's worth mentioning that the overwhelming majority of research on omega-3s and heart disease was done using the two omega-3s that are found in fish, EPA and DHA. But other studies have also found that ALA—the omega-3 found in plant foods such as flax and flaxseed oil—has benefits for the heart as well. One review of the literature pointed out that both *in vitro* (test-tube) studies and animal studies have shown that ALA can prevent ventricular fibrillation, the chief mechanism of cardiac death, and that it might be even more efficient at preventing this than EPA and DHA are. The review also noted that ALA was effective at lowering platelet aggregation, which is an important step in thrombosis (a stroke or nonfatal heart attack).[42]

Even if you're already on a statin drug and have decided to remain on one, fish oil can still help you. One study found that among more than 3,600 people with a history of cardiovascular disease—many of whom were on antiplatelet drugs, antihypertensive agents, and nitrates—daily fish oil supplementation led to a statistically significant 19 percent reduction in major coronary events compared to the control group.[43]

Omega-3 fats, particularly from healthy, wild fish, are your heart's best friend, whether you're recovering from a heart attack or hoping to prevent one. They lower triglycerides. And they lower blood pressure. And best of all, omega-3s are among the most anti-inflammatory compounds on the planet, meaning they have a beneficial effect on the root causes of heart disease.

We recommend that you take 1 to 2 g of fish oil daily, and that you eat cold water fish (such as wild salmon) as often as you can. (We both recommend Vital Choice, an impeccable source of wild salmon from pristine Alaskan waters that is reasonably priced and shipped in dry ice directly to your door.)

When you supplement with fish oil, remember that the total amount of omega-3s is not what's important. Bargain-basement omega-3 supplements often tout on their labels how much omega-3 they contain. This number by itself is meaningless. You want to know specifically how much EPA and DHA are contained within each capsule. These are the gold nuggets in the prospector's tin—you don't care about the *total* amount of stones in that pan, you care about the *gold*. EPA and DHA are the gold. Try to get at least 1 g daily of combined EPA and DHA. (For many of his patients, Dr. Sinatra prefers higher DHA, as it penetrates more into the heart, brain, and retina than EPA does, so he frequently uses squid or algae oil in addition to fish oil because of its higher DHA content.)

PANTETHINE: YOUR SECRET WEAPON

Pantethine is a metabolically active (and somewhat more expensive) form of vitamin B_5 (pantothenic acid). The blood tests of patients with dyslipidemia—a fancy way of saying that their blood levels of cholesterol are too high—significantly improve with pantethine supplementation. And although this can't be seen on a blood test, pantethine also reduces the oxidation of LDL.[44]

No fewer than twenty-eight clinical trials in humans have shown that pantethine produces significant positive changes in triglycerides, LDL cholesterol, and VLDL, along with increases in HDL cholesterol.[45] In all of these trials, virtually no adverse effects were noted. The mean dose of pantethine in these studies was 900 mg per day given as 300 mg three times daily. This appears to be the optimal dosage, and it is the one we recommend.

According to a review of the literature on pantethine published in *Progress in Cardiovascular Diseases*, Mark Houston, M.D., noted that in most studies, at the end of four months pantethine reduced total cholesterol by 15.1 percent, LDL by 20.1 percent, and triglycerides by 32.9 percent, with an increase in HDL of 8.4 percent.[46] Houston also noted that in studies of longer duration, there appeared to be continued improvement. (The only adverse reactions were mild gastrointestinal side effects in less than 4 percent of the subjects.) As previously stated, we recommend 900 mg of pantethine divided into three daily doses of 300 mg each.

OTHER SUPPLEMENTATION YOU SHOULD CONSIDER

Picking the "top" supplements for treating any health issue is always difficult. In trying to keep the list from being too overwhelming, you're always going to leave a few good things out. There's also the very real issue of compliance. Most people don't like to take a lot of pills, even if the pills in question are natural substances that will boost or protect their health. We consider the following supplements important, and we suggest that you read about what they do and consider using them in addition to the key supplements discussed above.

Vitamin C. Vitamin C is one of the most powerful antioxidants in the world, and because heart disease is initiated by oxidative damage (damage caused by free radicals), any help you can get in the antioxidant department is a good thing. And the evidence is not just theoretical: A large 2011 study published in the *American Heart Journal* found that the lower the level of vitamin C in the blood, the higher the risk for heart failure.[47] Take 1,000 to 2,000 mg a day.

Worth knowing: Vitamin C is extremely safe, and side effects are rare because the body can't store the vitamin. (In some cases, doses exceeding 2,000 mg a day can lead to a little harmless stomach upset and diarrhea.) The bigger danger is the fact that vitamin C increases the amount of iron absorbed from foods. People with hemochromatosis, an inherited condition in which too much iron builds up in the bloodstream, should not take more than 100 mg of supplemental vitamin C.

Curcumin. This extract from the Indian spice turmeric has multiple benefits, not the least of which is that it's highly anti-inflammatory. Scientific research has demonstrated its anti-inflammatory, antioxidant, anti-thrombotic, and cardiovascular protective effects.[48] Curcumin also reduces oxidized LDL cholesterol.[49] In animal studies, it was shown to protect the lining of the artery walls from damage caused by homocysteine.[50] The synergistic relationship of curcumin with resveratrol is especially important.

Resveratrol. Resveratrol is the ingredient in red wine that's best known for its "anti-aging" activity. It helps protect the arteries by improving their elasticity, inhibits blood clots, and lowers both oxidized LDL and blood pressure.[52] Not a bad résumé! It's both

NATURAL CLOT BUSTERS: NATTOKINASE AND LUMBROKINASE

Hyperviscosity refers to sticky, or sludgy, blood. When blood thickens, it bogs down as it moves through the blood vessels, causing platelets to stick together and clump. Blood vessels become more rigid, less elastic, and frequently calcified. The danger lies in the tendency to form clots that can block vessels leading to vital organs.

Nattokinase is extracted from the traditional fermented soy food natto, believed by many researchers to contribute to the low incidence of coronary heart disease in Japan. It provides a unique, powerful, and safe way to eliminate clots, or reduce the tendency to form clots, and thus decrease the risk of heart attack and stroke.[51]

Lumbrokinase, developed in both Japan and China, comes from an extract of earthworm, a traditional source of healing in Asian medicine. These two separate products of dynamic Asian research share a powerful and common property of great interest to anyone who wants to protect their cardiovascular system: They are natural clot eaters.

Here's how it works: Your body naturally produces *fibrin*, a fibrous protein formed from fibrinogen. (A fibrinogen test is one of the blood tests we recommend—see chapter 9— because it is a good marker of how much fibrin you're making.) Fibrin is both good and bad. Its clot-forming action is immediately activated when bleeding occurs, so that's a good thing. But excess fibrin activity can produce consistently thick blood, and that's a big problem.

To offset the danger—and to create thinner blood—the body produces another substance called *plasmin*, an enzyme whose job is to break down excess fibrin. A nice system of checks and balances. But if plasmin, the natural anticlotting agent, becomes overwhelmed and can't keep up with the job, there's trouble in River City. And that's where nattokinase and lumbrokinase come in. If blood clots in an already narrowed blood vessel, you're basically screwed. So if you can dissolve the clotted material, you can open arteries and improve blood flow. If you reduce the clot even just a tiny bit, you get a significant blood flow boost.

Nattokinase and lumbrokinase are natural blood thinners. They can literally turn your blood from the consistency of ketchup to the consistency of red wine! Best of all, they work pretty quickly, within minutes to hours.

If you take these supplements preventively, you may not form clots in the first place.

a strong antioxidant and a strong anti-inflammatory, inhibiting a number of inflammatory enzymes that can contribute to heart disease. It also inhibits the ability of certain molecules to stick to the arterial walls, where they can take up residence and contribute to inflammation.[53] The recommended daily dose is 30 to 200 mg of trans-resveratrol, the active component of resveratrol. Read labels carefully to see what percentage of the capsule is actually the "trans" variety, because that's the only kind you care about.

Cocoa flavanols. Plant chemicals in cocoa known as *flavanols* help the body synthesize a compound called nitric oxide, which is critical for healthy blood flow and healthy blood pressure. Nitric oxide also improves platelet function, meaning it makes your blood less sticky. It also makes the lining of the arteries less attractive for white blood cells to attach to and stick around. Researchers in Germany followed more than 19,000 people for a minimum of ten years and found that those who ate the most flavanol-rich dark chocolate had lower blood pressure and a 39 percent lower risk of having a heart attack or stroke compared to those who ate almost no chocolate.[54]

Cocoa flavanols now come in supplement form, so if you prefer not to eat a couple squares of dark chocolate a day, consider a supplement.

CONVINCING YOUR DOCTOR

If you show this chapter to your doctor, and he or she is still skeptical, we suggest you direct him or her to the superb review paper on nonpharmacological treatment for dyslipidemia written by Mark Houston, M.D., and published in *Progress in Cardiovascular Diseases*.[55] This paper has 421 citations and should go a long way toward reassuring him or her that there is plenty of research to support the use of these natural, non-toxic substances.

CHAPTER 8

STRESS:
THE SILENT KILLER

IF YOU LIKE DETECTIVE STORIES, YOU'RE GOING TO LOVE THIS.

Back around 2000, a story came out about how the population of gray tree frogs in many American lakes was being decimated. The general consensus was that this was due to the use of a common pesticide, carbaryl (known by the brand name Sevin), which was found in large quantities in all of the lakes where frogs were dying. Carbaryl was clearly the villain, and environmentalists demanded that the company making carbaryl be held accountable.

A familiar story, right?

But here's the thing: The manufacturers insisted that carbaryl wasn't harming the frogs. They had a ton of studies showing that if you took the little creatures out of their lake homes, put them in a lab, and exposed them to the pesticide, nothing happened to them.

But the tree frogs were still dying. And the environmentalists were positive it had something to do with their continued exposure to this pesticide.

So who was right?

As it turns out, they both were. The studies were accurate. Self-serving though it might have been, the big, bad industrial manufacturer had good science showing that frogs were not being knocked off by its chemical. And the environmentalists had *equally* good science showing that carbaryl was the likely suspect in this massive decimation of gray tree frogs, frogs that managed to survive just fine, thank you very much, as long as there wasn't any carbaryl around.

Enter Columbo in the form of Rick Relyea, Ph.D., a biochemical researcher from the University of Pittsburgh. Long story short, here's what he discovered: The pesticide, carbaryl, was indeed pretty innocuous to frogs (meaning it didn't kill them, at least) in the unnaturally tranquil setting of a lab. But most tree frogs don't live in a lab; they live in the wild, where there are constant dangers from predators. When the frogs pick up a predator signal, when they literally "smell danger," they secrete powerful stress hormones, just like our ancestors did when running from a wildebeest, or like we do when we're caught in traffic or miss a deadline. Expose a *stressed* frog to the pesticide, and you've got a dead frog. Neither stress hormones nor pesticides alone were enough to kill the average tree frog, but the *combination* of the two—stress hormones and pesticides—was lethal.[1]

Subsequent studies over the next decade looked at the interaction between these two stressors—chemicals and predators—and examined how they interacted in a number of different organisms, including salamanders.[2] Several of the studies tested different pesticide chemicals with and without "predator cues" (signals that trigger the release of stress hormones), and every study confirmed that the combination of a pesticide and predator cues was far more lethal than any of the chemicals alone.

The take-home point, and the reason for this story, is that environmental elements *interact* with physiological elements in ways that can cause serious problems. (In the case of the gray tree frog, the interaction was a death sentence.) Although certain environmental and physiological elements might not be detrimental by *themselves*, when they're combined they can sometimes spell big trouble.

And the element of our physiology that's most likely to cause major problems for the health of the heart happens, not coincidentally, to be the subject of this chapter: stress.

THE STRESS RESPONSE IN ACTION

Imagine, if you will, that you are a zebra grazing on the plains in the African Serengeti. Everything is peaceful, the grass is delicious, the sun is out, and all is well with the world. Suddenly you hear a faint rustling in the woods. You look up and see behind a bush the outline of a lion, a lion that is looking straight at you. You can almost see the thought bubble over its head: "Lunch!"

Your body switches into full alert, the equivalent of flipping to "red" in the Department of Homeland Security's threat advisory system. The moment you see the lion, your hypothalamus, a section of the brain that acts as a kind of "first responder" in emergency situations, sends a hormonal signal to your pituitary gland. Instantly, the pituitary relays the message to the adrenal glands, two little walnut-shaped glands that sit on top of the kidneys. Their job is to pump out hormones whose actions are your only hope of living long enough to eat lunch tomorrow rather than becoming lunch today. These hormones—cortisol and adrenaline, specifically—are known as the stress hormones, and whether you're a zebra running from a lion or a caveman running from a woolly mammoth, you have them to thank for your survival.

But these wonderfully adaptive, life-saving hormones have a dark side. They can, and do, contribute mightily to heart disease.

Let us explain.

Your stress hormones, also known as the "fight or flight" hormones, serve as a kind of turbocharger when you're in a threatening situation. Without them, you'd be unable to react quickly enough to protect yourself from a predator or any other kind of danger. Cortisol and adrenaline, working together, and working far more quickly than you can read these words, prepare the body for action. Adrenaline, for example, immediately raises your heart rate and blood pressure as your heart begins to furiously pump blood through the vascular system in a mad rush to get it to the organs and muscles that need it most. Cortisol, the main stress hormone, causes sugar to be released into the bloodstream so that it can be delivered to the muscle cells and burned for energy, which happens to be particularly useful if you're running for your life.

In response to these hormonal signals, the body diverts blood from wherever it's not needed and directs it to where it is needed. (After all, if you're running from a wild boar, it doesn't make much sense for your body to send a ton of blood to your fingers, ears, reproductive organs, or digestive system.) The whole system is exquisitely designed to deliver just the right amount of nutrients, oxygen, and blood to the places where it's most likely to contribute to your survival (the running muscles and the heart, for example).

This is the stress response in action. It's meant to be quick, instant, and effective, its purpose singular: keeping you alive in a life-and-death situation. In the case of the zebra, it lasts only as long as it takes to get away from the lion, after which the zebra's metabolism returns to normal, its heart rate slows down, and it goes back to grazing, blissfully forgetful that there was ever a problem in the first place.

Acute Versus Chronic Stress

This natural ability of animals to live in the moment as opposed to sitting around wondering whether there's going to be another lion behind the next bush is what the great neurobiologist Robert Sapolsky was referring to when he titled his masterpiece on stress physiology *Why Zebras Don't Get Ulcers*.

Sapolsky's zebras experienced *acute* stress, which is ultimately temporary (unless of course the zebra is a slow runner, in which case the point is moot). Acute stress passes quickly, allowing us to return to "normal" and go about our business. The far more dangerous kind of stress, the kind that directly affects heart disease, is *chronic* stress. And that's a whole different animal.

So here's the big difference between the *acute* stress experienced by the zebra and the *chronic* stress that damages your heart. Acute stress is immediate and attention-grabbing. Your brain registers the threat of the marauding lion, and your stress response is instantly activated. It's energetic, it's explosive, and it's wonderful—it's what saves your life in an emergency. But if you turn it on too often, too long, or for psychological reasons—essentially the definition of chronic stress—you set yourself up for getting sick.

When stress persists, as it often does in people today, especially in those with certain personality and character traits, the abundance of cortisol from the adrenal cortex begins to promote hardening of the arteries. Hypervigilance, or being constantly on guard (that sense of waiting for the other shoe to drop), may also create an overabundance of cortisol, thus turning a *psychological* coronary risk factor into a *physical* one. With this kind of chronic stress, we can overdose on our own adrenal hormones, making the

The common notion that stress is just a psychological state—that it's "all in your head"—is as outdated as the notion that cholesterol causes heart disease.

heart vulnerable to unexpected cardiac events, such as heart attacks or arrhythmias. Remember that this damage doesn't always occur immediately, but it will occur when the adrenal glands are pushed to the point of exhaustion. Overwork, prolonged stress, and exhaustion—all of which contribute to burnout—are harbingers of death by hormonal overdose. More on this in a moment.

Stress, Stress, Who's Got Stress?

If we asked you right now to sit down and list the top ten things in your life that you find stressful, we bet that none of you would have the slightest problem coming up with a list. (In fact, the challenge would be limiting it to only ten items!) We further bet that your list would be front-loaded with psychological stressors—deadlines, traffic jams, sick kids, money, relationships—all of which take a constant toll, physically and psychologically.

But the common notion that stress is just a psychological state—that it's "all in your head"—is as outdated as the notion that cholesterol causes heart disease. Stress has physical and physiological correlates. When you're under stress, your body releases specific hormones that have specific actions and measurable results.

The stress response can save your life. It can also kill you.

The Roseto Effect

Once upon a time, a country doctor was at a little tavern in Pennsylvania when in walked a doc from the "big city"; he was the head of medicine at the University of Oklahoma. The two physicians started talking shop over a couple of beers, and the local doc happened to casually mention a puzzling observation: Folks in his town were dying from heart disease at half the rate of the rest of the country.

Although this might sound like it's the opening scene for some kind of reverse horror story—instead of being struck by some weird, alien disease, towns-people seem to be mysteriously protected from the very diseases that kill their neighbors!—it's actually a true story. The meeting took place in the 1960s; the town was Roseto, Pennsylvania; and that chance meeting between two doctors at a local bar eventually led to an influx of medical researchers trying to understand the strange phenomenon, a phenomenon that ultimately became known as the "Roseto Effect." (Google it. Go on. We'll wait.)

In defiance of all logic, the residents of Roseto seemed to be eerily protected against heart disease. In Roseto the rate of death from heart disease was next to *zero* for men between the ages of fifty-five and sixty-four, not exactly an age group known to be immune to heart attacks. Men over the age of sixty-five did occasionally die from heart disease, but at a rate of about half the national average.

Okay, what could have been going on here? Tell the average American about the Roseto Effect, and he or she will probably say that the people of Roseto must have been living really healthy lives, going to the gym, eating low-fat diets, staying away from cholesterol, going easy on the salt, not eating red meat, and all that good stuff, right? That's got to be the answer.

Well, not exactly.

Roseto, Pennsylvania, was, to put it gently, a hardscrabble town. Life was anything but easy. The men spent their days doing backbreaking, hazardous labor in underground slate mines. Their traditional Italian food was Americanized in the worst possible ways. They fried everything in lard. Most, if not all, of the men smoked. If there was a contest for "most likely to die of heart disease," the men of Roseto could have won hands down.

So why weren't they dropping like flies?

That's exactly what the medical researchers wanted to know.

Here's what they found: Nearly all the houses in Roseto contained three generations of family members. Rosetans didn't put their elderly in assisted living homes; they incorporated them into community life. They treated them as wise village elders. Folks took evening strolls. They belonged to tons of social clubs. They participated in church and had community festivals. And remember those dinner tables piled high with the lard-fried food we mentioned a few paragraphs back? Those dinner tables happened to also offer enormous nourishment for, and nurturance of, the human spirit. They were family affairs where people connected, shared their experiences, and participated in family life in myriad ways.

Oh, by the way, the crime rate in Roseto—as well as the number of applications for public assistance—was zero.

What accounts for the Roseto Effect? Researchers now believe that the explanation can be summed up in two words: *community* and *connection*. These two things were (and are) such powerful protectors of health that they were apparently able to offset both cigarette smoking and a horrific diet.

Writing about the Roseto Effect in their classic book, *The Power of Clan*, Stewart Wolf, M.D., and sociologist John Bruhn correctly observed that the characteristics of tight-knit communities such as Roseto are *far* better predictors of heart health than cholesterol levels or even smoking. The social structures of communities such as Roseto are characterized by predictability and stability, with each person in the community having a clearly defined role in the social scheme of things. Everyone worked in Roseto, and they worked hard, all for a shared communal goal: creating a better life for their children. Being connected to other people in a close community makes you far less likely to be overwhelmed by the problems of everyday life. Being less likely to be overwhelmed by the problems of everyday life means you're *also* less likely to be a victim of chronic stress.

And chronic stress is one of the biggest contributors to heart disease.

The men of Roseto had a ton of physical stressors in their lives. Working in the slate mines is hardly a day at the beach, and smoking certainly qualifies as a major physical stressor. But because the men were generally protected from the constant, unending mental stress that many folks endure on a daily basis—protected, presumably, by their close-knit community and their secure, nurturing family ties—these physical stressors didn't seem to produce the collateral damage such stressors might be expected to produce. The absence of chronic mental stress seemed to afford the men some level of protection against heart attacks.

To understand why, we have to understand something about the stress response in general. And the best place to start is with a man named Hans Selye.

THE "INVENTION" OF STRESS

Selye didn't invent stress, but he sure put it on the map. Back in the 1930s, Selye was a young researcher and assistant professor at McGill University in Montreal, and he was just beginning his work in the field of endocrinology—the study of hormones and what they do. A biochemist working just down the hall from Selye had isolated a specific substance from the ovaries, and everyone was wondering what the heck that ovarian extract actually *did*. So Selye did what any ambitious, unknown researcher would do—he got a bucketful of this strange ovarian stuff and decided to test it out on his rats.

Every day Selye would inject the rats with this mysterious stuff. But the thing is, Selye was a klutz. He'd try to inject the rats, but he'd drop them, or miss them, or they'd run behind the refrigerator. Selye wound up spending half the day running around the lab with a broom trying to coax the rats out from their hiding places and herd the terrified animals back into their cages.

After a few months passed, Selye began examining the rats to find out what the heck this stuff he'd been injecting them with did. Lo and behold, all of them had ulcers. Not only that, but they also had greatly enlarged adrenal glands and shrunken immune tissues. Selye was delighted. Clearly he'd discovered something important and new about the ovarian extract his colleague had discovered: It gave you ulcers!

Selye was at heart a good scientist, even if he had absolutely no talent for handling animals. And a good scientist always runs a control group, which is exactly what Selye did. The control group, of course, was a group of rats identical to the first group in every way except that they were *not* injected with the mysterious ovarian extract.

When Selye examined the rats in the control group, he made an even stranger discovery than before: All of the control rats *also* had ulcers.

Hmm.

Here he had two groups of genetically identical rats. One group had been injected with a substance, and the other had not, yet both groups wound up with ulcers. Thus, Selye quickly reasoned that the ovarian hormone couldn't have been causing the ulcers. What *else* did the two sets of rats have in common?

The answer wasn't hard to figure out, especially for a research-trained scientist such as Selye. The one thing both groups of rats had in common was Selye.

Selye had properly concluded that the ovarian hormone couldn't possibly be responsible for the ulcers and swollen adrenal glands, because both groups of rats had developed ulcers, and only one of them had been exposed to the hormone. But perhaps his own inept handling of the rats—the incompetent injections, the dropping, the chasing, the running around—had something to do with it. Selye reasoned that the ulcers—as well as the shrunken immune tissues and enlarged adrenals—were some kind of response to *general unpleasantness*, which he came to refer to as *stress*.

So Selye set out to test his new theory. He created a high-stress environment. He put some of the animals up on the roof during the winter months. He put others in the basement next to the boiler. Others underwent stressful surgeries, or were subjected to very loud music, or were deprived of sleep.

Every one of them got ulcers. Every one of them had swollen adrenals.

From this early work, Selye eventually developed what's known as the General Adaptation Syndrome (GAS) theory of stress. The theory holds that the effect of stress on the body develops over three stages: alarm, resistance, and exhaustion. Here's how it works.

The Three Stages of Stress

In the *alarm* stage, you recognize that there's a danger. Your body secretes a bunch of adrenaline and

Selye eventually developed what's known as the General Adaptation Syndrome (GAS) theory of stress. The theory holds that the effect of stress on the body develops over three stages: alarm, resistance, and exhaustion.

cortisol to prepare you for action (i.e., fight or flight). Of course, if all this available energy is *not* used for physical action, big problems develop. For example, too much adrenaline will raise your blood pressure and ultimately damage the blood vessels of the heart and brain.

In the *resistance* stage, you deal with the stressor. If (hopefully) the situation resolves quickly, you return to something approaching a balanced state (what physiologists call *homeostasis*). Your stress hormones may come down, but you have also depleted some of your resources. More commonly, however, the situation persists, and now your body has to find a way to deal with it. Your body keeps trying to adapt and remains in a constant state of arousal. But you can't keep this up forever, with the stress pedal pressed to the metal and a ton of hormones pumping out into the bloodstream. If this continues too long, or if you repeat this process too often with too little recovery, you eventually move into the third stage.

This stage, aptly named the *exhaustion* stage, is also known as *burnout*. It's what we're referring to in this book when we talk about "maladaptation." Stress levels go up and stay up. These chronic stress levels deplete your immune system (one reason marathon runners are so much more susceptible to colds in the days following a race). Chronic stress levels also injure tissue cells, particularly in an area of the brain known as the *hippocampus*, which is involved with memory and cognition. (That's one reason you can't remember stuff you know when you're taking a very stressful exam.) Animal studies have demonstrated that the hippocampus actually shrinks under the weight of cortisol overload. And all of this has profound implications for high blood pressure and heart disease.

How You Cope with Stress Matters More Than the Stress Itself

So what's a stressor, anyway? It can be anything— and it's different for different people. Technically, a stressor is something to which special weight and significance has been attached. A stressor can be something as simple as the feeling of being overwhelmed. It can be the inability to give in to a situation (resistance), a fear of losing control, or a feeling of struggle or uncertainty. Often a stressor can't be changed or even controlled—a hurricane or natural disaster, for example. What *can* be controlled, however, is your behavioral response to the external stressor. As Werner Erhard once said, "Riding a raft down white water rapids, a master has no more control over the water than you do. The difference is that a master is *in control* of being *out of control* [Italics ours]."

Stressors come in all sizes, flavors, and packages. Hunger and deprivation are usually more significant stressors than a flat tire—except if you're a young woman who has to deal with a flat tire on a deserted country road late at night with no jack! A failing grade sounds like it would be a lot more important to a college student than, say, a bad haircut, unless perhaps the haircut damages an already low self-esteem. In these cases, the flat tire and the bad haircut can be considered strong external stressors in the person's life. How people respond to these (and other) stressors will determine their body's physiological reaction and, ultimately, their health.

When the promotion doesn't come, when the tire goes flat, when the haircut makes you look like Pee-wee Herman, you have only two choices—adapting or *not* adapting. You can adapt by "going with the flow," accepting the situation, or working to effect some kind of change. Or you can *maladapt* by preparing your body for "combat," either by withdrawing or pushing beyond normal expectations in an effort to make the stressor go away. When your coping styles are unhealthy and inappropriate—for example, abusing drugs or alcohol, overeating, or overworking—that's maladaptability. And these activities take an enormous toll on the body.

The big difference between stress in the caveman era and stress in the modern era is that the caveman's stress—and his adaptive responses—were largely physical. Ours are mental. We're not fighting off saber-toothed tigers, or running up trees to escape from bears, or in danger of being attacked by a neighboring tribe. Instead, we have to "fight back" mentally and keep "cool" at the same time, leaving the nervous system and the cardiovascular system in a state of constant and continuous "overpreparedness." It's this continual state of visceral vascular readiness that makes the heart so darn vulnerable. The chronic alarm reaction that develops is a harmful response in which the body continuously overdoses on its own biochemicals.

The biochemical alterations that occur in response to stress are powerful. When these responses are inappropriate or ineffective (e.g., screaming and pounding the wheel when you've been stuck for two hours in unmoving traffic on California's 405 freeway), you are *mal*adapting rather than adapting, and pathological changes can (and do) occur in the body. The disruption in hormonal secretions can be long term and even permanent.

Much of the answer in dealing with stress lies not in the stressors themselves, but in the way we *deal* with the stressors (which, like in-laws and taxes, have an annoying tendency to not go away). An important first step is to recognize the situations that create stress for you. These frequently include lack of communication, unfulfilled expectations, retirement, death of a loved one, job pressures, bad relationships, and, particularly important, dwelling upon past events or imagined future ones.

Dr. Jonny: Is It the Stress or Is It the Response?

I grew up in a large, seven-room co-op in Jackson Heights, Queens (New York City). Many years ago, when my parents were in their late sixties, they went on a weeklong vacation to Bermuda. When they got back, the apartment was essentially empty.

Burglars had cased the joint and done a darn good job of it. No one saw or heard a thing, including their very friendly neighbors who would have called the police in a heartbeat had they suspected anything fishy was going on. The burglars clearly knew when people would be around and were exquisitely well prepared. They stripped the house as quickly and efficiently as a school of piranha might strip the meat from the carcass of a dead cow.

That house contained just about every material thing of any value that my parents had jointly collected over thirty-five years of marriage.

So that's what happened. A pretty big stressor, wouldn't you say?

My mother's response was one of her finer moments and one I will always remember.

"You know," she said, "the important things—our health, our family, our love—they didn't take. Sure, I'm sad to see all this stuff go. But you know what? It's kind of exciting in a way. Now we have the opportunity to create something completely new. We can design new rooms, get some new furniture, which I've been wanting to get anyway, and basically start again."

By shifting the way she reacted to this event, she turned it from a potential tragedy and enormous stressor into something that oddly enough sounded like an adventure.

What happened couldn't be changed. But how she reacted was in her control. Her reaction is what determined the toll this stressor would take on her. It was her reaction—not the stressor itself—that determined the result.

And the result—thanks to her attitude and serenity—was that minimal damage was done to her health.

You can't control the "event" (i.e., what actually happens), but you can control the "story" (i.e., what you make it mean). By making this event mean opportunity rather than tragedy, my mother probably saved herself quite a lot of physical damage, and in the long run that probably extended her life.

STRESS AND YOUR HEART

When you're under constant (chronic) stress, you secrete *more* hormones, such as epinephrine and the glucocorticoids, which prepare the body to fight or flee. At the same time, you make *less* of other hormones, such as growth hormone. Why? Because at this point, at least from the body's point of view, these hormones are a big waste of time.

When your life is at stake, or your body *thinks* it is, your body does an instant evaluation (like a triage nurse) and decides what's essential and what's not. When you're running for your life, it doesn't make much sense to invest energy in reproductive or digestive functions, and it doesn't make sense to increase circulation to the stomach or the ears. What *does* make sense is keeping you alive, so the body diverts blood from the gut and sends it to the legs (so you can run faster). It doesn't bother with little extras, such as growth hormone or sex hormones, because if you're not going to be around past dinnertime, what's the point? Instead, it mobilizes all of its resources to combat the immediate life-threatening problem at hand.

This "triage" phenomenon was first noted around 1833 by a bunch of physician scientists treating a man with a gunshot wound.[3] When the docs were about to patch him up, they noticed, not surprisingly, that he had a significant amount of red and rosy blood flow beneath where his guts were exposed. Then, for some reason—who knows, maybe he didn't like the doctors' aftershave—the guy got pissed off and angry. His body treated his anger and pissed-off-ness as an emergency, and his stress response kicked in immediately.

Suddenly that red and rosy blood they were seeing in his guts turned pink and pale. It was almost as if all that deep red blood had disappeared!

So what happened?

What the docs were witnessing was a vivid visual example of the triage phenomenon described earlier. Stress hormones divert blood flow from the areas that aren't immediately necessary to your survival and send it to where it can do the most good in an emergency—the heart, lungs, and running muscles. That's why the blood in the guts of the guy with the gunshot wound changed color.

So your body perceives a life-threatening emergency (and remember, your body makes no distinction between an "old-school" emergency, such as an attacking lion, and the modern version of the same thing, such as being stuck for hours on the freeway). But releasing stress hormones that divert blood from nonessential to essential areas is only the beginning. You also need to get *more* blood into your system, or at least make sure you don't lose any of the blood you already have! (Remember, from an evolutionary and historical point of view, most life-threatening "emergencies" carried with them the distinct possibility of blood loss!)

Now what does your body do? It makes more of a certain type of red blood cell called a *platelet*. Platelets stick together and form clots, which, when you think about it, is a pretty spiffy protection against the possibility of bleeding out.

So stress hormones trigger the production of platelets, a good thing in the short run when your body is anticipating the possibility of a major bloodletting wound, but not such a good thing in the long run. When stress hormones are constantly in the "on" position, you're *overproducing* platelets. Inevitably, the platelets begin to stick together, and your blood thickens. They combine with other red and white blood cells, as well as with a compound called *fibrin,* to form a kind of "super clot" called a *thrombus.* When a thrombus blocks an artery that leads to the heart muscle, you have a heart attack.

Okay, so what else does your body have to do in a life-threatening emergency to ensure that you stay alive? Divert blood from nonessential areas to essential, check. Make sure you don't lose any more blood than you absolutely have to by making more platelets so that you can clot more easily, check. But wait! What about *replacing* any blood that you might lose in battle? You're going to need replacement blood, and where the heck is that going to come from?

Glad you asked.

Heart Attacks Waiting to Happen

Because there are no blood transfusions available in the African Serengeti, you're going to have to make your own blood. The first thing you'll need is water, which is found in the kidneys! The kidneys are sitting around, peacefully filtering water and getting ready to send it out into the universe in the form of urine, but now, with the new demand for water, your stress hormone-fueled body runs down to the kidneys and says, "Wait! Hold the presses! Don't send that water out into the universe, because we're gonna need it right here to make more blood!" And because the kidneys really don't speak English, this message is

sent to them via a hormone aptly named the *anti-diuretic hormone,* or ADH, which tells the body to reabsorb water from the kidneys and put it into circulation to increase blood volume.

Brilliant. And it all makes total sense from the point of view of survival.

But what happens when you do this chronically?

Let's take a look.

See, if you increase the volume of your blood pressure for thirty seconds while you run from a lion, you are one smart dude, from an evolutionary point of view at least. But elevate it for weeks, and you have chronic hypertension. And this is exactly the state that many of us are in today—heart attacks waiting to happen. According to the World Health Organization (WHO), hypertension is one of the most important causes of premature death worldwide, and it's certainly one of the most important risk factors for heart disease.[4] Let's take a look at why.

Stress and Blood Pressure: The Missing Link to Heart Disease

When blood pressure increases, the heart starts pumping blood with more force, pushing the blood vessels outward in response to the sheer power of it. (Imagine a garden hose hooked up to a fully opened fire hydrant. The garden hose would look like it's about to burst!)

In response to this distending, the blood vessels build up more muscle around them (more layers of rubber on the garden hose), which now makes the vessels more rigid. This in turn requires even *more* pressure to get the blood through them, which means—not surprisingly—your blood pressure goes even higher.

If blood pressure is increased, the heart muscles pay the price. Because blood is being pumped out with more force, it slams back with more force as well. And the area that takes the brunt of this returning blood under high force is the left ventricle. The muscle there begins to enlarge—a condition known as *left ventricular hypertrophy*—and that sets the heart up for irregularities.

Now we'll discuss how this can cause inflammation and trigger the whole chain of events that leads to heart disease, a chain of events in which cholesterol is the most minor of players.

Coming out of your heart is one huge blood vessel called the *ascending aorta*. After a certain distance, this vessel splits into two, a process called *bifurcation*. Each of these two vessels eventually splits into two *more* vessels, which keep bifurcating until you're down to the little capillaries. Now when your blood pressure goes up, the bifurcation—the point where the vessel divides into two—is exactly the spot that gets the brunt of this bashing by the increased force, or blood pressure. Eventually you start to get what's known in physics as *fluid turbulence*. (Think of a tube with fluid moving through it with more and more force; the fluid starts to resemble a miniature version of the water sloshing around a tunnel at a water park.) As the fluid—blood, in this case—slams into the weak spots with increasing force, you get little bits of scarring and tearing, which soon become inflamed. These spots of vessel damage attract more inflammatory cells (such as oxidized LDL cholesterol), which gets into the inflamed areas, sticking to them. Before you know it, you've got plaque.

You've also got damaged blood vessels. Healthy coronary blood vessels *vasodilate* (open) when you need more blood (e.g., when you're running from a saber-toothed tiger). That makes sense—water flows more freely through a fire hose than through a garden hose, and blood flows more easily through a dilated (open) vessel than a constricted (closed) one. But when the coronary blood vessels are damaged, they no longer vasodilate. Just when you need them to open up the most, they actually *close up*, or constrict. Now the heart doesn't get enough blood or oxygen, and you have something called *cardiac ischemia* (lack of oxygen to the heart). The heart muscle isn't getting enough energy, and it hurts. The all-too-familiar name for this pain is *angina*.

And at the core of all this is inflammation.

"Twenty years ago, if you wanted to measure one thing to see how the cardiovascular system was doing, you'd measure your cholesterol," Sapolsky said. "In recent years people have realized that cholesterol is important, but that *other* things are more important. If you have undamaged vessels there's no place for cholesterol to stick to," he explained. "If you don't have inflammation, there's no problem."[5]

VOODOO DEATH

A man wakes in the morning feeling unwell and complains of pain and distress in his chest and abdominal area. He is sweating profusely and gasping for air. His alarmed wife calls 911, but the man dies before the paramedics arrive.

Frequently, the first symptom of heart disease, at least the first symptom that gets *noticed,* is sudden death. (Sudden death tends to get people's attention.) Unfortunately, there is no chastisement, no warning to mend our ways, no trade-off or time to bargain with fate. The heart, omnipotent organ that it is, demonstrates its power over us with one unforgiving defensive maneuver—it attacks us.

Clinical studies have found that from 40 to 50 percent of the time, the first recognized symptom of heart disease is a fatal heart attack, also known as sudden cardiac death (the number one killer of people between the ages of thirty-five and sixty). The big problem with cardiac disease is that it happens with little or no warning. It's literally ominous in its silence. Ninety percent of individuals with heart disease are asymptomatic.

Many of us have heard stories about "voodoo death" (sudden death related to psychogenic stress), a concept researched in detail by the American physiologist Walter B. Cannon, who first introduced the word *homeostasis* and coined the term *fight or flight.* Cannon traveled around the world studying voodoo death in places such as Africa, the Pacific Islands, and Australia. According to Cannon, voodoo death defies the imagination of modern Western man. He cited a case in which a Maori woman died within a day after discovering that she had eaten a piece of fruit that came from a "tabooed" place.

Well, unless you believe that the fruit was cursed or had magical powers, there's clearly another explanation, and it's this: the person's *belief* that the curse was inescapable. A common feature of such a belief, shared by many who believe in the supernatural, is a heightened emotional response. The stress hormones go crazy. The heart pumps blood like sailors bailing out a sinking ship—quickly and furiously. Blood pressure goes through the roof, causing vascular injury. The possessed woman, and other members of her family, believed that she was doomed to die. She had to deal with the sheer, unmitigated terror of the curse itself, compounded by the fact that she was physically and emotionally isolated. She was all alone in a terrible struggle that eventually ended in death.

But how and why did she die?

Did the social isolation or despair cause a loss of hope and a willingness to die? Or was it the curse itself? Many voodoo deaths are commonly preceded by alienation, isolation, and lack of social support for the person enduring the experience. In the cases that he observed, Cannon concluded that the victims of voodoo death were overcome by terror at the exact moment that they found themselves without the safety net of a supportive environment. The combo was lethal. The victims accepted their deaths as a way to escape an intolerable, miserable situation.

But with all that, there's still no perfect explanation for the physical mechanism of death. What went wrong? Did these people's cholesterol levels suddenly jump?

Here's what Cannon concluded: The overwhelming stimulation of the sympathetic nervous system provokes lethal electrical instability in the heart. In modern terms, doctors would describe this whole "sudden death syndrome" as the result of *malignant arrhythmia culminating in ventricular fibrillation*, or *acute coronary spasms and myocardial infarction*—in other words, a heart attack.

What's important here is not the exact *way* that the heart fails, but the fact that its breakdown—whatever the specifics—are *precipitated* by a profound loss of hope. Interestingly, Cannon observed that this profound loss of hope was so deep that all attempts to revive these individuals were fruitless.

Once again, we see that psychological belief can determine physical destiny, or at least have a profound influence on it.

Experimental research has demonstrated the impact of acute psychological stress on sudden cardiac death. In one study, 91 percent of patients who experienced sudden cardiac death but were then successfully resuscitated reported that they were experiencing acute psychological stress at the time of their "sudden death" experience. A typical scenario: A middle manager is winding down after a busy week. The economy is in recession. The guy has to cut costs. His overhead is ridiculously high. There's a real potential of losing his job, and with the loss of his job would come a loss of self-esteem. He is not involved in a loving relationship and is isolated and depressed. He's exercising at his local gym when he hears unexpected and disturbing news. He drops dead suddenly from a massive coronary.

It's not the stressor, per se, that killed him. Under other circumstances—or in another person— disturbing news would be, well, *disturbing*. Not fatal.

Much like people who catch colds easily because their immune systems are weak, he is far more susceptible to being hit like a sledgehammer by news that would merely shake a less vulnerable person. In his weakened, vulnerable state, the disturbing news acts like the pesticide carbaryl on a stressed-out frog—it kills him.

We hope we've convinced you that stress isn't just "in your head," and that the mind and the body operate very much as an integrated unit. A trauma to the body can cause enormous amounts of psychic pain and ultimately even lead to depression or fibromyalgia. And a trauma to the psyche has significant repercussions for the body. They can't be separated, nor should they be. Both are part of the whole person. This is why medicine that looks at the entire person, and how everything is connected, is aptly called *holistic* medicine. (Dr. Sinatra and Dr. Jonny share this orientation; Dr. Sinatra has been practicing "integrative" [holistic] medicine for decades, and Dr. Jonny's Ph.D. is in *holistic nutrition*.)

In this next section, we're going to talk specifically about stress and the impact it can have on your heart and your health. And we'll make recommendations for how you can reduce stress with an easy exercise that anyone can do.

HOW THOUGHTS AND FEELINGS AFFECT YOUR HEART

An essential part of our prescription for heart health involves monitoring and reducing stress, and that means exploring (and expressing) your thoughts and your feelings.

If you want proof that what you think about affects your heart, try this exercise: Sit quietly and peacefully until you feel your breathing calm and your heart rate steady. Concentrate on peaceful words and images. Imagine yourself in a safe, warm, engulfing place—perhaps a favorite beach or even an imaginary tropical island. Stop reading and breathe deeply for a few minutes before continuing to the next paragraph.

Now that you're in this "state," think about something that really disturbs you, maybe a situation at work, or at home, or with your kids or mate. Maybe some incident that caused a great deal of distress in your life, such as a mugging, or the theft of your car, or the death of a loved one. It can even be something that didn't affect you directly—a real-life disaster such as Hurricane Katrina or the BP oil spill. Stop reading for another minute and really feel whatever comes up for you when you think of that disturbing event or situation.

Okay, what happened? Your heart rate probably went up, as did your blood pressure. You might have been able to hear your own heartbeat as it pounded in your ears. You might have felt anxiety and distress mounting in your body. Yet absolutely nothing happened physically. All that changed was your mental state, but this had a noticeable effect on a variety of physical measures.

Years ago, the great neuroscientist Antonio Damasio did a clever experiment that demonstrated how dramatically thoughts affect your body's physiological reactions. He asked Herbert von Karajan, the legendary conductor of the Berlin Symphony, to sit quietly in a chair while hooked up to a variety of devices that monitored heart rate, blood pressure, and brain waves. After getting baseline measurements, he gave von Karajan the score to a Beethoven symphony and asked the conductor to go through it, imagining that he was conducting the orchestra through each passage, but without any significant physical movement. Damasio measured the exact same changes in brain waves, blood pressure, and heart rate that he had observed when von Karajan actually conducted that same symphony. By merely thinking about and imagining the score, von Karajan's body had responded exactly as it did when he was actually conducting the score.

Overdosing on Adrenaline

Your nervous system can be conveniently described as having two parts, *voluntary* and *involuntary*, which pretty much cover the two major classes of functions that the nervous system performs.

The voluntary nervous system refers to those bodily functions that are under conscious control (doing the tango, knitting, walking, filing your nails, filing your taxes, playing golf, or talking, for example). The involuntary nervous system—technically called the *autonomic nervous system*—is not under conscious control and includes the lion's share of our nervous system and functions (heartbeat, digestion, hair growth, hormone secretion, biochemical release—all the things your body does automatically without your thinking about them). Many of our functions—breathing, for example—run automatically (such as when we sleep), except when we consciously take charge of them (for example, when we "breathe deeply" or "hold our breath"). If this weren't the case, we'd be like the proverbial centipede trying to tell each leg where to go.

Our involuntary functions—those that are for the most part automatic—are very sensitive to our emotions. When we're startled or frightened, the diaphragm, our main breathing muscle, automatically flattens (inhales) and then stays flattened until the emergency is over, and we exhale with a "sigh of relief." Unfortunately, this is also the case with chronic anxiety. People suffering from anxiety—along with women in labor, or even people with chronic respiratory disease—are taught how to take voluntary control of their diaphragms, inhaling, sighing, or humming to promote exhalation.

The heart is even more vulnerable to our emotions.

Our emotions affect the heart through the autonomic nervous system, which is divided into two opposite and opposing branches. These branches are the *sympathetic nervous system* and the *parasympathetic nervous system*. Ideally, they work together to create a nice state of balance called homeostasis.

The sympathetic system is what prepares us for fight or flight. It's basically responsible for everything that happens once the "warning light" is turned on signaling an emergency. It's the sympathetic nervous system that's responsible for you swerving to avoid an oncoming car or quickly scaling the nearest tree when a wild boar starts charging your campsite. The sympathetic system is in charge of increasing your heart rate and blood pressure while at the same time suppressing "nonemergency" functions such as digestion. The parasympathetic system, on the other hand, is responsible for slowing down. It lowers pulse rate, lowers blood pressure, and stimulates gastrointestinal movements.

Like our ancient ancestors did, we rely on the sympathetic nervous system for extra energy in situations of physical and emotional stress, including combat and athletic events. But such high arousal without an outlet for expression can be damaging. Emotional and psychological arousal (such as fear, dread, worry, and anger) can generate cardiac arrhythmias and coronary artery spasms. They can (and do!) increase blood pressure. And they can even provoke heart attacks and sudden cardiac death.

How does this happen? What life-and-death communications travel between the nervous system and the heart? How can they produce such physiological and pathological responses to both real—and imagined—events?

Well, just as two ordinarily happy partners can have some knock-down, drag-out arguments, in a very real sense the brain and heart can also have some "lethal conversations." Obviously we don't mean that the two organs sit down and have a nice chat over a latte at Starbucks—the communication takes place through the nervous system by way of chemical messengers (hormones!) that literally serve as harbingers of death. Yes, we can even overdose on our own adrenaline in situations that involve fear, horror, excessive arousal, or deep despair and depression. The body can commit suicide by overstimulating the heart. And the heart running wildly in panic mode terminates with ventricular fibrillation.

So the brain and the heart are in constant communication. There's definitely a heart-brain "hotline." Identifying people at risk for sudden death depends on identifying not only the traditional risk factors for heart disease but also psychological and emotional elements.

Thoughts, unconscious and conscious, appear to be critical factors that link our "personalities" with the centers of the brain that control the functions of the heart. These are the hidden emotional risk factors for heart disease. And they're far more important than cholesterol is!

Denial Ain't a River in Egypt

Some people truly don't feel the pain of their symptoms because, frankly, they're living in denial, which, for our purposes, we'll define as a state of being cut off from the awareness of what is happening to your body. Living in denial—out of touch with your body and its feelings—often leads to disaster. You fail to admit that a problem exists. Or you believe your symptoms are "nothing," or something very "minor." (Steve has seen this situation time and time again in many coronary-prone patients who told him they were experiencing indigestion when in fact they were having a heart attack.)

Take, for example, the case of Jim.

Jim was a banker, opening up a checking account for a new client, as he had done many times in the past. The client had a bunch of questions, all of which Jim answered patiently. But the client persisted with more questions and concerns. Jim had another client waiting and began to feel trapped.

He probably should have told his client that he had someone else waiting and that they'd have to continue another time. But instead—as is typical in many type-A men—he withheld his emotions and frustrations. He was feeling so much stress that he had to wipe the sweat off his brow.

Jim totally denied this bodily sensation, as well as all the other obvious messages his body was sending him. His hands began to sweat. He had difficulty breathing. He became dizzy, and he experienced chest pains.

Thinking the pain was just indigestion, Jim didn't let anyone around him know how he was feeling. Fifteen minutes later, Jim was brought to the emergency room after suffering a heart attack.

Thus, a seemingly everyday occurrence ended in tragedy. But why? Why does a man put so much strain on his body that he ends up in total collapse?

The answer is simple. Jim was living in denial.

Living with awareness about your body is really the key to preventing ill health. Jim denied all the signals his body was sending him. (Although we can't know for sure, it's a safe bet to say that Jim's life-long habit of repressing his feelings was a strong contributing factor to his heart attack.) Instead, he pushed beyond his normal expectations and almost died in the process. Jim was really out of touch with his body. He really didn't listen to any of the "conversations" that went on between his brain and his heart. The mind saying one thing while the body is saying another is at the root of what cardiologists call *silent myocardial ischemia* (a lack of blood flow to the heart, which often results in damage to the heart muscle). The EKG tells us the heart is in trouble, even though the patient has no sensation. But the body is telling the truth, as the heart reveals its distress.

No one questions that there are strong behavioral and psychological factors that frequently precipitate cardiac arrest. It's no coincidence that sudden psychological or emotional stress frequently occurs just prior to a heart attack. It's well documented that Monday morning, the day most people go back to work after a weekend away, is the most common time for sudden cardiac death. Approximately 36 percent of all sudden deaths occur on Monday! And interestingly, the second most common time is Saturday. Why? Could it be the result of psychologically and emotionally gearing up (Monday) or gearing down (Saturday)? Is the office a safe place? Or is it a place of combat and stress (especially for the heart)? Look, some people may loathe going to work, but others may loathe going home. Whatever the stress is, the heart will reveal it. And the heart will tell the truth about it.

STRESS AND CHOLESTEROL

Your doc may tell you to fast before certain blood tests, but we'll bet that no doc ever told you to meditate before taking a cholesterol test. Now granted, we don't think cholesterol test results are important (*unless* you get the particle size test we recommended

 Dr. Sinatra:

I remember the unfortunate case of a fifty-two-year-old diabetic woman who had spontaneously bled into her eye and required emergency surgery. Two years before, she had sustained a heart attack but had since enjoyed a good quality of life. She was not experiencing any symptoms of chest pain or shortness of breath, and there were no other obvious signs of heart problems. She was admitted to the hospital and underwent immediate surgery that was, unfortunately, unsuccessful.

Upon learning of the loss of her eyesight, she became deeply saddened and depressed. (Who wouldn't be?) I remember seeing her in the hospital ward and feeling her depth of sorrow. Sitting in a wheelchair, she was despondent that she couldn't see. She talked in a monotone voice and kept her head down. She said that she had lost all hope and had nothing to look forward to.

She died a day later.

earlier). But your doctor undoubtedly *does*. And he or she would probably be surprised to learn that stress can actually influence those cholesterol test results. After all, how could stress—which clearly originates in the brain—influence something like cholesterol in the bloodstream?

Glad you asked. Here's what Dr. Sinatra has to say:

Some years ago, I was asked to submit to a fasting serum cholesterol test for an insurance evaluation. Because I was performing three cardiac catheterizations that day, I asked that blood be drawn prior to 7:30 in the morning.

At that time, my blood cholesterol was 180 mg/dL, a number my doctors and I were utterly delighted with. After performing two of the three cardiac catheterizations, both of which went smoothly, I tackled the third case, which was anything but routine. This was an individual with complex congenital heart disease. The cardiac catheterization itself was further complicated by the fact that during the procedure, the patient suffered cardiac arrest. The patient actually stopped breathing, though, luckily, he was successfully resuscitated. The procedure took a grueling five hours, and it required multiple catheters and multiple pharmacological interventions.

Man, I really sweated during that case, even though, thankfully, it all ended well.

When the procedure was over, it was approximately three in the afternoon, and I hadn't eaten all day. As I was walking to the cafeteria, I passed the blood lab where I had blood drawn earlier that morning. Because I had a strong belief in the effect of psychological stress on the body, I was curious to see whether the day's activities had produced any changes in my own blood. So I asked my colleagues to perform a second blood test.

My blood cholesterol had risen to 240 mg/dL, a number that would cause virtually any conventional practitioner to put me on a statin drug immediately.

I had been fasting for nearly 20 hours at this point, and there was absolutely no dietary variable that could have caused this jump of 33 percent in my cholesterol. Obviously, my body reacted to the stressful events of the day by producing an excessive amount of cholesterol.

The connection between stress and elevated cholesterol is well documented. In 2005, researchers conducted a study of about 200 middle-aged government workers in London.[6] First the workers gave blood samples and "rated" their levels of stress. Then they were given two paper and pencil tests, both designed to be somewhat stressful. In the first test, they were shown mismatched words and colors. For example, the word "red" would be written in blue letters. The participants had to name the color in which the words appeared (in this case "blue"). It's a confusing and annoying test and makes people uneasy. In the second test, the participants were told to trace the outline of a star in a mirror, under a deadline. (Try it sometime—it'll make you crazy.) Afterward, the participants gave blood again, had their cholesterol checked, and rated their stress levels.

Three years later everyone had their cholesterol levels measured again.

The first finding was interesting on its own: Cholesterol rose for everyone after doing the stress-inducing paper and pencil tests. But it rose for some people a lot more than it did for others. Let's call them the "high reactors."

Now check this out: Three years later, the high reactors had the highest cholesterol levels.

The researchers created three "thresholds" for cholesterol: low, medium, and high. After the three years, those who hit the "high cholesterol" threshold included 16 percent of those who had initially shown little cholesterol reaction to the stress tests and 22 percent of those who had initially shown a "moderate" cholesterol reaction to the stress tests.

But a whopping 56 percent of those who initially had the biggest change in their cholesterol after the stress tests were now in the "high cholesterol" group! And this was even after making adjustments for weight, smoking, hormone therapy, and alcohol use.

The short stress tests were excellent predictors of how people—and their cholesterol levels—responded to stress. "The cholesterol responses we measured in the lab probably reflect the way people react to challenges in everyday life," said lead researcher Andrew Steptoe, D.Sc. "The larger cholesterol responders to stress tasks will be large responders to emotional situations in their lives," he added. "It is these responses in everyday life that accumulate to lead to an increase in fasting cholesterol . . . three years later. It appears that a person's reaction to stress is one mechanism through which higher [cholesterol] levels may develop."[7]

Stress and Depression

Stress is certainly a trigger for depression, and the relationship between depression and heart disease is well established. Individuals who suffer from mood disorders are twice as likely to have a heart attack when compared to people who are not depressed.

One researcher who has spent much of his career investigating the relationship between depression and heart disease is Alexander Glassman, M.D., a professor of psychiatry at Columbia University and chief of clinical psychopharmacology at New York State Psychiatric Institute. In a number of published studies, he has shown that medically healthy but clinically depressed patients are at increased risk of both cardiovascular disease and cardiac death. Depression following a heart attack especially increases the risk of death.[8] "It is now apparent that depression aggravates the course of multiple cardiovascular conditions," he wrote.[9]

The Stress of Sorrow

If we look at those suffering a bereavement, sudden death is two to ten times higher than in the general population. It's even worse if a man loses his wife than if a woman loses her husband. In general, women adapt better than men do. Women express feelings more often. They find joy in sharing those feelings, especially with other women. They form networks and nurture each other. Men, on the other hand, build walls. They hold feelings in. They keep secrets and sometimes have a really hard time communicating.

📄 Dr. Sinatra:

As trite as it sounds, love heals.

In my "Healing the Heart" workshops, we see profound cholesterol lowering when a patient experiences contact and connectedness in a supportive environment. In these four- to seven-day workshops, cholesterol levels have been lower in every one of our participants, with some losing as much as 100 mg/dL of cholesterol in just a few days!

The dramatic reduction in cholesterol supports the notion that emotional contact can positively affect our health.

Once, during a workshop, a physician from Greece was asked about the relative lack of heart disease in Crete and Greece. He immediately responded by speaking of the healing powers of nurturing relationships, particularly among the males. He described how men in Crete spend quality time with one another, talking over lunch about real feelings. The typical topics discussed when American men get together—sports, politics, and money—just aren't central in their conversations. They talk about feelings. They talk about their families. They talk about their dreams and even their spiritual beliefs. And they rarely wear "social masks." Instead, they argue, cry, support, and even hold each other. The Greek doctor felt that such camaraderie—occurring often over games of chess or during two-hour lunches—is a major factor in the reduction of coronary heart disease.

Maybe part of the "secret" of the Mediterranean diet isn't the diet at all. Maybe it has something to do with how the people in the Mediterranean live.

> When you support and nurture yourself, your positive self-esteem reflects itself in the healing of your body.

Although digging into your emotions and allowing yourself to be vulnerable can be difficult if you are unaccustomed to such soul-searching, we invite each of you to consider looking more deeply into your emotional self. Such introspection can initially be painful, but it is well worth the effort in the long run. When you support and nurture yourself, your positive self-esteem reflects itself in the healing of your body. Such nurturing and protective influences have been validated in studies time and time again.

Animals and the Stress of Heartbreak

If you're an animal lover like we are, you might not want to read the next few paragraphs. We're going to tell you about a horrible and sad study that nonetheless dramatically illustrates the role of psychological stress in heart disease and death. (Don't say we didn't warn you.)

Baboons are some of the most lovable creatures on earth. They sleep and travel in groups of about fifty individuals. They're highly social and very connected. Adults sit in small groups grooming one another while the youngsters romp and play. They forage for about three hours in the morning, rest during the afternoon, and then forage again later on before returning to their sleeping places. Before bed, they spend more time grooming each other, which not only keeps them clean and free of external parasites, but also serves to strengthen their bonds. And they're ambassadors for "family values"—they mate for life.

Early in the twentieth century, Soviet experimenters performed the following experiment. They reared eighteen baboon couples together, and then, after the bonds were strongly established, they removed the male from the cage and replaced him with a new male. The ex-mate was placed only a few feet away in another cage, fully able to observe his former partner and her new "mate."

Within six months, every one of the eighteen "ex-husbands" died.

Technically, they died of strokes, hypertension, and heart attacks. Less technically, we could say they died of heartbreak. Either way, the acute psychological stress of being trapped, heartbroken, and, most important, helpless to do anything about it, overwhelmingly resulted in death.[10]

📄 Dr. Jonny:

Warren Buffett is a particular hero of mine, but not because he's the richest dude in America. Rather, I admire him because, by all accounts, he is remarkably down-to-earth, unpretentious, compassionate, and unafraid of expressing his feelings—not exactly a constellation of traits most of us associate with incredible wealth and power.

Much of this probably has to do with Susie.

Susie met Buffett in 1950, and they were married two years later. "She put me together," he said.[11] Susie was big on civil rights and fairness. She was involved in helping the cause of integration in Omaha back in the 1960s and influenced Buffett so much that he became active in overturning anti-Semitic membership rules at the fancy Omaha Club.

She humanized him.

Prior to meeting Susie there was little time in Buffett's life for anything but moneymaking. Although they eventually separated, they shared a great love, and it was probably the most transformative relationship of Buffett's life. Susie even introduced him to her friend Astrid, who, with Susie's blessing, eventually became his mistress and, after Susie's death, his second wife.

Seven years after Susie's death, Buffett was the subject of a *Time* cover story by Rana Foroohar.[12] When discussing Susie, he burst into tears. Foroohar reported that it took several moments for him to recover. She put her hand on his arm. "Eventually," she said, "we moved on to an easier subject—his investments."

Few men of Buffett's station in life would allow themselves to feel vulnerable enough to break down and cry in front of a reporter when talking about the love of their life. In fact, few men of any station in life would feel free enough—and be in touch with their feelings enough—to do so.

Buffett eats a horrific diet of fast food, is reported to drink about 60 ounces (1.7 liters) of Coca-Cola a day, and has never been seen at a gym. Yet at eighty-one, he's sharp, active, involved, and engaged.

He's also healthy.

Could his dyed-in-the-wool optimism coupled with his ability to express his feelings easily and relate to people deeply be profoundly protective of his heart?

Food for thought.

PUTTING IT ALL TOGETHER– A SIMPLE AND EASY BLUEPRINT FOR A HEALTHY HEART–AND LIFE!

IN THIS CHAPTER, we're going to make specific suggestions about what you can do right now to prevent a first (or second) heart attack and keep your heart healthy for many decades.

We're going to advise you about which tests you should ask your doctor for and why. We'll recommend which foods you should incorporate into your diet, if you haven't already.

And we're also going to discuss the emotional and psychological risk factors for heart disease, which need to be taken just as seriously as the physical ones. We'll give you specific tools to help lower these risk factors.

THE TESTS YOU SHOULD ASK YOUR DOCTOR FOR

We hope by now you're convinced that total cholesterol is a meaningless number and should be the basis for absolutely nothing in your treatment plan. The old division into "good" (HDL) cholesterol and "bad" (LDL) cholesterol is out of date and provides only marginally better information than a "total" cholesterol reading. As we've said, both good and bad cholesterol have a number of different components (or subtypes) that behave quite differently, and the twenty-first-century version of a cholesterol test should always tell you exactly which subtypes you have. Anything less is not particularly useful and should never be the sole basis on which a treatment plan or a statin drug is recommended. That's why the LDL particle size test is the first test we recommend.

1. Particle Size Test

Although LDL cholesterol is known as the "bad" cholesterol, the fact is that it comes in several shapes and sizes, as does HDL cholesterol, the so-called "good" kind. These different subtypes of cholesterol behave very differently. Seen under a microscope, some LDL particles are big, fluffy, and harmless. Some are small, dense, "angry," and much more likely to become oxidized, slipping through the cells that line the walls of the arteries (the endothelium) and beginning the inflammatory cascade that leads to heart disease.

Tests are now available that measure LDL particle size, and that's the information you really want to have. If you have a pattern A cholesterol profile, most

of your LDL cholesterol is the big, fluffy kind, which is great; but if you have a pattern B profile, most of your LDL cholesterol is composed of the small, dense, atherogenic particles that cause inflammation and ultimately plaque. (Fortunately, you can change the distribution from small to buoyant by following the dietary and supplement recommendations in this book.)

One widely used test is called the **NMR LipoProfile**, and it analyzes the size of LDL particles by measuring their magnetic properties. Others—including the **Lipoprint** and the **Berkeley** (from the Berkeley HeartLab) use electrical fields to distinguish the size of the particles. Another test known as the **VAP** (Vertical Auto Profile) separates lipoprotein particles using a high-speed centrifuge.[1] And still another is the **LPP** (or Lipoprotein Particle Profile). Any of these newer cholesterol tests can be offered by your doctor.

Taking a statin drug, or any other medication, based solely on the standard cholesterol test is a really bad idea. Ask your doctor for one of the newer particle tests. If he objects, make sure he has a darn good reason. It's the only cholesterol test that matters.

2. C-Reactive Protein (CRP)

CRP is a marker for inflammation that is directly associated with overall heart and cardiovascular health. In multiple studies, CRP has been identified as a potent predictor of future cardiovascular health—and, in our opinion, one that is far more reliable than elevated cholesterol levels. Biological characteristics that are associated with high CRP levels include infections, high blood sugar, excess weight, and hypercoagulability of blood (sticky blood).

Fortunately, there is a simple test that your doctor can conduct to find out how much CRP is in your blood. Just make sure the high-sensitivity test **(hs-CRP)** is used. This test doesn't take much time: Typically, blood is drawn from a vein located either on your forearm or on the inside of your elbow. The blood is then analyzed in several tests to determine the level of CRP present. (Dr. Sinatra's recommendation for an optimal CRP level is less than 0.8 mg/dL.)

3. Fibrinogen

Fibrinogen is a protein that determines the stickiness of your blood by enabling your platelets to stick together. You need adequate fibrinogen levels to stop bleeding when you've been injured, but you also want to balance your fibrinogen levels to support optimal blood circulation and prevent unnecessary clotting. (In women younger than forty-five, Dr. Sinatra has seen far more heart attacks caused by improper blood clotting than by anything else.) Normal levels are between 200 and 400 mg/dL, and they may be elevated during any kind of inflammation.

Fibrinogen has been identified as an independent risk factor for cardiovascular disease and is associated with the traditional risk factors as well. In one study, fibrinogen levels were significantly higher among subjects with cardiovascular disease than among those without it.[2]

There are two ways to test for fibrinogen. The first is the **Clauss method** and the second is a newer test called the **FiF** (immunoprecipitation functional intact fibrinogen) test, which was developed by American Biogenetic Sciences.[3] The FiF test is the better one because it shows a stronger association with cardiovascular disease than the Clauss method does.[4] If the FiF test isn't available, use the Clauss method—it still has a strong association with cardiovascular disease, even if it's not quite as accurate as the newer test.

If you have a family history of heart concerns, you must check your serum fibrinogen level. Women who smoke, take oral contraceptives, or are postmenopausal usually have higher fibrinogen levels.

Worth noting: This test hasn't caught on with many doctors because there are no direct treatments for elevated levels. But supplements such as nattokinase, discussed in chapter 7 on supplements, can work well to "thin" the blood and prevent unwanted clotting. Adding omega-3 fatty acids to your diet may also help.

4. Serum Ferritin

Ever wonder why so many vitamin manufacturers offer multiple vitamins "without iron"? Here's why: Iron is one of those weird substances where if you don't have enough you can have some real problems (e.g., iron-deficiency anemia), but if you have too much, look out! Iron is highly susceptible to oxidation. (Imagine someone leaving a barbell from your gym outside in the rain for a couple of days. It's going to rust like crazy. That's oxidation.)

Iron levels in the body are cumulative (stored in the muscles and other tissues), and unless iron is lost through menstruation or by donating blood, over the years toxic levels can build up in the system. Although this danger always exists for men, it becomes a real risk for women after menopause. Both of us are adamant that no one but premenopausal women should ever take vitamins with iron, or supplemental iron of any kind, unless prescribed by a doctor.

Iron overload—technically called *hemochromatosis*—can actually contribute to heart disease. Researchers measure iron in the blood by measuring a form of it called *ferritin*. A 1992 study by Finnish researchers examined the role of iron in coronary artery disease. After studying 1,900 Finnish men between the ages of forty-two and sixty for five years, the researchers found that men with excessive levels of ferritin had an elevated risk of heart attack, and that every 1 percent increase in ferritin translated into a 4 percent increase in heart attack risk.[5]

Those with high levels of ferritin were more than twice as likely to have heart attacks than those with lower levels. The authors of this study concluded that ferritin levels may be an even stronger risk factor for heart disease than high blood pressure or diabetes is.[6] It's certainly a more important risk factor than high cholesterol.

If your ferritin levels are high, consider donating blood every so often, or ask your doctor to consider a therapeutic phlebotomy. (Dr. Sinatra's recommendation for an optimal serum ferritin level is less than 80 mg/L for women and less than 90 mg/L for men.)

Worth noting: One consideration regarding supplemental vitamin C is that it helps the body absorb iron better. If you have a problem with iron levels, keep your supplemental vitamin C to less than 100 mg a day.

5. Lp(a)

Lp(a) is a type of cholesterol-carrying molecule that contains one LDL (low-density lipoprotein) molecule chemically bound to an attachment protein called *apolipoprotein(a)*. In a healthy body, Lp(a) isn't much of a problem. It circulates and carries out repair and restoration work on damaged blood vessels. The protein part of it promotes blood clotting. So far, so good.

The problem is, the more repair you need on your arteries, the more Lp(a) is utilized, and that's when things get ugly. Lp(a) concentrates at the site of damage, binds with a couple of amino acids within the wall of a damaged blood vessel, dumps its LDL cargo, and starts to promote the deposition of oxidized LDL into the wall, leading to more inflammation and ultimately to plaque.

Also, Lp(a) promotes the formation of blood clots on top of the newly formed plaque, which narrows the blood vessels further. If the clots are large enough, they can block an artery. (Most heart attacks are due to either a large clot developing in vessels with moderate-to-severe narrowing or a plaque rupture that blocks the artery.)

Elevated Lp(a) is a very serious risk factor. A very high percentage of heart attacks happen to people with high Lp(a) levels. Dr. Sinatra thinks Lp(a) is one of the most devastating risk factors for heart disease and one of the hardest to treat.

One reason doctors aren't running out to test for Lp(a) all the time is that there are no real pharmaceutical interventions that work to lower it. In addition, Lp(a) levels are largely genetically determined and not very modifiable by lifestyle choices. However, your Lp(a) level can give you a good idea of your real risk for heart disease, and a high level may serve as a wake-up call to inspire you to work harder to improve your heart health using the strategies, foods, supplements, and lifestyle changes suggested in this book. That said, Dr. Sinatra feels that Lp(a) can be lowered with a combination of 1 to 2 g of fish oil, 500 to 2,500 mg of niacin (not the slow-release kind), and 200 mg of lumbrokinase.

Worth noting: Statin drugs can sometimes raise Lp(a) levels! This is mentioned on the warning labels of statin drug ads in the Canadian edition of the *New England Journal of Medicine*, but such labeling is not required by the Food and Drug Administration, so you won't see it in ads published in the United States.[7]

6. Homocysteine

Homocysteine is an amino acid by-product that causes your body to lay down sticky platelets in blood vessels. Having some homocysteine is normal, but an excess might affect your cardiovascular health. Evidence shows that homocysteine contributes to atherosclerosis, reduces the flexibility of blood vessels, and helps make platelets stickier, thus slowing blood flow. Net result: There's a direct correlation between high homocysteine levels and an increased risk of heart disease and stroke.

Elevated homocysteine strongly predicts both a first and a recurring cardiovascular incident (including death).[8] Too much homocysteine adversely affects the function of the endothelium, the all-important lining of the artery walls. It also increases oxidative damage and promotes inflammation and thrombosis—a regular evil trifecta for heart disease.[9] One study looked at more than 3,000 patients with chronic heart disease and found that a subsequent coronary event was 2.5 times more likely in patients with elevated levels of homocysteine. What's more, each 5 μmol/L of homocysteine predicted a 25 percent increase in risk![10]

Fortunately, there's an easy way to bring down homocysteine levels. All you have to do is give the body the three main nutrients it needs to metabolize homocysteine back into harmless compounds. The three nutrients are folic acid, vitamin B_{12}, and vitamin B_6. All it takes is about 400 to 800 mcg of folic acid, 400 to 1,000 mcg of B_{12}, and 5 to 20 mg of B_6. If you've had a heart attack or other cardiovascular event; if you have a family history of early heart disease; or if you have hypothyroidism, lupus, or kidney disease, consider asking your doctor to test your homocysteine levels. Finally, if you take drugs that tend to elevate homocysteine—theophylline (for asthma), methotrexate (for cancer or arthritis), or L-dopa (for Parkinson's)—you should be tested. (Dr. Sinatra's recommendation for an optimal homocysteine level is between 7 and 9 μmol/L.)

7. Interleukin-6

Interleukin-6 is important because it stimulates the liver to produce CRP. And we are learning that this inflammatory cytokine has a strong association with not only heart disease but also asthma. (Asthma is the result of airways swelling and constricting, so it makes sense that an inflammatory agent is behind the curtains here as well.) The Iowa 65+ Rural Health Study demonstrated that elevated levels of interleukin-6 and CRP were associated with an increased risk for both cardiovascular disease and general mortality in healthy older people.

Interleukin-6 may be an even better marker for inflammation than CRP is because these "precursor" levels rise earlier. If you're concerned about inflammation and its effect on your heart, ask your doctor to do an interleukin-6 test. (Dr. Sinatra's recommendation for an optimal interleukin-6 level is 0.0 to 12.0 pg/mL.)

8. Coronary Calcium Scan

Calcium is great—as long as it stays in the bones and teeth. One place you don't want it is in the coronary arteries.

Coronary calcification is one of the major risk factors that predicts coronary heart disease and future heart attacks.[11] The more calcium present, the greater the risk of suffering a heart attack. Men develop calcifications about ten to fifteen years earlier than women do. Calcification can be detected in the majority of asymptomatic men over fifty-five years of age and in women over sixty-five.

As far back as 1991, cardiologist Stephen Seely, M.D., published a paper in the *International Journal of Cardiology* titled "Is Calcium Excess in the Western Diet a Major Cause of Arterial Disease?" He pointed out that cholesterol only makes up 3 percent of arterial plaque while calcium makes up 50 percent![12]

The Florida cardiologist Arthur Agatston, M.D., is best known for his wildly popular South Beach diet, but what many people don't know is that he also developed a widely accepted test for coronary calcification known as the **Agatston test**. Individuals who score less than 10 on the Agatston test have minimal calcification; those with Agatston scores of 11 to 99 have moderate calcification; those with scores of 100 to 400 have increased calcification; and those with scores above 400 have extensive calcification.

It is well established that individuals with Agatston scores above 400 have an increased occurrence of coronary procedures (bypass, stent placement, and angioplasty) and events (myocardial infarction and cardiac death) within the two to five years following the test. Individuals with very high Agatston scores (over 1,000) have a 20 percent chance of suffering a heart attack or cardiac death within a year. Even among patients over the age of seventy who frequently have calcification, an Agatston Score above 400 was associated with a higher risk of death.[13]

The American Heart Association and the American College of Cardiology provide guidelines for coronary calcification testing, available online, www.ahajournals. org/misc/sci-stmts_topindex.shtml. These guidelines

◀ WHAT YOU NEED TO KNOW

Ask your doctor for the following tests, which are more important than the standard test for cholesterol:

- LDL particle size
- Hs-CRP
- Fibrinogen
- Serum ferritin (iron)
- Lp(a)
- Homocysteine
- Interleukin-6
- Coronary calcium scan

Eliminate these foods:

- Sugar
- Soda
- Processed carbs
- Trans fats
- Processed meats
- Excess vegetable oils

Eat more of these foods:

- Wild salmon
- Berries and cherries
- Grass-fed meat
- Vegetables
- Nuts
- Beans
- Dark chocolate
- Garlic and turmeric
- Pomegranate juice, green tea, and red wine
- Extra-virgin olive oil

Make these lifestyle changes to reduce stress:

- Meditate or practice deep breathing.
- Express your emotions.
- Play.
- Cultivate intimacy and pleasure.
- And most of all . . . enjoy your life!

currently suggest—and we agree—that screening for calcification is of value for an individual who is considered to be at intermediate ten-year risk, which means that he or she has a 10 to 20 percent likelihood of experiencing a cardiac event within the next ten years.[14]

EAT THIS, DUMP THAT

This section is divided into two parts—what to eat and what *not* to eat for optimal heart health. Fortunately, the list of what not to eat is fairly short, so let's get that one out of the way first. We call it the "Dump It!" list and provide you with specific "fast action plans" to help you remove these nutritionally empty, heart-unfriendly foods from your diet. The second section is called "Eat This!" and reveals some of the healthiest foods on the planet.

Dump It: Sugar

As we've said throughout this book (see chapter 4), sugar is a far worse threat to your heart than fat ever was.

The 2010 Dietary Guidelines for Americans suggest that no more than 25 percent of your calories should come from added sugars, but we think that's a ridiculously high amount. (The American Heart Association recommends no more than 5 percent.) Research by Kimber Stanhope, Ph.D., at the University of California, Davis, has shown that when people consume 25 percent of their calories from fructose or high-fructose corn syrup, several factors associated with an increased risk for heart disease—including triglycerides and a nasty little substance called *apolipoprotein B*—escalate.[15]

(Remember, it's the fructose in sugar that's the problem. High-fructose corn syrup is 55 percent fructose, and regular sugar is 50 percent fructose, so for all intents and purposes, they have the same bad effect on your heart and your health.)

Fast Action Plan: Cut out soda. Soda is probably the worst offender in this category, but not by much. Fruit juices are loaded with sugar and only marginally better than soda. "Energy drinks" aren't any better. Most are loaded with sugar, and the sugar-free versions are loaded with chemicals. Many processed carbs (see below) are also full of sugar, and virtually all cakes, candies, pastries, doughnuts, and other sources of empty calories are also sugar heavyweights.

Dump It: Processed Carbohydrates

Processed carbs include almost any carbohydrate food that comes in a package: cereals, pasta, bread, minute rice, you name it. These foods are almost always high-glycemic, meaning they quickly and dramatically raise your blood sugar, which is exactly what you do not want. A 2010 study in the *Archives of Internal Medicine* demonstrated that women who ate the highest amount of carbohydrates had a significantly greater risk of coronary heart disease than those who ate the lowest amount, and that carbohydrates from high-glycemic carbs were particularly associated with significantly greater risk for heart disease.[16] (This association was not confirmed for men in this particular study, but we suspect that future studies will discover that it's true for both sexes.)

CORNFLAKES A GREAT BREAKFAST? THINK AGAIN!

If any of you out there still think cornflakes are a great, wholesome breakfast, read on.

A landmark research study conducted by Michael Shechter, M.D., of Tel Aviv University's Sackler School of Medicine and the Heart Institute of Sheba Medical Center, with collaboration from the Endocrinology Institute, shows exactly how high-carbohydrate foods increase the risk for heart problems.[17]

Researchers looked at four groups of volunteers who were given different breakfasts. The first group was given a cornflake mush mixed with milk, not unlike the typical American breakfast. The second group was given a pure sugar mixture. The third group was given bran flakes. And the fourth group was given a placebo (water).

Over four weeks, Shechter applied a test that allows researchers to visualize how the arteries are functioning. It's called *brachial reactive testing*, and it uses a cuff on the arm (similar to those used for measuring blood pressure) that can visualize arterial function in real time.

The results were dramatic. Before any of the patients ate, their arterial function was basically the same. After eating, all had reduced functioning except for the patients in the water-drinking placebo group. Enormous peaks indicating arterial stress were found in the high GI groups: the cornflakes and sugar groups.

"We knew high glycemic foods were bad for the heart. Now we have a mechanism that shows how," Shechter wrote. "Foods like cornflakes, white bread, French fries, and sweetened soda all put undue stress on our arteries. We've explained for the first time how high-glycemic carbs can affect the progression of heart disease."

During the consumption of foods high in sugar, there appears to be a temporary and sudden dysfunction in the endothelial walls of the arteries. Endothelial health can be traced back to almost every disorder and disease in the body. According to Shechter, it is the "riskiest of the risk factors."

Shechter recommended sticking to foods such as oatmeal, fruits and vegetables, and legumes and nuts, which all have a low glycemic index. Exercising every day for at least thirty minutes, he added, is an extra heart-smart action to take.

There's no two ways about it—high-glycemic carbohydrates are inflammatory. As researchers from Harvard Medical School and the Harvard School of Public Health noted, quickly digested and absorbed carbs (i.e., those with a high glycemic load) are associated with an increased risk of heart disease.[18]

These same researchers examined the diets of 244 apparently healthy women to evaluate the association between glycemic load and blood levels of CRP (C-reactive protein, the systemic measure of inflammation discussed earlier in this chapter). They found "a strong and statistically significant positive association between dietary glycemic load and [blood levels of] CRP."[19] And that's putting it mildly. Women whose diets were highest in glycemic load had almost twice the amount of CRP in their blood as women whose diets were lowest in glycemic load (3.7 for high-glycemic load ladies, 1.9 for low-glycemic load ladies). The difference in inflammation levels was even more pronounced for overweight women. Among women with a body mass index (BMI) greater than 25, those whose diets were lowest in glycemic load had an average CRP reading of 1.6, but those whose diets were highest in glycemic load had a CRP reading more than three times that amount (average measurement: 5.0 mg/L).[20]

Full disclosure: We don't much buy into the argument that "whole grains" eliminate all the problems associated with processed carbs, and here's why: Number one, most commercial products that are made with whole grains don't contain all that much of them. Number two, whole grains raise blood sugar almost as much as processed grains do. Number

three, whole grains still contain gluten, which can be very inflammatory for people who are gluten-sensitive. That said, real whole grain products (Ezekiel 4:9 breads, for example) are way better than their processed counterparts. But be a careful consumer—just because a label says "wheat" instead of "white," don't assume it's good for you.

Fast Action Plan: Reduce (or eliminate) consumption of processed carbohydrates. At the same time, increase non-processed carbohydrates such as vegetables and low-sugar fruits. Replace your bagel and orange juice with some eggs, veggies, and a slice of avocado. Have berries for dessert. When eating out, say "no" to the breadbasket.

Dump It: Trans Fats

According to findings presented at the annual meeting of the American Heart Association in 2006, women who ate the most trans fats were more than three times as likely to develop heart disease as women who ate the least.[21] Harvard researcher Charlene Hu examined data from the long-running Nurses' Health Study, which has followed 120,000 female nurses for more than thirty years. His research shows that for each 2 percent increase in trans fat calories consumed, the risk for coronary heart disease roughly doubles![22] Trans fats raise LDL cholesterol levels, which doesn't mean very much by itself, but at high intakes they also reduce HDL levels, which definitely isn't good.[23]

The worst offenders include nondairy "creamers," most margarines, cake mixes, ramen noodles, soup cups, virtually all packaged baked goods (e.g., Twinkies,

THE "NO TRANS-FATS!" SCAM

When the government mandated that trans fats be listed on the nutrition facts label of food, big food lobbyists sprang into action. They somehow created a loophole that lets manufacturers use trans fats while legally claiming "no trans fats!" on their packaging. Here's how:

Manufacturers can claim "no trans fats" as long as there is less than half a gram of the stuff per serving. Sounds reasonable, until you remember how clever and ruthless Big Food can be. By making "serving sizes" ridiculously small, and by keeping trans fats to just under half a gram per "serving," they were able to technically comply with the rules. But the end result is that if each artificially small "serving" contains, say 0.4 g of trans fats, you could quite easily consume a gram or two of the stuff just by eating what most people would consider a "normal" serving size. Do that a few times a day and before you know it you've raised your heart disease risk by quite a few percentage points.

What to do? Simple. Ignore the "no trans fats!" legend on the front of the package and read the ingredients list instead. No matter what the label says, if the list of ingredients contains partially hydrogenated oil or hydrogenated oil, the product has trans fats. Period. (Typically, you'll see partially hydrogenated soybean oil in the ingredients list, but it could be any type of oil at all. What you're looking for are the keywords *hydrogenated* and *partially hydrogenated*.)

chips, and crackers), doughnuts, many breakfast cereals, "energy" bars, cookies, and definitely fast food. (Just for example, a medium order of fries contains an incredible 14.5 g of trans fat, and a Kentucky Fried Chicken Original Recipe chicken dinner has 7 g. The ideal intake for humans is 0 g.)

Worth knowing: There is one exception to the don't-eat-trans-fats rule, and that's something called *conjugated linoleic acid*, or CLA. CLA is a trans fat that's not man-made; rather, it's made naturally in the bodies of ruminants (cows). Factory-farmed meat doesn't have any, but grass-fed meat—and products that come from pasture-raised animals–do. CLA has both anticancer and antiobesity properties. CLA is good for you, unlike hydrogenated or partially hydrogenated oils–the very definition of man-made trans fats–which are definitely *not* good for you.

Fast Action Plan: Stop eating fast food. On all packaged foods from the supermarket, check the ingredients list for "partially hydrogenated" or "hydrogenated" oils. If either of those is listed, don't eat it. Look in particular at margarines, cookies, cakes, pastries, doughnuts, and, as mentioned, fast food.

Dump It: Processed Meats

Processed meats contribute to both inflammation in general and heart disease specifically.

Harvard researchers investigated the effect of eating processed meat versus unprocessed meat. Processed meat was defined as any meat preserved by curing, salting, smoking, or with the addition of chemical preservatives, such as those found in salami, sausages, hot dogs, luncheon meats, and bacon. (Previous studies had rarely separated processed meat from unprocessed meat when investigating the relationship between disease and meat eating.) The researchers analyzed twenty studies that included a total of 1,218,380 people from ten countries on four continents (North America, Europe, Asia, and Australia). They found that each 1.8-ounce daily serving of processed meat (about one hot dog or a couple slices of deli meat) was associated with a 42 percent higher risk of developing heart disease. (In contrast,

no relationship was found between heart disease and nonprocessed red meat.[24])

Although the study didn't identify which specific ingredients in processed meat could be responsible for the association, many health professionals believe that the high levels of sodium and nitrates might be responsible." When we looked at average nutrients in unprocessed red and processed meats eaten in the United States, we found that they contained similar average amounts of saturated fat and cholesterol. In contrast, processed meats contained, on average, four times more sodium and 50 percent more nitrate preservatives," said Renata Micha, a research fellow in the department of epidemiology at the Harvard School of Public Health and lead author of the study. "This suggests that differences in salt and preservatives, rather than fats, might explain the higher risk of heart disease and diabetes seen with processed meats, but not with unprocessed red meats."[25]

Fast Action Plan: Cut out processed (e.g., deli) meats.

Dump It: Excessive Omega-6 Fats

Vegetable oils (corn, canola, and soybean) are mostly made up of pro-inflammatory omega-6 fats, and you should reduce (not necessarily eliminate) your consumption of them while increasing your consumption of anti-inflammatory omega-3 fats.

This is the one recommendation that comes with an asterisk. Omega-6 fats, the ones that are most prevalent in vegetable oils, are not in and of themselves "bad." But they *are* pro-inflammatory, and they need to be balanced by an equal (or near-equal) intake of anti-inflammatory omega-3s. (You can review this information in chapter 5, "The Truth about Fat.") The optimal ratio of omega-6 to omega-3 in the human diet is no higher than 4:1, and many believe the ideal ratio is 1:1. In the average Westernized diet, the ratio is anywhere between 15:1 and 25:1, which creates a highly inflammatory state in the body. Because heart disease is primarily a disease of inflammation, such a state should be avoided as much as humanly possible.

And by the way, it's not just the oils you use for cooking that tip the scales into inflammation land. Omega-6 fats are everywhere in the food supply—you can't swing a rope without hitting a food product loaded with omega-6s. Nearly all processed foods contain them. They're used almost exclusively in restaurants, for frying, sautéing, and baking, so virtually anything you order from the menu has got a ton of omega-6 fats.

So choose your omega-6 fats carefully and use them sparingly. (The best choices are cold-pressed, unrefined oils—sesame oil is a particularly good choice.) Use highly processed supermarket oils (such as corn oil) infrequently or not at all. When you sauté food, try substituting monounsaturated fats such as olive oil and macadamia nut oil for high omega-6 oils such as canola or soybean. And, above all, increase your intake of omega-3 fats to help balance your intake of omega-6s (see the "Eat This!" section below).

Fast Action Plan: Never use generic processed oils such as Wesson or Crisco. Cut down on corn oil, safflower oil, soybean oil, and canola oil (see Dr. Sinatra's personal story on canola oil in chapter 5). Whenever possible, use olive oil, sesame oil, or macadamia oil. And pay attention to the "Eat This!" section in this chapter on omega-3s.

THE "EAT THIS!" LIST

Both of us are frequently interviewed about the best foods for health. Virtually every reporter either of us has ever spoken with winds up asking, "How much of this food do you need to eat to get its benefits?" It's a reasonable question, but there's almost never a perfect answer. We know of no study, for example, that has systematically tested the effects of eating five portions of blueberries a week as opposed to three, or compared eating two portions of salmon per week with eating it daily. Our recommendation is to put these foods in heavy rotation in your diet, enjoying them as frequently as you like.

Here are the foods you want to include in your diet on a regular basis.

Eat This: Wild Alaskan Salmon

Salmon is one of the best sources of anti-inflammatory omega-3s. But not all salmon is created equal. Wild Alaskan salmon is far superior to the farm-raised variety. (According to independent lab tests by the Environmental Working Group, seven out of ten farmed salmon purchased at grocery stores were contaminated with polychlorinated biphenyls [PCBs] at levels high enough to raise health concerns.) Wild salmon is far cleaner, and it has the added benefit of containing one of the most powerful antioxidants on the planet, *astaxanthin*. A 4-ounce serving also contains 462 mg of heart-healthy potassium, the same amount in a medium banana.[26]

Both of us have been buying our salmon from a wonderful company called Vital Choice for many years. Vital Choice is run by third-generation Alaskan fishermen who are scrupulous about using sustainable fishing and equally scrupulous about testing their fish thoroughly for contaminants and metals. They ship in dry ice, and they have the best fish we've ever tasted.

Fast Action Plan: Eat wild salmon twice a week.

Eat This: Berries

All berries are loaded with natural anti-inflammatory properties and natural antioxidants. They're also very low in sugar. Blueberries contain a beneficial compound called *pterostilbene*, which helps prevent the deposit of plaque in the arteries and also helps prevent some of the damage caused by oxidized cholesterol.[27] Raspberries and strawberries contain another substance, *ellagic acid*, which offers similar protection against oxidized LDL.[28] And all berries– blueberries, raspberries, strawberries, and others– contain *anthocyanins*, plant compounds that help lower inflammation (see "Cherries" below).

Fast Action Plan: Eat berries three (or more) times a week.

Eat This: Cherries

Cherries and cherry juice have long been known to be effective against the pain of gout, and scientists believe that the compounds in cherries responsible for this are *anthocyanins*. Anthocyanins act like natural COX-2 inhibitors. "COX" stands for *cyclooxygenase*, which is produced in the body in two forms called COX-1 and COX-2. COX-2 is used for signaling pain and inflammation.

The popularity of arthritis drugs such as Vioxx and Celebrex was based on their unique ability to block the pain and inflammation messages of COX-2 while leaving the non-inflammatory COX-1 alone. Unfortunately, there were some really unpleasant side effects associated with Vioxx, and it was taken off the market. But anthocyanins produce a similar effect with none of the problems of such drugs. Cherries (along with raspberries) have the highest yields of pure anthocyanins. In one study, the COX inhibitory activity of anthocyanins from cherries was comparable to that of ibuprofen and naproxen. Researchers feel that in addition to helping with pain and inflammation, consuming anthocyanins on a regular basis may help lower heart attack and stroke risk.

Fast Action Plan: Eat cherries two (or more) times a week.

Eat This: Grass-Fed Beef

We're not anti-meat guys, but we are very much against factory-farmed meat. The majority of the meat we consume, unfortunately, is feedlot-raised meat from factory farms. It's loaded with antibiotics, steroids, and hormones; it's very high in inflammatory omega-6 fats; and it contains virtually no anti-inflammatory omega-3s.

Grass-fed meat is a whole different "animal." (Okay, bad pun, sorry, we couldn't resist.) Raised on pasture, it contains less omega-6s plus a fair amount of omega-3s, resulting in a much better omega-6: omega-3 ratio. Grass-fed meat is almost always raised organically, and, in any case, it never has hormones, steroids, or antibiotics. If you eat meat, grass-fed is the only way to go.

Fast Action Plan: Eat only grass-fed meat when you eat meat.

Eat This: Vegetables (and Some Fruit)

No matter what kind of diet you're on—from vegan to Atkins—you can probably benefit from eating more vegetables than you already do. The entire vegetable kingdom is loaded with natural anti-inflammatories, antioxidants, and other plant compounds, such as flavonoids, that are good for your heart.

In two long-running Harvard-based research projects, the Nurses' Health Study and the Health Professionals Follow-up Study, the higher the average daily consumption of vegetables and fruits, the lower the chances of developing cardiovascular disease. Compared with those in the lowest category of fruit and vegetable intake (fewer than one and a half servings daily), those averaging eight or more servings per day were a whopping 30 percent less likely to have had a heart attack or stroke.[29]

Although all vegetables and fruits probably contributed to this stunning effect, the researchers felt that the most outstanding contributors were the green, leafy veggies (such as spinach and Swiss chard) and the cruciferous ones (broccoli, Brussels sprouts, kale, cabbage, and cauliflower). (In the fruit department, citrus fruits such as oranges, lemons, limes, and grapefruit were particularly protective.[30])

When researchers took the Harvard studies mentioned above and combined them with several other long-term studies both in Europe and the United States, they found a similar protective effect. Individuals who ate more than five servings a day of vegetables and fruits had a roughly 20 percent lower risk of coronary heart disease,[31] and a similar reduction in the risk of stroke.[32]

The reason we're not as over-the-top enthusiastic about fruit is that despite its terrific benefits, it still contains sugar, which can be a problem for many folks. For the large number of people whose blood sugar rises when they merely look at a candy bar, unlimited fruit is a bad idea. Low-sugar fruits (such as apples, grapefruit, cherries, berries, and oranges) are fine in moderation. Vegetables, on the other hand, can be virtually unlimited.

Fast Action Plan: Eat 5 to 9 half cup servings of vegetables and fruit a day.

Eat This: Nuts

Although an apple a day may indeed keep the doctor away, the same can also be said of a handful of nuts. People who eat nuts regularly are less likely to have heart attacks or die from heart disease than those who don't. Five large studies—the Adventist Health Study, the Iowa Women's Health Study, the Nurses' Health Study, the Physicians' Health Study, and the CARE Study—have all found a consistent 30 to 50 percent lower risk of heart attacks or heart disease associated with eating nuts several times a week.[33]

FIGHT HEART DISEASE WITH FOOD

In a fascinating and much-discussed article that appeared in the December 16, 2004, issue of the *British Medical Journal*, researchers put forth an idea called the *polymeal*.[34] They examined all of the research on foods and health to see whether they could put together the ideal meal (the polymeal) that, if you ate it every day, would significantly reduce your risk for cardiovascular disease. They came up with a theoretical meal that, eaten daily, would reduce cardiovascular risk by a staggering 75 percent (there's not a pill in the world that can do that!).

The ingredients of the polymeal?

Wine, fish, almonds, garlic, fruits, vegetables, and dark chocolate.

One of the many reasons for the protective effect of nuts may be an amino acid named *arginine*. Remember our earlier discussion about the endothelium, (the inner lining of the arterial walls)? Arginine has a role in protecting this inner lining, making the arterial walls more pliable and less susceptible to atherogenesis. Arginine is needed to make an important molecule called *nitric oxide*, which helps relax constricted blood vessels and ease blood flow.[35]

In addition, nuts are a great source of numerous *phytonutrients*—bioactive chemicals found in plants. These compounds have powerful health benefits, not the least of which is their antioxidant activity, which is linked to the prevention of coronary heart disease. And if you're worried about calories, consider this: In the Nurses' Health Study out of Harvard, nut consumption was inversely related to weight gain.[36] Several large studies, including the Physicians' Health Study (22,000 men) and the Adventist Health Study (more than 40,000 people), have demonstrated a link between nut eating and a reduction in heart disease.[37] Just keep portions reasonable—an ounce or so a day is great.

Fast Action Plan: Eat 1 ounce of nuts five times a week.

Eat This: Beans

Fact number one: Fiber is good. (High-fiber diets have been associated with lower rates of a host of diseases, including heart disease.) Fact number two: We don't get enough of it. (Most health organizations recommend a daily intake of 25 to 38 g daily; the average American gets 11 g.) Fact number three: Beans are a fiber heavyweight.

Case closed.

One study found that one serving of beans on a daily basis lowered the risk of a heart attack by 38 percent.

Regarding heart disease, the big selling point of beans used to be that they lowered cholesterol.[38] That's definitely true, but, as you've learned, it's not nearly as important as whether they actually lower *heart disease*. And they do. One study found that one serving of beans on a daily basis lowered the risk of a heart attack by an eyebrow-raising 38 percent![39] Another study found that individuals eating beans and legumes at least four times a week had a 22 percent lower risk of heart disease than individuals consuming beans/legumes less than once a week.[40]

Their high fiber content alone would make beans a top food for the heart, but beans offer a lot more than fiber. The U.S. Department of Agriculture ranking of foods by antioxidant capacity lists small red dried beans as having the highest antioxidant capacity per serving size of any food tested. In fact, of the four top-scoring foods, three were beans (red beans, red kidney beans, and pinto beans). Many bean varieties have a lot of folic acid (especially adzuki beans, lentils, black-eyed peas, and pinto beans). Folic acid is one of the key players in bringing down the inflammatory compound *homocysteine*, itself a risk factor for heart disease.

Fast Action Plan: Eat a serving of beans or lentils at least four times a week. (One serving is $\frac{1}{2}$ cup to 1 cup cooked beans.)

Eat This: Dark Chocolate

Study after study is confirming that plant chemicals in cocoa-rich dark chocolate called *flavanols* can lower blood pressure and reduce inflammation. A 2011 study in the *British Medical Journal* found that high levels of chocolate consumption are associated with a one-third reduction in the risk of developing heart disease. The highest levels of chocolate consumption were associated with a 37 percent reduction in cardiovascular disease and a 29 percent reduction in stroke when compared to the lowest levels.[41]

Flavanol-rich cocoa lowers blood pressure.[42] And the Zutphen Elderly Study of 470 elderly men found that those who ate the most cocoa had literally half the risk of dying from heart disease than men who ate the least.[43]

Now the thing about chocolate is that all the good stuff is found in the cocoa that it's made from, so you really want high-cocoa chocolate. We're not talking about the candy bars you get at the 7-Eleven here; we're talking about a cocoa-rich chocolate that contains all the flavanols that have been found to be so healthy. White chocolate and milk chocolate have hardly any flavanols to speak of, so it's got to be dark. Many dark chocolate bars will now tell you their cocoa content in percentage form—look for at least 60 percent cocoa. (The higher the cocoa content, the less sweet the bar.)

You'll also find that this kind of chocolate is easy to eat in small quantities—it's not so sweet that it causes you to crave more and more of it, and it's easy to be satisfied with just a square or two, which is all you need for the health benefits.

Fast Action Plan: Eat one to two squares of dark chocolate four to six days a week.

Eat This: Turmeric

Turmeric is the spice that makes curries yellow. It occupies a place of distinction in both Ayurvedic and Chinese medicine, largely because of its phenomenal anti-inflammatory properties. (It also has anticancer activity and is very helpful for the liver.) The active ingredients in turmeric are a group of plant compounds called *curcuminoids* (collectively known as *curcumin*). In addition to being anti-inflammatory, curcumin is a powerful antioxidant. Because oxidized LDL is a big player in the cascade that leads to inflammation and heart disease, turmeric's antioxidant properties are a big benefit.

Fast Action Plan: Put turmeric at the front of your spice cabinet and use it often. It goes well on veggies, eggs, sautéed dishes, meats, fish, and poultry.

Eat This: Pomegranate Juice

Pomegranate juice is one of the few "trendy" health foods that actually lives up to its hype. Researchers at the Technion-Israel Institute of Technology in Haifa suggest that long-term consumption of pomegranate juice may help slow aging and protect against heart disease.

In a study published in the *American Journal of Cardiology*, forty-five patients with heart disease drank either 8 ounces of pomegranate juice or 8 ounces of a placebo drink for three months. The pomegranate juice drinkers had significantly less oxygen deficiency to the heart during exercise, suggesting that they had increased blood flow to the heart.

Pomegranate juice has the ability to inhibit the oxidation of LDL cholesterol.[44] (Remember that LDL cholesterol is only a problem when it's oxidized!) And an impressive number of studies have demonstrated a beneficial effect of pomegranate juice on cardio-vascular health, including one that showed 30 percent reduced arterial plaque.[45] Pomegranate juice also enhances the activity of nitric oxide, a molecule essential for cardiovascular health.[46]

One caution: Avoid "juice blends" and "juice cocktails," because these have much less pomegranate juice in them and much more sugar. We like pure pomegranate juices such as Just Pomegranate, which are admittedly expensive but contain absolutely nothing but pure pomegranate juice. Another popular brand we like a lot is Pom Wonderful.

Fast Action Plan: Put pomegranate juice in "heavy rotation" on your menu: 4 to 8 ounces a day, or as often as you like.

Eat This: Red Wine

For years, it was believed that the reason the French could "get away" with eating high-fat foods—while still having remarkably lower rates of heart disease than Americans—was because of their regular consumption of red wine, which contains numerous compounds that protect the heart. Chief among these is *resveratrol*, a polyphenol (plant compound) that's found in the skins of dark grapes and is highly concentrated in red wine. Resveratrol is a potent antioxidant that can prevent harmful elements in the body from attacking healthy cells. Red wine has been shown to be cardioprotective in quite a number of studies.[47] And resveratrol isn't the only reason. Other compounds in red wine such as flavonoids inhibit the oxidation of LDL cholesterol, which is pretty darn important because oxidized LDL cholesterol initiates and intensifies the inflammatory process.[48] Red wine also limits the tendency of compounds in the blood to clot and increases HDL cholesterol to boot.[49] Interestingly, in one study, moderate consumption of red wine was associated with lower levels of three markers we told you about earlier: CRP, fibrinogen, and interleukin-6.[50] It's hard to think of a more heart-healthy drink.

Worth noting: The dark side of alcohol is well known, and we don't have to recount it here. If you're not a drinker, please don't start because of the benefits of red wine. Not everyone can handle alcohol, and if you suspect you're someone who doesn't do well with it, for goodness' sake, don't drink it! (With all the talk about how the wine-drinking French have the lowest rates of heart disease in western Europe, it's frequently forgotten that they also have the highest rates of liver cirrhosis!) The key to enjoying wine's beneficial effects is moderate consumption, defined as about two glasses a day for men and about one a day for women, about three to four times a week. Also worth mentioning is that alcohol increases the risk for breast cancer in women who aren't consuming enough folic acid, so make sure you're getting at least 400 mg of folic acid a day through food or supplementation.

Fast Action Plan: If you are a drinker, have a glass of red wine with dinner. (If you're not, don't start!)

Eat This: Green Tea

Apart from water, tea is probably the most consumed beverage in the world, and it's also one of the healthiest. That's because it's absolutely loaded with protective plant-based chemicals known as *polyphenols*. Green tea in particular has gotten a ton of attention in the media, largely for the anti-cancer action of one of its compounds, *epigallocatechin gallate* (EGCG).

But green tea also contributes to cardiovascular health. Although much has been written about its cholesterol-lowering effect, we find it much more interesting that green tea lowers fibrinogen, a substance in the body that can cause clots and strokes. In an article in the journal *Circulation* titled "Effects of Green Tea Intake on the Development of Coronary Artery Disease," researchers from the department of medicine at Chiba Hokusoh Hospital, Nippon Medical School, Chiba, Japan, concluded that "the more green tea patients consume, the less likely they are to have coronary artery disease."[51]

Worth knowing: Just because green tea gets the lion's share of attention from health writers doesn't mean there's not great stuff in other teas, such as black, oolong, white, and yerba matte. At Boston University's School of Medicine, Joseph Vita, M.D., conducted a study in which sixty-six men either drank four cups of black tea a day or took a placebo. The researchers showed that drinking black tea can help reverse an abnormal functioning of blood vessels that can contribute to stroke or heart attack. Best of all, improvement in the functioning of the blood vessels was visible within two hours of drinking just one cup of black tea![52]

"What we found was that if you take a group of people with heart disease who have abnormal blood vessel function to begin with and asked them to drink tea, their blood vessels improved," said Vita.[53]

Fast Action Plan: Remember, any form of tea contains caffeine, so drink in moderation. Make a big pitcher of green tea and keep it in the fridge. Drink it in the earlier part of the day, up to two glasses.

Eat This: Olive Oil

Olive oil is the primary fat used in the Mediterranean area and the one most associated with what's been called the Mediterranean diet. (There is no single "Mediterranean diet," but all variations of it contain high amounts of fish, fruits, vegetables, nuts, wine, and olive oil.) There are countless studies on the Mediterranean diet and heart health and virtually all of them show enormous benefits for the heart and the brain. These studies have left olive oil with an unimpeachable reputation as one of the healthiest fats for the heart.

Research in the *Archives of Internal Medicine* concluded that greater adherence to the traditional Mediterranean diet (including plenty of olive oil and other monounsaturated fats such as nuts and avocados) was associated with significant reduction in mortality among people who had been diagnosed with heart disease.[54] Another study in the same journal compared two groups of people with high blood pressure.[55] One group was given sunflower oil, a typical high omega-6 oil used in Western diets, and one group was given the good stuff: extra-virgin olive oil. The olive oil decreased the second group's blood pressure by a significant amount; it also decreased their need for blood pressure meds by a whopping 48 percent. As the English might say, "Not too shabby."

Like red wine and green tea, olive oil contains polyphenols that are anti-inflammatory and act as powerful antioxidants. (Researchers have isolated one in particular, *oleocanthal*, which acts similarly to ibuprofen.[56]) Because so many of these polyphenols have significant health benefits, some people believe that the fat in olive oil may not be the only reason olive oil is so darn healthy. They think that the main health benefits of olive oil come from the fact that it is a delivery system for these powerful polyphenols. Either way, the stuff is great, and you should make it a part of your heart-healthy diet.

Worth knowing: All olive oil is not created equal. Unfortunately, commercial manufacturers, trying to ride the health hype on olive oil, have rushed to market all kinds of imitation and inferior products that say "olive oil" on them but are highly processed and refined and have questionable benefits. That's why you want "extra-virgin" olive oil, which is the least processed, the most like what you'd get if you walked around barefoot in barrels of olives. It's made without the use of heat, hot water, or solvents, and it is left unfiltered. (The first pressing produces the best stuff, known as "extra-virgin.")

Once you begin machine harvesting and processing with very high heat, you start damaging the delicate compounds in olive oil responsible for all those great health benefits. The antioxidant and anti-inflammatory polyphenols are water soluble and can be washed away with factory processing. That's one reason that factory-produced olive oil has a shorter shelf life—no antioxidants to protect it. Real olive oil—the extra-virgin kind, made with care and love and the absence of high heat and harsh chemicals—lasts for years.

Fast Action Plan: Switch to extra-virgin olive oil. Use it for salad dressing, low-heat stir-fries, and sautées.

Eat this: Garlic

Garlic is a global remedy. More than 1,200 (and counting) pharmacological studies have been done on garlic, and the findings are pretty impressive. In addition to lowering lipids and preventing blood coagulation, it has antihypertensive, antioxidant, antimicrobial, and antiviral properties. Garlic has been shown to lower triglyceride levels. It can also reduce plaque, making it a powerful agent for cardiovascular health.

In one study, subjects receiving 900 mg of garlic powder for four years in a randomized, double-blinded, placebo-controlled study had a regression in their plaque volume of 2.6 percent; meanwhile, a matched group of subjects given a placebo (an inert substance) saw their plaque increase over the same time period by 15.6 percent![57]

One of the active ingredients in garlic—*allicin*—also has significant antiplatelet activity. That means it helps prevent platelets in the blood from sticking together. To understand just how important that is, consider that many heart attacks and strokes are caused by spontaneous clots in the blood vessels. The anticoagulant effect of garlic is an important health benefit.

Worth knowing: The preparation of garlic is critical for it to release its health-providing benefits. If for any reason you had the impulse to swallow a garlic clove whole, not much would happen. The garlic clove has to be crushed or chopped—the more finely the better—for the compounds in it to mix together to create *allicin*, the active ingredient responsible for the health benefits. Allicin starts degrading immediately after it's produced, so the fresher it is when you use it, the better. (Microwaving destroys it completely.) Garlic experts advise crushing a little raw garlic and combining it with cooked food. If you add it to food you're sautéing, do it toward the end so the allicin is freshest.

Fast Action Plan: Start cooking with garlic.

THE "HIDDEN RISK FACTORS" FOR HEART DISEASE

Everyone reading this book needs to know this: You can prevent and even heal heart disease through diet, exercise, and/or nutritional supplements.

But if you're interested in doing that—and we're pretty sure you are, or you wouldn't be reading this—diet, exercise, and supplements are only a part of the picture. The many hidden emotional and psychological risk factors that are hardly ever addressed by conventional medicine are equally important—and sometimes even more so. They include suppressed anger, rage, the loss of love (what Dr. Sinatra calls "heartbreak"), and the emotional isolation that results from lack of intimacy with other people; we've touched on some of this in the previous chapter on stress.

Opening your heart to your feelings and learning how to express them in a healthy way will do far more for your heart and your overall health than you might imagine. Here are some specific ways you can accomplish this.

Breathe Deeply

When people are subjected to chronic stress, they oftentimes become tense and rigid. They take shallow breaths. Improper breathing can, over the course of time, result in actual physical changes in the body, such as a more rigid upper body, including the chest and shoulders. High chest breathing tends to be rapid and shallow and is frequently associated with emotional upset, physical tension, or ordinary mental stress. Slow, rhythmic, deep abdominal breathing, however, is physiologically more suited to the body and has the added benefit of allowing a greater intake of oxygen.

Proper breathing has been the subject of many stress-management programs. It's the first place you start when you learn to meditate, and it's a principle focus of yoga. In Gestalt psychotherapy, deep breathing is used as a vehicle to loosen up the energy of the chest and to free emotions.

A more prolonged form of deep breathing is meditation, which has an impressive amount of research showing that it lowers blood pressure effectively. Cardiologist Herbert Benson, M.D., has been doing pioneering research on meditation and deep breathing for decades. An associate professor of medicine at Harvard Medical School and founder of the Benson-Henry Institute for Mind Body Medicine at Massachusetts General Hospital, he coined the term "the Relaxation Response" to refer to a physical state of deep rest that changes the physical and emotional responses to stress. And it's all based on deep breathing and calming the mind.

Benson was able to show time and again that the relaxation response decreases the heart rate, lowers blood pressure, slows the rate of breathing, and relaxes the muscles. It also increases levels of nitric oxide—a molecule that's important for circulation and improved blood flow. Tai chi, meditation, yoga, and mindfulness are all able to elicit the relaxation response.

According to the Benson-Henry Institute, between 60 and 90 percent of all doctor visits are for complaints related to, or affected by, stress. "Scores of diseases and conditions are either caused or made worse by stress," Benson has said. "These include anxiety, mild or moderate depression, anger, hostility, hot flashes of menopause, infertility, PMS, high blood pressure, and heart attacks. Every one can be caused by stress or exacerbated by it. And to the extent that that's the case, the relaxation response is helpful." [58]

HOW TO DO "THE RELAXATION RESPONSE"

Allow ten to twenty minutes to try this simple technique:

• Sit quietly in a comfortable position.

• Close your eyes.

• Deeply relax all your muscles beginning at your feet and progressing up to your face. Keep them relaxed.

• Breathe through your nose. Become aware of your breathing. As you breathe out, say the word *one* silently to yourself. For example, breathe in . . . out, (one), in . . . out (one), etc. Breathe easily and naturally.

• Continue for ten to twenty minutes.

• You may open your eyes to check the time, but don't use an alarm. When you finish, sit quietly for several minutes at first with your eyes closed and later with your eyes open. Don't stand for a few minutes.

"Don't worry about whether you are successful in achieving a deep level of relaxation. Maintain a passive attitude and permit relaxation to occur at its own pace. When distracting thoughts occur, try to ignore them by not dwelling upon them and return to repeating *one*."

—From *The Relaxation Response* by Herbert Benson, M.D., used with permission

NOTE: Try not to do this within a couple hours of eating. According to Benson, the digestive process seems to interfere with eliciting the relaxation response.

See the sidebar on how you can do the relaxation response.

How Crying and Laughing Can Help
Next to love, crying is perhaps the most healing activity for the heart. It frees the heart of muscular tension and rigidity. Sobbing enhances oxygen delivery. Man is the only primate able to weep for emotional reasons. Weeping is nature's way of releasing the pain of heartbreak and preventing death. Any expression of feeling will help to heal your heart. Despite what we're taught, it's not weak to show your feelings. In fact, it's far healthier than "stuffing" your feelings and seething silently.

Laughing is a way of experiencing strong feelings, just as crying is. (In fact, strenuous laughter often turns into tears.) When you laugh fully, breathing increases, freeing up the rigidity in the chest, diaphragm, and even deep down in the psoas muscles. As a spontaneous release of energy, laughter has the potential to be extremely therapeutic.

Laughing Your Way to Health
Over the course of his lifetime, Norman Cousins, the legendary journalist and editor of the *Saturday Evening Post*, suffered from a number of serious medical conditions, including heart disease and ankylosing spondylitis, a disease characterized by chronic inflammation along the axial skeleton. At one point, doctors gave him little hope of surviving. He ignored their doomsaying and developed his own program for recovery that involved love, hope, faith, and, courtesy of the Marx Brothers films he loved to watch, an awful lot of laughter.

Although he eventually died of heart failure at age seventy-five, Cousins lived far longer than his doctors predicted, a full thirty-six years after first being diagnosed with heart disease. (Cousins also did research on the biochemistry of human emotions at the School of Medicine at the University of California, Los Angeles, and wrote two important books on emotion, healing, and illness—*Anatomy of an Illness* and *The Healing Heart*.)

Sex: The Advantages of Intimacy
Have you ever wondered why some elderly people look much younger than their stated age while some younger people look so much older? This observation was studied by a Russian gerontologist who examined 15,000 individuals over the age of eighty in provinces of the former Soviet Union. He found several common denominators or markers for longevity. People who lived the longest reported working outdoors, high levels of physical activity, and a diet high in vegetables, fruits, and fresh whole grains. But several of the common denominators involved relationships, intimacy, and sexuality.

Many of these individuals continued to have an active sex life well into their eighties and nineties. And why not? Aging couples who are committed to one another's pleasure can adapt sexually to the aging process. On an emotional level, sexuality provides a sense of security, connectedness, and emotional intimacy. When sexuality is an expression of love, the energies of the partners can fuse in harmony like two tuning forks vibrating with the same frequency. Feelings of warmth, connectedness, and emotional intimacy can help open our hearts.

EXPRESSING EMOTIONS (ESPECIALLY FOR MEN!)

Showing and expressing feelings can be a huge challenge for some people, particularly men. But getting in touch with your feelings doesn't have to be embarrassing at all. You don't have to get up in front of some encounter group and spill your guts to strangers. All it may take is a pencil and paper.

A writing exercise developed by social psychologist James Pennebaker has been tested in dozens of studies in which subjects were assigned to write about either mundane activities, such as running errands, or personal traumas. The technique is pure simplicity. You write your deepest thoughts and emotions about any event, situation, person, or even trauma for about fifteen minutes on four consecutive nights. Pennebaker has found that people who do this simple, private exercise show improvements in immune system functioning, are less likely to visit doctors, get better grades in school, and miss fewer days of work.[59]

The Power of Touch and Massage

Touch therapy or massage appears to be associated with a decreased heart rate, decreased blood pressure, and increased endorphin release, resulting in an increased sense of relaxation and heightened well-being. In humans, massage can be considered a tranquilizer with absolutely no side effects!

Remember the parasympathetic (slowing down) and the sympathetic (speeding up) nervous systems? Massage activates the parasympathetic system and provides a nice, healing balance to the typical sympathetic overdrive experienced by type-A, coronary-prone individuals.

Play

Play is one of the most healing things you can do for your heart health and your emotional well-being. And most adults have no idea how to do it. Sure, we talk about "playing" tennis or golf, but sports are different—though enjoyable, they're not healing because they involve performance, competition, and the need to win! (Just ask Dr. Jonny how he feels after losing a tennis match!)

Play is totally different. True play is spontaneous and has no agenda, rules, or regulations, or even a desired outcome. When we play, we are totally free. That is, we do things solely for joy and pleasure. When we play, we become totally absorbed in what we are doing; we are taken out of our heads (and down into our bodies). Time stops for us.

Think of how completely absorbed five- or six-year-olds become when they're painting a picture. Within minutes, nothing else matters to them but the colors, the feel of the brush on the paper, the way the paint drips and blobs and runs, the way the colors mix, and how closely they can match the picture with the image in their minds. Being carried away by their imaginations and getting their inspirations down on paper is, for a short time, the single most important thing in the world to them. Everything else falls away—worries, fears, wants, needs, hunger—and is replaced by a sense of total involvement, excitement, satisfaction, and gratification.

If you can play even partially this way, it can completely cut you free from stress and worry and help heal your mind and heart. Because of this nearly miraculous benefit of play, we encourage you to play like children. If, like most adults, you've forgotten how, observe children and see what they do.

Remember, play has no outcome, no goal. You need to play for play's sake alone, and, when you play, try to bring out the little child inside you. Once you connect with your inner child—believe us, we all have one—it will bring you to another level of healing.

Final Words

Foods can fuel your heart, supplements can support it, and exercise can strengthen it. But never neglect the "hidden" emotional and psychological risk factors that contribute to the development of heart disease as surely as smoking, a high-sugar diet, stress, high blood pressure, and lack of exercise do.

Building and maintaining strong emotional connections with other people is one of the best stress-management strategies on the planet. It's also one of the best ways to keep your heart healthy and your soul nourished. Next to exercise, it's the closest thing we have to a panacea. It also makes life a lot more rich, a lot more fun, and a lot more gratifying.

Enjoy the journey.

· SECTION 2 ·

How to Eat Well for a Long and Healthy Life

100 DELICIOUS AND NUTRITIOUS RECIPES YOUR HEART WILL LOVE

A collection of nutritionally balanced dishes rich in heart-healthy essential nutrients, low in sugar, and bursting with flavors to suit any tastes and desires

GOOD START BREAKFASTS

Quick Weekday Breakfasts
Get-Up-And-Go Banana Berry Quinoa Porridge
Melt-in-Your-Mouth Baked Granola
Protein-Powered Muesli with Coconut and Raisins
Regenerating Herb Scrambled Eggs
Fortifying Flourless Chicken Flapjacks

Leisurely Weekend Breakfasts
Brain-Boosting Salmon Eggs Benedict
Strengthening Sun-Dried Tomato and Feta-Chive Omelet
Hearty Mediterranean Frittata
Super-Energizing Baked Beans
Zesty Digestive Herb and Cheddar Breakfast Muffins

MIDDAY MEALS AND ANYTIME SNACKS

Salads for all Seasons
Almighty Avocado and Black Bean Salad
Mood-Boosting Chicken and Pineapple Coleslaw with
  Coconut-Lime Dressing
Vitalizing Broccoli and Cauliflower Salad
Cardioprotective Salmon Caesar Salad
Energizing Thai Spice Chicken Salad
Pumping Jumping Bean Salad

Delicious Dressings
Simply Nourishing Salad Dressing
Cardioprotective Caesar Salad Dressing
Energizing Thai Spice Salad Dressing
Holy-Moly Guacamole Dressing

Lunch Box-worthy Meals
Stress-Less Turkey, Avocado, and Veggie Nori Wrap
Gluten-Free Mediterranean Veggie Pizza
Vibrant Avocado and Veggie Salsa Collard Wraps
Feel-Good Turkey or Salmon Tomato Panini

Heartwarming Soups & Broths

Nutritive Chicken Stock
Digestive Vegetable Stock
Heart-Protective Carrot Ginger Soup with Chives
Love-Your-Heart Red Lentil Soup
Immune-Boosting Basque Bean and Cabbage Soup
Build-Me-Up Butternut and Macadamia Nut Bisque

Satisfying Snacks

Low-Carb Herbed Cheddar Crackers
Blood-Sugar Balancing Butternut & Leek Pies
High-Energy Chicken & Cauliflower Croquettes
Turkey, Lamb, or Beef Koftas with a Heart-Healthy Kick
Spiced Honey-Glazed Nuts
Calming Coconut-Date Balls
Detoxifying Lima Bean Blinis with Artichoke Herbed Dip

ON THE DINNER MENU

Meatless Main Dishes

Spicy Moroccan Tempeh with Lentils
Hi-Fibe Red Bean Burgers
Protein-Packed Vegetarian Shepherd's Pie
Nutrient-Rich Roasted Quinoa with Mushrooms, Cumin,
  and Coriander
High-Fiber Butternut Gnocchi with Herbed
  Cream Sauce
Revitalizing Vegetable Biryani
Comforting Cheddar and Broccoli Quiche with
  Quinoa Crust
Strengthening Spinach, Feta, and Rice Casserole
Immune-Boosting Thai Tempeh Cakes with
  Sweet Spicy Dipping Sauce
Stress-Less Shiitake and Asparagus Risotto

BEEF, SEAFOOD, AND POULTRY MAINS

Beef

Easy Beef Sauté with Fresh Herbs
Favorite Sweet, Spicy, and Crunchy Meatloaf
Nice and Spiced Beef or Chicken Stir-Fry

Seafood

Fisherman's Omega-3 Fish Fingers
Mega-Omega Spice-Crusted Salmon
Tantalizing Thai Fish Cakes
Soul-Warming Tuna Lasagna
Healing Baked Halibut or Salmon and Shiitake
Spicy Shrimp and Tomato Kebabs with
  Herbed Lima Beans

Poultry

Mighty Moroccan Chicken Tagine
Metabolism-Boosting Chicken Curry Feast
Tantalizing Chicken Satay with Powerful Peanut
  Coconut Sauce
Supercharged Chicken or Turkey Meatloaf
Anti-Inflammatory Turmeric Turkey Burgers

Vegetables, Grains, and Beans on the Side

Get-Up-and-Go Indian Chickpea Delight
Fragrant Cauliflower-Quinoa Risotto
Luscious Lima Bean Mash
Anti-Ox Pumpkin and Cauliflower Mash
Sautéed Shiitake Mushrooms with a Kale Kick
Zesty Broccoli with Garlic and Ginger
Balancing Basmati Almond Rice
Sumptuous Spinach and Swiss Chard with Pine Nuts
Cardioprotective Green Beans
Sustaining Ginger-Sesame Carrots

NOURISHING ACCOMPANIMENTS AND MENU ENHANCEMENTS

Choice Condiments
Mediterranean Black Olive Tapenade
Super-Healthful Hummus
Bone-Strengthening Lemon Tahini
Heart-Healthy Almond Mayonnaise

Succulent Sauces
Punchy Peanut-Coconut Sauce
Spice-it-Up Sweet Chili Sauce
Health-Giving Hollandaise Sauce
Antioxidant BBQ Sauce

Powerful Preserves & Fabulous Ferments
Antioxidant Ginger, Date, and Orange Chutney
Berry-Buzz Jelly
Immune-Building Lemon Ginger Butter
Bone-Building French Cream
Restorative Cucumber-Yogurt Raita
Immune-Boosting Yogurt
Probiotic Fruit Chutney

SWEET ENDINGS: DESSERTS AND OTHER DELIGHTS

Cookies, Cakes, & Breads
Hearty Hazelnut Rounds
Luscious Lemon-Pineapple Yogurt Cake
Health-Gratifying Grapefruit and Orange Cake
Almighty Almond and Walnut Pumpernickel Bread
Powerhouse Pumpkin, Spice, and Almond Bread
Nourishing Crusty Onion and Parmesan Rolls

Puddings & Pies
Fortifying Fig and Minty Blueberry Brûlée
Energy-Giving Coconut, Almond, and Raisin Custard
Blueberry and Apple Crumble Gone Nuts
Berry-Beneficial Blueberry and Pecan Pie
Anti-Ox Orange Mousse
Soothing Pear, Date, and Almond Pudding with
  Grapefruit Cream Sauce
Sweet Brown Rice Pudding with an Antioxidant Twist
No-Bake Superfood Fudge Brownies

· GOOD START · BREAKFASTS

Breakfast is the most important meal of the day because it sets the pace for your metabolism, making it more or less efficient. Eating breakfast allows you to restock the energy stores that have been depleted overnight and begin the day with a tank full of the right fuel. All of the recipes in this chapter include a variety of healthy proteins and fats, and low-on-the-glycemic-index carbohydrates to ensure a steady supply of fuel. These recipes provide you with the nutrition necessary for energy production and keep you nourished and satisfied. You may even lose a few inches around your waist, too!

You'll find a ready selection of quick weekday breakfasts that take little time to prepare when you're adhering to a busy schedule. Weekends often afford us some extra time to spend in the kitchen, and you'll find recipes that take a little longer to make but offer a combination of choices and flavors to suit any taste sensations and desires. Variety is the spice of life, and you will thrive when you start your day out with a heart- and brain-healthy breakfast.

GET-UP-AND-GO BANANA BERRY QUINOA PORRIDGE

If you've never tried quinoa for breakfast, you're in for a treat. Quinoa is great combined with the sweet taste of fruit and spices or served with more savory items such as vegetables and herbs. It is a dieter's dream because it is satisfying, filling, rich in fiber, and full of all nine essential amino acids that make it a complete protein. Quinoa is digested slowly and has a low glycemic index, helping keep your blood sugar levels stable for hours. Quinoa dates back several thousand years, when the Incas discovered and prized it because they believed it increased the stamina of their warriors.

- **4 cups (680 g) quinoa**
- **1 cup (160 g) dates**
- **1 banana**
- **1 cup (145 g) berries, fresh or frozen**
- **1 teaspoon ground nutmeg**
- **1 teaspoon ground cinnamon**
- **1 cup (120 g) chopped walnuts**

Soak the quinoa overnight in filtered water and drain the next morning. Soak the dates overnight in 1½ cups (355 ml) filtered water. The next morning, drain the dates but reserve the soak water. Blend the quinoa, dates, soak water, banana, berries, nutmeg, and cinnamon in a blender until smooth. Sprinkle with walnuts and serve cold or at room temperature.

Yield: 12 servings

Note: Quinoa is a flavorful source of plant-derived calcium, so it helps regulate contraction of the heart and facilitates nerve and muscle function. It also contains impressive amounts of potassium, magnesium, and zinc.

Reasons to Crave Quinoa

If you're looking for a high-protein substitute for cereal, look no further. Although quinoa is technically a seed, it cooks up like a grain and is a terrific substitute for wheat. The protein quality and quantity in quinoa is often superior to that of the more common cereal grains—certainly superior to wheat—and, according to the Food and Agricultural Organization of the United Nations, the nutritional quality of quinoa is comparable to dried whole milk. It's also high in iron (about 8 mg per ½ cup) and has a hefty 5 grams of fiber to boot!

[NUTRITIONAL ANALYSIS]

Per serving: 336.5 calories; 10.2 g fat; 10.1 g protein; 55.1 g carbs; 6.5 g fiber; 15.3 mg sodium.

MELT-IN-YOUR MOUTH BAKED GRANOLA

If you love the crunch, texture, and flavor of granola, look no further than this delicious treat. This granola is high in heart-healthy fiber and flavors, sprinkled with a wide range of nutrients that are fun to eat.

- 6 cups (480 g) rolled oats
- 3 cups (360 g) rye flakes
- 2 cups (160 g) shredded coconut
- 1 cup (145 g) sunflower seeds
- 1 cup (144 g) sesame seeds
- 1 cup each almonds (145 g), pecans (110 g), and walnuts (120 g), chopped
- ¾ cup (90 g) barley malt powder
- ⅔ cup (160 ml) coconut oil
- 1 cup (235 ml) pure maple syrup
- 1 teaspoon vanilla extract
- 1 tablespoon (15 ml) pure almond extract
- ¼ teaspoon pure maple extract
- 1 cup (145 g) raisins

Preheat the oven to 375°F (190°C, gas mark 5)..In a large bowl, combine the oats through the walnuts. Set aside.

In a separate bowl, stir together the barley malt powder, oil, maple syrup, and vanilla, almond, and maple extracts. Add the wet mixture to the dry mixture and mix well. (For granola that sticks together more, use a food processor to combine the wet and dry mixtures.) Spread the combined mixture onto a large baking sheet and bake for 50 minutes, or until the mixture is lightly browned. Let cool for 30 minutes.

Mix in the raisins and serve immediately or store in an airtight, sealable container for future breakfasts. It will keep for 10 days or slightly longer if refrigerated.

Yield: 24 servings

Note: Oats are naturally high in iron, an essential mineral for healthy red blood cells to reduce your risk of iron-deficiency anemia.

————————[NUTRITIONAL ANALYSIS]————————

Per serving: 387.3 calories; 23.7 g fat; 7.8 g protein; 39 g carbs; 7.4 g fiber; 5.8 mg sodium.

PROTEIN-POWERED MUESLI WITH COCONUT AND RAISINS

Loaded with fiber and rich in antioxidants, this sublimely tasty muesli is nutrient rich, crunchy, and flavorful. It will satisfy your appetite and keep your system working like a well-oiled machine for hours. Enjoy this dish as part of a nourishing breakfast or filling snack.

2 cups (160 g) rolled oats

1 cup (120 g) rye flakes

1 cup (160 g) dried dates, chopped

1 cup (145 g) raisins

1 cup (145 g) almonds, chopped roughly

½ cup (60 g) walnuts, chopped roughly

½ cup (55 g) pecans, chopped roughly

½ cup (72 g) sunflower seeds

⅓ cup (27 g) shredded coconut

1 teaspoon pure vanilla extract

¼ teaspoon ground nutmeg

½ teaspoon ground cinnamon

4 cups (946 ml) apple cider

1 banana

1½ cups (220 g) blueberries

In a large bowl, combine the oats through the cinnamon. Mix well. Place the mixture in an airtight, sealable container and stir in the apple cider. Cover, refrigerate overnight, and serve in the morning with chopped banana and blueberries.

Yield: 8 to 10 servings

Note: Nuts and seeds provide protein, essential fatty acids, and several antioxidant vitamins and minerals.

———————[**NUTRITIONAL ANALYSIS**]———————
Per serving: 455.5 calories; 20.9 g fat; 9.4 g protein; 63.2 g carbs; 9.7 g fiber; 16.1 mg sodium.

REGENERATING HERB SCRAMBLED EGGS

In addition to containing all nine essential amino acids that make up protein, eggs contain choline, a nutrient important for neurotransmitter function, the nervous system, and the cardiovascular system. This delicious and nutritious combination of garlic and fresh herbs, coupled with the additional nutrients in the greens they are served over, provides fiber and potent antioxidant activity that strengthen your entire system.

4 eggs

1 clove garlic, minced

1 tablespoon (4 g) chopped fresh parsley

½ teaspoon chopped fresh basil

Pinch of salt, Celtic or sea

Pinch of cayenne pepper (optional)

2 tablespoons (28 ml) Bone-Building French Cream (page 277)

2 to 3 finely chopped scallions

1 tablespoon (15 ml) extra-virgin olive or coconut oil

2 cups mixed lettuce greens (110 g), romaine lettuce (110 g), or spinach (60 g)

Whisk the eggs in a medium bowl with the garlic, parsley, basil, salt, cayenne, and cream. Stir in the scallions. Heat the oil in a medium skillet over medium heat. Pour in the egg mixture and scramble with a spatula, slowly turning and breaking up the egg mixture until it reaches desired doneness. Turn the off heat before most of the moisture has evaporated. Serve over mixed lettuce greens, romaine lettuce, or spinach.

Yield: 2 servings

———————[**NUTRITIONAL ANALYSIS**]———————
Per serving: 258 calories; 19.7 g fat; 13.7 g protein; 3.5 g carbs; 1.5 g fiber; 221 mg sodium.

FORTIFYING FLOURLESS CHICKEN FLAPJACKS

Good-choice breakfasts contain a full profile of essential amino acids that turn on brain neurotransmitters and provide energy to help carry you over the morning hungries. These delicious chicken pancakes are no exception! They will keep your weight in check and your heart healthy thanks to vitamins B_6 and B_3, both of which are known for their energy-giving benefits. Vitamin B_6 in particular assists the heart by keeping homocysteine levels low, thereby reducing damage to the walls of the blood vessels. Apart from the delicious taste sensation, the addition of turmeric, avocado, and spinach in this dish will ensure the healthy functioning of your digestive and immune systems.

1 cooked chicken breast, chopped

3 eggs

½ teaspoon ground turmeric

1 tablespoon (15 ml) coconut or grapeseed oil

2 cups (110 g) salad greens or raw or lightly steamed spinach

½ avocado, pitted, peeled, and sliced

3 to 4 tablespoons Simply Nourishing Salad Dressing (page 217)

Blend the chicken, eggs, and turmeric in a food processor until completely smooth. (The mixture will look just like thick pancake batter.)

In a medium skillet, melt the oil over medium-high heat. Pour ¼ cup of the chicken mixture into the skillet. You may need to spread the batter a bit so that it is not too thick. Cook for 1 to 2 minutes on each side (these pancakes cook much faster than regular flour pancakes, so watch them closely).

Serve over a bed of fresh salad greens or spinach and top with avocado slices. Drizzle with the dressing.

Yield: 4 to 5 pancakes

Note: Organic, free-range, hormone- and antibiotic-free chicken does not contain chemicals that may, over time, cause harm.

──────[**NUTRITIONAL ANALYSIS**]──────
Per serving: 217.1 calories; 14.6 g fat; 14.6 g protein; 4.5 g carbs; 1.2 g fiber; 94 mg sodium.

BRAIN-BOOSTING SALMON EGGS BENEDICT

You have nothing to fear and much to gain when it comes to eating eggs. They are a good source of high-quality protein and vitamins D, B_2, B_5, and B_{12}, as well as iodine, selenium, and tryptophan, all of which help improve overall health. In this dish, the addition of omega-3 fatty acids in the salmon and abundance of vitamin K in the spinach greatly contribute to a healthy metabolism, nervous system, and brain function. Flavorful and delicious in every way.

1 tablespoon (15 ml) extra-virgin olive or coconut oil

1 salmon fillet (4 ounces [115 g])

5 cups (150 g) spinach

1 tablespoon (15 ml) vinegar (e.g., apple cider or white)

4 eggs

Health-Giving Hollandaise Sauce (page 273)

Dash of black pepper

Preheat the oven to warm. In a medium-size pan, melt the oil over medium heat and sauté the salmon for about 4 minutes on each side until just cooked through. Keep it warm in the oven.

While the salmon is cooking, place a steamer basket in a small saucepan, add the spinach, and steam lightly for about 3 minutes, or until wilted. Place the spinach in the oven with the salmon to keep it warm.

Fill a medium-size skillet halfway with water and add the vinegar. Heat the water until simmering and then crack the eggs into the pan, one at a time, being careful not to break the yolks. The eggs will be done when the whites have become solid, about 4 to 5 minutes.

Remove the spinach and salmon from the oven and divide among 4 plates, placing the spinach on first, topped with the salmon, and then a poached egg. Serve with hollandaise sauce and sprinkle with freshly ground black pepper.

Yield: 4 servings

Note: Choose organically farmed, free-range eggs because they provide a higher quality nutrient content and lack the harmful growth hormones that can compromise your health.

————[**NUTRITIONAL ANALYSIS**]————

Per serving: 161.2 calories; 8.4 g fat; 13.4 g protein; 2 g carbs; 0.8 g fiber; 100.7 mg sodium.

STRENGTHENING SUN-DRIED TOMATO AND FETA-CHIVE OMELET

This easy and delicious omelet is packed with heart-healthy goodness. Tomatoes are loaded with lycopene, a natural pigment produced by plants and a potent antioxidant that offers cardiovascular benefits. The inclusion of feta cheese adds a bold and tangy flavor and supplies key vitamins D and B$_{12}$ plus calcium and iron, all of which support overall metabolism.

4 eggs, separated

1 tablespoon (15 ml) Bone-Building French Cream (page 277)

1 clove garlic, minced

1 tablespoon (3 g) chopped fresh chives

¼ teaspoon salt, Celtic or sea

Dash of black pepper

1 teaspoon coconut oil or extra-virgin olive oil

¼ cup (28 g) oil-packed and drained sun-dried tomatoes, sliced, divided

¼ cup (37 g) sheep or goat feta cheese, sliced, divided

In a medium bowl, whisk the egg yolks, cream, garlic, chives, salt, and pepper until light and fluffy. In a separate bowl, whisk the egg whites until stiff, about 3 to 5 minutes, and then fold them into the other whisked ingredients.

Heat a nonstick saucepan over medium heat with the oil. Pour in half the egg mixture, swishing it around to leave a thin layer of egg on the sides of the pan. Cook for a few minutes and then add half the sun-dried tomatoes and half the feta on top of one side of the omelet. Using a spatula, flip the other side of the omelet on top of the filling. Cook for a few more minutes. Place the omelet aside and keep warm. Repeat the process for the other omelet.

Serve immediately. These omelets can be served with any other fillings desired and go well with Spice-It-Up Sweet Chili Sauce (page 152).

Yield: 2 omelets

Note: No other system in the body has greater need for antioxidant protection than the cardiovascular system. And when it comes to heart health, tomatoes are loaded with three important cardioprotective antioxidants: vitamins C, E, and lycopene, a powerful carotenoid.

————[**NUTRITIONAL ANALYSIS**]————

Per serving: 278.3 calories; 18 g fat; 18 g protein; 9.7 g carbs; 2.1 g fiber; 494.1 mg sodium.

HEARTY MEDITERRANEAN FRITTATA

Load up on fresh vegetables that pack a wallop of vitamins, minerals, antioxidant nutrients, and fiber that explode with flavor and a cheesy texture with each bite. This is a delicious breakfast or any-time dish combining elements of the heart-healthy Mediterranean diet.

1 tablespoon (15 ml), plus 1 teaspoon extra-virgin olive oil, butter, or ghee

1 cup each chopped broccoli florets (71 g) and bell pepper (150 g)

2 cups (60 g) chopped spinach

½ cup (50 g) pitted and halved black olives

⅔ cup (110 g) chopped onion

1 clove garlic, minced

2 tablespoons (5 g) chopped fresh or 1 teaspoon dried basil

8 eggs, lightly beaten

¼ cup (60 ml) Bone-Building French Cream (page 277)

¼ teaspoon salt, Celtic or sea

Dash of black pepper

1 teaspoon dried oregano

½ cup (50 g) grated Parmesan cheese

½ cup (55 g) oil-packed and drained sun-dried tomatoes, sliced

Preheat the oven to 350°F (180°C, gas mark 4). Grease a 9-inch (23-cm) baking dish with the tea-spoon of oil. Evenly arrange the broccoli, bell pepper, spinach, and olives in the dish.

In a medium saucepan, add the remaining tablespoon of oil or ghee and sauté the onion and garlic until tender, about 3 minutes, over medium to high heat. Add the basil and sauté until wilted, about 30 sec-onds. Remove from the heat and let cool. Whisk the eggs with the cream, salt, and pepper until creamy. Add the oregano, Parmesan, and sun-dried tomatoes, blend together, and then pour over the vegetables. Bake for 30 minutes, or until the frittata is firm to the touch. Let cool for 10 minutes before serving, or serve cold.

Yield: 4 to 6 servings

Note: A five-year Spanish study conducted on 7,500 people and published in April 2013 in the New England Journal of Medicine *concluded that people who ate a Mediterranean diet (which focuses on olive oil, nuts, produce, and seafood) had a 30 per-cent reduction in stroke and other cardiovascular diseases compared to control subjects, who were low-fat dieters.*

─────[**NUTRITIONAL ANALYSIS**]─────

Per serving: 252 calories; 15.5 g fat; 13.7 g protein; 11.3 g carbs; 2.3 g fiber; 302.1 mg sodium.

SUPER-ENERGIZING BAKED BEANS

The humble baked bean is the perfect breakfast food. Navy beans, used in this recipe, are a nutritional powerhouse of plant protein, fiber, iron, magnesium, copper, and calcium that supports cellular energy and an overall healthy metabolism. The pureed tomatoes are tasty and also a good source of the antioxidant lycopene. You'll love the savory and flavorful addition of the herbs and spices that enhance the cardioprotective benefits of this dish.

2 cups (416 g) dried navy beans

2 tablespoons (28 ml) extra-virgin olive oil or ghee

2 cups (320 g) chopped onions

1 clove garlic, minced

2 cups (248 g) tomato puree

½ cup (170 g) organic honey

2 tablespoons (28 ml) apple cider vinegar

¼ teaspoon ground nutmeg

½ teaspoon ground cinnamon

3 bay leaves

½ teaspoon each ground turmeric and cumin

¼ teaspoon each salt, Celtic or sea, and black pepper

Soak the beans overnight. Drain and rinse under cold water. Add the beans to a large pot, cover with water, and bring to a boil. Reduce the heat to a simmer and cook for up to 2 hours.

Preheat the oven to 300°F (150°C, gas mark 2).

Drain the beans and place them in a large casserole dish. In a small skillet, heat the oil or ghee and sauté the onions and garlic until browned, about 3 or 4 minutes. Add the onions and garlic to the beans and mix together. Add all the other ingredients and stir to combine. With the lid on, bake the beans for 3 hours, stirring frequently. Check the moisture level and add water if needed. After 3½ hours, remove the cover and bake for another 30 minutes.

Serve with Zesty Digestive Herb and Cheddar Breakfast Muffins (page 89). Refrigerate the beans in an airtight jar, where they will keep for up to 1 week.

Yield: 1 quart or 8 servings

Note: The insoluble fiber in baked beans is not fully digested but moves into the large intestine or colon, where friendly bacteria thrive on it to produce beneficial B-complex vitamins, enzymes, and short-term fatty acids.

———————[NUTRITIONAL ANALYSIS]———————

Per serving: 314.8 calories; 4.2 g fat; 12.4 g protein; 56.1 g carbs; 14.1 g fiber; 16.6 mg sodium.

ZESTY DIGESTIVE HERB AND CHEDDAR BREAKFAST MUFFINS

These wholesome almond flour muffins are high in plant protein and fiber as well as calcium and heart-protective vitamin E. Almond flour imparts a satisfying taste to baked goods and is more filling than grain-based flours, so you will probably eat less. The fresh ginger and orange zest will help give your digestive system a boost and keep your metabolism running smoothly.

1 teaspoon butter or extra-virgin olive oil

1 whole egg

2 eggs, yolks and whites separated

¼ cup (56 g) butter, softened

¼ cup (60 g) Immune-Boosting Yogurt (page 278)

1 teaspoon organic honey

1 tablespoon (6 g) minced fresh ginger, peeled

1 teaspoon grated orange peel

¼ teaspoon salt, Celtic or sea

½ cup (60 g) grated Cheddar cheese

2 cups (230 g) almond flour

1 teaspoon baking soda

2 hard-boiled eggs, peeled

Preheat the oven to 325°F (170°C, gas mark 3). Lightly oil a large, 6-hole muffin tin using 1 teaspoon butter or oil.

In a large bowl, combine the whole egg with the two egg yolks, butter, yogurt, honey, ginger, orange peel, and salt and whisk until light and fluffy, about 3 minutes. Add the Cheddar and combine well. In a separate bowl, mix the almond flour with the baking soda and add to the egg mixture. Beat the 2 egg whites until stiff, about 3 or 4 minutes, and gently fold into the dough. Chop the hard-boiled eggs into large chunks and fold into the mixture. Evenly distribute the dough among the muffin tin holes and bake for 30 minutes, or until the muffins feel spongy. Let cool for 10 minutes before serving warm with butter or alongside your favorite breakfast dishes.

Yield: 6 servings

Note: Almond flour is heavier and coarser than wheat flours, causing baked goods not to rise as much. They usually rise in the oven and then sink when cooled.

────[NUTRITIONAL ANALYSIS]────
Per serving: 420.8 calories; 33.5 g fat; 14 g protein; 10.7 g carbs; 4.1 g fiber; 368.5 mg sodium.

· MIDDAY MEALS ·
AND ANYTIME SNACKS

Including plenty of antioxidant vitamin- and mineral-laden foods, the raw, lively salads and energy-sustaining soups and sandwiches in this section are vital to your heart- and brain-healthy diet. These recipes contain foods to balance your metabolism, boost your immune system, and fight stress, thereby warding off the tendency to reach for high-glycemic carbohydrate foods. Many of the recipes contain heart-strengthening minerals such as potassium and magnesium, plus ample amounts of vitamins A, C, and E. In addition, you'll find vitamin B–complex-rich foods to strengthen your blood vessels, arteries, and heart, plus lots of fiber to keep your metabolism efficient. I recommend eating at least one raw salad every day—notice what happens to your health when you do. You'll be pleasantly delighted, I am certain.

Experiment until you find the right balance of foods that makes you feel best, as no two people are identical. Gradually you will learn how to eat to protect your heart and improve your entire health. Your taste buds will enjoy the journey, also.

ALMIGHTY AVOCADO AND BLACK BEAN SALAD

Apart from their smooth nutty flavor, avocados are rich in monounsaturated fat, which is easily burned for energy. They are an excellent source of fiber, folate, vitamins E, C, B_6, and B_5, and potassium, all of which have cardioprotective benefits. Black beans are high in plant protein and fiber plus an impressive array of essential antioxidant vitamins and minerals that reduce inflammation and benefit the whole body. This combination together with the herbs and spices in this salad is a dieter's dream dish.

2 cups (388 g) dried black beans

1½ tablespoons (1.5 g) chopped fresh cilantro

1½ tablespoons (6 g) chopped fresh parsley

1 tablespoon (15 ml) fresh lime juice

¼ teaspoon salt, Celtic or sea

¼ teaspoon black pepper

½ cup (90 g) chopped tomatoes

½ cup (73 g) diced avocado

2 tablespoons (12 g) chopped scallions

1 teaspoon chopped green chile pepper, seeded

4 cups (220 g) salad greens

Soak the beans overnight. Drain, rinse, and place into a medium-size pot. Cover with water, bring to a boil, and reduce to a simmer. Cook for up to 2 hours, until the beans have softened. Drain.

Whisk together the cilantro, parsley, lime juice, salt, and pepper in a large bowl. Add the beans, tomatoes, avocado, scallions, and pepper, and toss well. Cover and chill for 2 hours. Combine with the salad greens shortly before serving.

Yield: 4 servings

Note: One cup of avocado has 23 percent of the recommended daily value of folate. Studies have shown that folate improves heart health and is protective against strokes.

[NUTRITIONAL ANALYSIS]

Per serving: 183.9 calories; 2.8 g fat; 19.3 g protein; 50 g carbs; 34.7 g fiber; 176.1 mg sodium.

MOOD-BOOSTING CHICKEN AND PINEAPPLE COLESLAW WITH COCONUT-LIME DRESSING

Delight your taste buds as you improve your health with the delicious combination of spices and nutrients in this dish. Coleslaw is made from one of the most powerful health-promoting vegetables in the food kingdom—cabbage. Cabbage is rich in fiber and vitamins A, C, and K, all of which are natural antioxidants that help prevent heart disease. The addition of chicken to this dish adds complete protein along with vitamins B_6 and B_3, which support energy metabolism throughout the body.

FOR THE COLESLAW:

1 pound (455 g) chicken breast

1 cup (235 ml) filtered water

1 cup (110 g) carrots, peeled and grated

3½ cups (315 g) savoy cabbage, thinly sliced

1 cup (155 g) diced fresh pineapple

2 scallions, chopped

¼ cup each chopped fresh cilantro (4 g) and mint (24 g)

FOR THE DRESSING:

1 cup (235 ml) coconut milk

¼ cup (60 ml) fresh lime juice

2 tablespoons (28 ml) fish sauce

1 tablespoon (20 g) organic honey

To make the coleslaw: Place the chicken and 1 cup (235 ml) filtered water in a saucepan over medium heat and steam until cooked through, about 15 to 20 minutes. Let it cool, then shred. Place the chicken in a large bowl and combine with the remaining coleslaw ingredients.

To make the dressing: In a separate bowl, whisk together all the dressing ingredients and pour over the top of the chicken.

Yield: 4 servings

Note: Apart from its high content of vitamin C, fiber, potassium, and other nutrients, cabbage has the fewest calories and least fat of any vegetable. Store cabbage whole in the refrigerator, which will help to retain its vitamin C content.

————[NUTRITIONAL ANALYSIS]————
Per serving: 314 calories; 14.9 g fat; 28.3 g protein; 18.6 g carbs; 3.9 g fiber; 799.2 mg sodium.

VITALIZING BROCCOLI AND CAULIFLOWER SALAD

Together, these two superfoods, broccoli and cauliflower, will provide your body with its daily dose of fiber, antioxidants, and essential vitamins and minerals. Botanically, they are part of the cruciferous family of vegetables, which are loaded with B-complex vitamins like niacin, riboflavin, pantothenic acid, thiamine, and folate, as well as vitamin K, potassium, calcium, magnesium, and iron. The nutrients are made even more bioavailable by steaming them first, which we've done here. The antioxidants in the spices combine to make this salad a winner when it comes to providing sustained energy, and the natural flavor companions in this stunning dish are simply delicious.

1½ cups each cauliflower (150 g) and broccoli florets (107 g), chopped into bite-size pieces

1 cup (130 g) chopped carrots

3 tablespoons (45 ml) Bone-Building French Cream (page 277)

2 tablespoons (28 ml) apple cider vinegar

1 teaspoon organic honey

¼ teaspoon salt, Celtic or sea

½ teaspoon ground fresh ginger, peeled

½ teaspoon ground cumin

¼ teaspoon each ground coriander and nutmeg

Dash of cayenne pepper

2 tablespoons (12 g) chopped scallions

Place the cauliflower, broccoli, and carrots in a vegetable steamer and steam for about 3 minutes. Rinse under cold water, drain well, and place in a large bowl.

In a separate bowl, combine the cream, vinegar, and honey and mix well. In a third bowl, combine the salt, ginger, cumin, coriander, nutmeg, and cayenne and add to the cream mixture. Pour this over the cooled vegetables and garnish with the scallions. Serve.

Yield: 4 servings

Note: To ensure freshness and higher nutrient content, purchase whole rather than precut broccoli and cauliflower and store it in the refrigerator. Once cooked, you should consume it within a couple days to avoid spoilage.

[NUTRITIONAL ANALYSIS]

Per serving: 69.1 calories; 3.8 g fat; 2.4 g protein; 8.1 g carbs; 2.9 g fiber; 157.3 mg sodium.

CARDIOPROTECTIVE SALMON CAESAR SALAD

Adding salmon to a traditional Caesar salad increases the flavor and omega-3 fatty acid content by a mile. The protein in salmon is easy to digest and absorb, which speeds up your metabolism and keeps blood sugar levels in check. The eggs, romaine lettuce, and dressing meld nicely in this dish to satisfy your palate, all the while contributing to a healthy lifestyle.

FOR THE SALAD:

2 salmon fillets (4 ounces [115 g] each)

½ teaspoon salt, Celtic or sea

¼ teaspoon black pepper

4 cups (220 g) romaine lettuce, washed, roughly shredded

4 hard-boiled eggs, shelled and cut into quarters

Cardioprotective Caesar Salad Dressing (page 214)

Rub the salmon with the salt and pepper and steam it, covered, in a small skillet over medium heat, with a little water (about ½ cup [120 ml]) for about 10 minutes, until just cooked through. Set aside and let cool. Cut into slices. Place the romaine lettuce into a large bowl and add the salmon and quartered eggs. Toss with the dressing and serve immediately.

Yield: 4 servings

Note: Omega-3 essential fatty acids not only strengthen your heart muscle but help your brain work better and improve memory.

Salmon: High Quality Protein and Nutrition

Salmon is a superb source of omega-3 fatty acids, which strengthen your heart muscle and help your brain and memory function better. It's also a great source of high-quality protein. One 3-ounce serving of wild salmon gives you more than 18 g of protein, plus 360 mg of potassium and almost half the Daily Value (DV) of the important cancer-fighting mineral, selenium. It also contains more than half the DV for vitamin B_{12} and 30 percent of the DV for niacin.

Although we'll eat farm-raised salmon in a pinch, our first choice—by far—is wild Alaskan salmon. Here's why. Farm-raised salmon are raised on grain—hardly their natural diet—and have higher amounts of inflammatory omega-6 fatty acids. Like factory-farmed cattle, they're also frequently given antibiotics. And farm-raised salmon are a significant source of PCBs. Whenever possible, opt for wild Alaskan salmon.

──────[NUTRITIONAL ANALYSIS]──────

Per serving: 177.5 calories; 5.3 g fat; 18.3 g protein; 2.1 g carbs; 1 g fiber; 272 mg sodium.

ENERGIZING THAI SPICE CHICKEN SALAD

There's something balanced about Thai food because of the sweet, salty, and sour combination of flavors in the dishes. It's also one of the healthiest cuisines because of the wide use of fresh medicinal herbs. This recipe is no exception.

FOR THE MARINADE:

1 teaspoon salt, Celtic or sea

6 cloves garlic

2 tablespoons (28 ml) fresh lemon or lime juice

1 cup (16 g) chopped fresh cilantro

1 teaspoon black pepper

FOR THE SALAD:

2 cups (140 g) finely shredded cabbage

1½ cups (83 g) mixed lettuce greens

1 cup (40 g) shredded fresh basil

1 fresh red chile pepper, minced

2 chicken breasts (4 ounces [115 g] each)

FOR THE DRESSING:

See Energizing Thai Spice Salad Dressing (page 218)

To make the marinade: Place all the marinade ingredients into a food processor and blend until minced.

To make the salad: Combine the cabbage, mixed lettuce greens, basil, and pepper in a large bowl. Set aside.

Place the chicken and marinade in a saucepan with ½ cup (120 ml) filtered water and simmer, covered, for about 20 minutes, or until the chicken is cooked through. Let cool. Shred the cooled chicken by hand. Toss with the dressing and serve immediately over the mixed greens.

Yield: 4 servings

Note: Cilantro is one of the richest herbal sources for vitamin K and a good source of potassium, calcium, iron, and magnesium, all of which support healthy metabolism and cellular energy.

---[NUTRITIONAL ANALYSIS]---

Per serving: 99.8 calories; 2.2 g fat; 15.8 g protein; 4.2 g carbs; 1.8 g fiber; 371.5 mg sodium.

PUMPING JUMPING BEAN SALAD

Keep your blood sugar balanced while you enjoy the delicious nutty flavors of this legume-filled salad, which is high in plant protein and fiber and loaded with health-supportive nutrients to give you energy. The pine nuts are high in vitamins E and K, copper, magnesium, and iron, all of which are heart healthy.

FOR THE SALAD:

1 can (13¾ ounces [390 g]) garbanzo beans, drained and rinsed

½ cup (80 g) chopped red onion

1 cup (120 g) diced celery stalks

1 cup (130 g) diced carrots

½ cup (30 g) chopped fresh parsley

1 cup (135 g) seeded and diced cucumber

1 cup (150 g) diced red bell pepper

½ cup (70 g) pine nuts

For the dressing:

Simply Nourishing Salad Dressing (page 217)

Combine all the salad ingredients in a large bowl and toss with Simply Nourishing Salad Dressing. Cover and chill for 1 hour before serving.

Yield: 4 servings

Note: If using dry beans, soaking them for several hours before cooking or consuming them helps to break down the antinutrients and hard-to-digest components of the legume and at the same time, release the beneficial nutrients. This recipe, which calls for canned beans, was adapted from one that came from my book Foods That Fight Fibromyalgia.

Recipe Variations

Bean recipes are very tolerant to substitutions but color, texture, and flavor are also criteria to consider. For the Pumping Jumping Bean Salad, you might switch out the garbanzo beans for black beans if you prefer a meatier texture and a flavor that has been compared to mushrooms. To turn up the heat on a summer's day, you may like to add some fresh mango, lime juice, fresh cilantro, and a jalapeño.

————————[NUTRITIONAL ANALYSIS]————————

Per serving: 235 calories; 13.4 g fat; 8.2 g protein; 26.5 g carbs; 7.3 g fiber; 411.9 mg sodium.

SIMPLY NOURISHING SALAD DRESSING

This dressing provides a good balance of essential fatty acids and tastes delicious. Make it in bulk and keep a fresh supply on hand to add to raw salads or drizzle it over your favorite steamed veggies.

1 clove garlic, minced

4 tablespoons (60 ml) extra-virgin olive oil

2 to 4 tablespoons (28 to 60 ml) flaxseed oil

2 tablespoons (28 ml) fresh lemon or lime juice

2 tablespoons (28 ml) apple cider vinegar

1 teaspoon dry mustard powder

¼ teaspoon salt, Celtic or sea

Dash of black pepper

Dash of cayenne pepper (optional)

Place all the ingredients into a food processor and blend until smooth, or place all the ingredients in a jar with a tight-fitting lid and shake vigorously until well blended. Taste, and adjust seasonings as desired. Serve over mixed lettuce leaves or other favorite salad ingredients.

Yield: 1 cup

Note: Flaxseed oil is easily oxidized and therefore should never be heated, always refrigerated, and purchased in opaque bottles that have been refrigerated.

CARDIOPROTECTIVE CAESAR SALAD DRESSING

The anchovies in this tasty dressing deliver health benefits in the form of essential fatty acids, protein, calcium, and magnesium, all of which combine to keep your heart in good shape. The other ingredients simply add to the nutritional profile and pack a flavorful punch.

5 anchovies

1 egg

¼ teaspoon dry mustard powder

1 tablespoon (15 g) Dijon mustard

1 clove garlic

¾ cup (175 ml) extra-virgin olive oil

2 tablespoons (28 ml) fresh lemon or lime juice

Place the anchovies, egg, mustard powder, Dijon mustard, and garlic into a food processor and blend until smooth. Add a little of the oil, about 2 tablespoons (28 ml), and blend again. Keep adding the oil slowly while still blending. Then add the lemon or lime juice and keep blending until the dressing starts to thicken. Refrigerate in an airtight container. Serve over top of the Cardioprotective Caesar Salad (page 217).

Yield: 1 cup

Note: Anchovies packed in cans or jars are frequently high in sodium. The best way to eliminate some of the excess salt is to rinse or soak them first in cold water.

[NUTRITIONAL ANALYSIS]

Per tablespoon: 60.7 calories; 6.9 g fat; 0 g protein; .2 g carbs; 0 g fiber; 35.4 mg sodium.

[NUTRITIONAL ANALYSIS]

Per tablespoon: 98.2 calories; 10.9 g fat; 0.7 g protein; 0.1 g carbs; 0 g fiber; 72.4 mg sodium.

ENERGIZING THAI SPICE SALAD DRESSING

Fragrant and full of flavor—these are some of the words used to describe this delectable dressing. The kaffir lime leaf adds an unmistakable, refreshing taste that is used in many Thai dishes and provides an array of digestive nutrients. The spices in this dish will dress up any raw salad greens with delightful flavors.

1 tablespoon (15 ml) fish sauce

1 tablespoon (4 g) lemongrass

1 kaffir lime leaf

1 clove garlic

1 tablespoon (20 g) organic honey

1 teaspoon grated fresh ginger, peeled

2 tablespoons (28 ml) fresh lime juice

½ cup (8 g) chopped fresh cilantro

1 teaspoon Spice-It-Up Sweet Chili Sauce (page 272)

5 tablespoons (75 ml) filtered water

Place all the ingredients into a food processor and process until finely minced. Serve over Energizing Thai Spice Chicken Salad (page 95). Refrigerate in an airtight container.

Yield: ⅓ cup

Note: Kaffir lime leaves are used in many Thai dishes, where they not only add aromatic fragrance but are believed to brighten a person's mental outlook as well.

HOLY-MOLY GUACAMOLE DRESSING

A member of the fruit family, avocados are considered one of the healthiest foods on the planet. They contain more than twenty-five nutrients, including essential fatty acids, vitamins C, E, K, and the heart-healthy minerals magnesium, selenium, and zinc. This delicious guacamole has zingy flavors to match the nutrient density and antioxidants in it.

1 avocado, pitted and peeled

1 small tomato, diced

¼ cup (60 ml) lemon or lime juice

1 tablespoon (1 g) chopped fresh cilantro

1 spring onion, chopped

1 clove garlic, chopped

¼ teaspoon cayenne pepper

Place all the ingredients in a blender or food processor and blend until coarse in texture. Spread the dressing over toast or crackers, or serve on top of mixed salad greens.

Yield: 1 cup

Note: A firm, green avocado can be ripened more quickly by placing it in a paper bag or fruit basket at room temperature. The used ripe portion should be stored in the refrigerator, where it will maintain freshness for several days. Sprinkle with lemon juice to avoid brown spots.

———[NUTRITIONAL ANALYSIS]———

Per tablespoon: 5.8 calories; 0 g fat; 0.1 g protein; 1.5 g carbs; 0 g fiber; 88 mg sodium.

———[NUTRITIONAL ANALYSIS]———

Per tablespoon: 21.3 calories; 1.7 g fat; 0.3 g protein; 1.8 g carbs; 0.9 g fiber; 1.8 mg sodium.

STRESS-LESS TURKEY, AVOCADO, AND VEGGIE NORI WRAP

Turkey is high in protein and the amino acid trypto-phan, which produces the feel-good neurochemical serotonin. In addition to being deliciously tasty, nori seaweed is a great way to obtain natural iodine, a trace mineral that stimulates the thyroid to produce hormones required for healthy metabolism. Adding avocado is simply icing on the nutrient-rich cake, or wrap, as the case may be.

4 raw nori sheets

4 romaine lettuce leaves

4 tablespoons (60 g) Bone-Strengthening Lemon Tahini (page 271), divided

4 slices turkey (1 ounce [28 g] each)

1 cup (50 g) alfalfa sprouts

1 carrot, peeled and julienned

½ cup (75 g) cherry tomatoes, halved

1 avocado, peeled, pitted, and sliced into quarters

¼ cup (60 ml) filtered water

Lay out 1 nori sheet and place 1 lettuce leaf across the end. Spread 1 tablespoon (15 g) of the tahini on top of the lettuce leaf. Layer the lettuce leaf with 1/4 of the sprouts, carrot, tomatoes, and avocado on top (ensure vegetables are distributed evenly). Dip your fingers in the water to dampen them and begin rolling the nori sheet into a wrap. The water will make it easy to stick together. Repeat the process with the other 3 sheets.

Yield: 4 wraps

GLUTEN-FREE MEDITERRANEAN VEGGIE PIZZA

Rich in flavor and Mediterranean goodness, this pizza is made with heart-healthy olive oil, protein-rich nuts, and colorful, fiber-rich vegetables that will sustain you for hours. Feel free to add chicken or shrimp on top if you want extra protein.

FOR THE CRUST:

½ cup (80 g) brown rice flour, plus a little extra for dusting

½ cup (68 g) whole grain sorghum flour

½ cup (58 g) almond meal

¼ cup (26 g) ground flaxseed

½ teaspoon salt, Celtic or sea

¼ teaspoon garlic powder

2 tablespoons (30 g) Bone-Strengthening Lemon Tahini (page 271; optional)

2 tablespoons (28 ml) filtered water

2 tablespoons (28 ml) extra-virgin olive oil

FOR THE TOPPING:

1 to 2 tablespoons (15 to 28 ml) extra-virgin olive oil

½ red onion, thinly sliced

1 cup (150 g) chopped red bell pepper

1 tablespoon (4 g) oregano, fresh or dried, chopped finely

1 small zucchini, sliced into thin strips

2 cloves garlic, chopped finely

1 cup (70 g) portobello mushrooms, chopped into ¼-inch (6-mm) cubes

---

[NUTRITIONAL ANALYSIS]

Per serving: 139.8 calories; 8.5 g fat; 7.6 g protein; 8.7 g carbs; 3.7 g fiber; 278.1 mg sodium.

[NUTRITIONAL ANALYSIS]

Per slice: 139.4 calories; 7.4 g fat; 3.7 g protein; 16 g carbs; 2.2 g fiber; 122.4 mg sodium.

Dash each of cayenne and black pepper

3 tablespoons (45 g) Mediterranean Black Olive Tapenade (page 270)

1 cup (115 g) shredded mozzarella

4 ripe tomatoes, thinly sliced (or use sun-dried tomatoes if preferred)

1 cup (100 g) grated Parmesan cheese

Preheat the oven to 400°F (200°C, gas mark 6).

To make the crust: Combine all the crust ingredients in a bowl and mix thoroughly. Cover the dough and refrigerate overnight, or about 8 to 12 hours. The next day, remove the dough from the refrigerator and let it sit at room temperature for 1 hour before using. Prepare the surface of a baking sheet with a light rub of coconut or olive oil. Lay a few overlapping pieces of waxed paper on a countertop to cover a large rolling area and lightly dust the surface with brown rice flour. Place the dough on top. Dust a rolling pin with more flour and roll the dough into a $\frac{1}{8}$-inch (3-mm) layer to fit the size of your baking sheet. Reshape and patch rolled areas as needed.

To transfer the dough to the baking sheet, lay the sheet face down on top of the dough. Slide one hand underneath the waxed paper and place the other hand on top of the baking sheet. Quickly flip the two over and peel away the waxed paper. Bake for 20 minutes.

To make the toppng: In a large saucepan, heat the oil over medium heat. Add the onion, pepper, and oregano and sauté for 5 minutes. Stir in the zucchini, garlic, and mushrooms and sauté for 5 more minutes. Remove from the heat and add the cayenne and black peppers.

When the crust is ready, remove from the oven and evenly spread black olive tapenade over it. Sprinkle mozzarella over the crust. Top with the tomatoes. Layer the cooked vegetables on top and sprinkle with Parmesan and mozzarella cheeses. Bake for 10 minutes, or until the cheeses melt and brown slightly. Cut into slices with a pizza roller and serve hot with a tossed green salad or refrigerate and serve cold.

Yield: 1 pizza (8 slices)

Recipe Variation

The crust for this pizza is more of a crackerlike flat bread, so be sure to roll it thinly enough so that it bakes nice and crispy. If you want a more puffy, doughy texture, add 1 teaspoon of xanthan gum, and, after the refrigeration stage, add $\frac{1}{4}$ teaspoon of instant yeast dissolved in 1 tablespoon (15 ml) water to the dough.

VIBRANT AVOCADO AND VEGGIE SALSA COLLARD WRAPS

Why use bread when you can use the tasty collard green to wrap your veggies? High in heart-healthy vitamin C and soluble fibers, collard greens are renowned for their ability to strengthen immunity.

FOR THE SALSA:

1 cup (180 g) diced tomatoes

1 clove garlic, minced

½ medium shallot, minced

½ jalapeño pepper, deseeded and minced

1 tablespoon (15 ml) fresh lime juice

FOR THE WRAPS:

4 large collard greens, without rips or holes

2 avocados, peeled and pitted

¼ teaspoon salt, Celtic or sea

4 raw nori sheets, cut in half

2 cups (110 g) mixed baby greens

2 cups (100 g) sprouts (mung bean, sunflower, or your favorite)

2 cups (220 g) shredded carrots

To make the salsa: Combine all the salsa ingredients together in a medium bowl. Refrigerate for a minimum of 30 minutes before serving to allow the flavors to meld.

To make the wraps: Blanch the collard greens by dipping each leaf in boiling water for 10 seconds, then immediately submerging in a bath of ice water. Dry them thoroughly before using. Lay 1 leaf at a time flat on a cutting board and cut off the end stem so that it's flush with the leaf edge. Repeat with the remaining leaves and set aside.

In a medium bowl, mash the avocados with a fork. Add the salsa and salt and mix together. To assemble the wraps, take a leaf and lay it on a flat surface with the lighter side facing up and the spine vertical to you. Lay a nori strip horizontally across each leaf, about 2 inches (5 cm) up from the bottom end. Spread the avocado salsa along the nori, leaving about an inch (2.5 cm) from each horizontal side. Layer with baby greens, sprouts, and carrots. Using your fingers, pack the ingredients together and roll the collard green tightly over the filling. Cut the wrap on a diagonal in half to serve. Repeat the process for the remaining wraps.

Yield: 4 wraps

Note: Wash collard greens thoroughly before cooking or eating them, as they tend to collect dirt and soil.

───**[NUTRITIONAL ANALYSIS]**───

Per serving: 205.9 calories; 11.4 g fat; 7.3 g protein; 22.6 g carbs; 8.1 g fiber; 298.9 mg sodium.

FEEL-GOOD TURKEY OR SALMON TOMATO PANINI

Turkey or salmon with summer-ripe tomato slices in-between a creamy spread full of Parmesan and fresh basil combine to make this savory hot sandwich your favorite go-to snack or mealtime solution. The fresh tomatoes, basil, and avocados are a treasure of anti-oxidants such as vitamin A and C that provide support at the cellular level, which is increased further with the addition of lime juice. The wholesome goodness is further enhanced by protein with the addition of turkey or salmon. Make double the amount and save one for later.

3 tablespoons (42 g) Heart-Healthy Almond Mayonnaise (page 271)

2 tablespoons (30 g) Immune-Boosting Yogurt (page 158)

2 tablespoons (10 g) shredded Parmesan cheese

2 tablespoons (5 g) chopped fresh basil

1 teaspoon lemon or lime juice

Dash of freshly ground black pepper

4 slices gluten-free bread or Nourishing Crusty Onion and Parmesan Rolls (page 285)

4 slices deli turkey or ½ cup (112 g) canned red salmon

4 tomato slices

½ avocado, pitted, peeled, and mashed

1 teaspoon extra-virgin olive oil

In a small bowl, combine the mayonnaise, yogurt, Parmesan, basil, lemon or lime juice, and black pepper. Spread about 2 teaspoons of the mixture on each slice of bread. Divide the turkey or salmon and tomato, place on top of the bread, and cover with sliced avocado. Place the remaining bread on top.

In a medium skillet, heat the olive oil over medium heat. Place the 2 panini in the pan and cook until golden brown on one side, about 2 minutes. Reduce the heat to low and flip the panini. Cook until the second side is golden, about 1 to 3 minutes. Alternatively, place the sandwiches under the grill for 5 minutes. Cut in half diagonally and serve immediately.

Yield: 2 sandwiches

Note: Grass-fed, organically raised turkey, as opposed to factory farmed, offers substantially higher nutritional content and conveys the most health benefits.

[NUTRITIONAL ANALYSIS]

Per serving (with salmon): 565.9 calories; 36.7 g fat; 20.4 g protein; 42.4 g carbs; 2.5 g fiber; 653.4 mg sodium.

NUTRITIVE CHICKEN STOCK

In addition to being simple, easy, and cost effective, preparing your own chicken stock provides your body with many essential minerals and vitamins to rejuvenate your entire system. Enjoy this tasty, nourishing stock on its own as a broth or use it as a base when cooking grains, legumes, or any other recipe that calls for stock or water.

4 quarts (3.8 L) filtered water

1 chicken carcass

1 pound (455 g) chicken thighs, with bones

1 cup (160 g) onions, peeled and chopped into chunks

1 cup (120 g) diced celery

1 cup (130 g) diced carrots

4 cloves garlic, chopped

2 bay leaves

2 sprigs fresh thyme, chopped, or 1 teaspoon dried thyme

1 bunch parsley stems, chopped

2 tablespoons (28 ml) apple cider vinegar

Place the water, chicken carcass, and thighs in a large stockpot and bring to a boil over high heat. Reduce the heat to low and skim off the foam that rises during the first 10 to 15 minutes of simmering. Add the remaining ingredients. Simmer for 2½ to 3 hours. Turn the heat off and let stand, cooling, for 1 to 2 hours. Pour through a strainer, pushing with the back of a spoon to extract as much liquid as possible. Discard the vegetables and meat and other solids or fat from the surface of the stock, then transfer the stock to a variety of container sizes, including ice-cube trays. The stock can be refrigerated and used within 3 days, or it can be frozen for up to 3 months.

Yield: 3 quarts (2.8 L)

Recipe Variation

Change the chicken to beef if you want to include more red meat in your diet or if the dish you are preparing calls for beef stock.

[NUTRITIONAL ANALYSIS]

Per cup: 83 calories; 2.7 g fat; 11 g protein; 3.4 g carbs; 1.3 g fiber; 60.8 mg sodium.

DIGESTIVE VEGETABLE STOCK

Vegetable stock is loaded with healing nutrients that will alkalize your system, making it easier to cleanse and detoxify and boost your metabolism. Enjoy this tasty, nourishing stock on its own as a broth or use it as a base when cooking grains, legumes, or any other recipe that calls for stock or water.

- **2 quarts (1.9 L) filtered water**
- **2 cups (260 g) chopped carrots**
- **4 cups (480 g) diced celery**
- **1 parsnip, chopped**
- **1 cup (160 g) chopped onion**
- **2 leeks, white and light green parts only, trimmed, rinsed, and thinly sliced**
- **1 bunch parsley stems, chopped**
- **3 cloves garlic, chopped**
- **1 tablespoon (5 g) whole black peppercorns**
- **2 sprigs fresh thyme, chopped, or 1 teaspoon dried thyme**
- **2 bay leaves**

Pour the water into a stockpot and add the remaining ingredients. Bring to a boil over high heat, then reduce the heat to low and simmer the stock, uncovered, for 1 hour. Turn the heat off and let cool for 1 to 2 hours.

Pour through a strainer, discarding the vegetables and solids. Allow the stock to cool at room temperature. Spoon into smaller containers, including ice-cube trays. Refrigerate a portion for upcoming use and store the rest in the freezer, where it will keep for up to 3 months.

Yield: 2 quarts (1.9 L)

Recipe Variation

The recipe can be varied according to taste. For example, you can add more root vegetables in the winter such as potatoes and turnips, or add more herbs.

The Culinary Advantages of Using Stock

You may think it's not necessary to use vegetable stock if you're making a vegetarian or vegan dish that includes the same vegetables, but that's not the case. Using stock creates a much more richly flavored dish that can't be replicated by increasing the quantity of vegetables cooked in it.

———————[**NUTRITIONAL ANALYSIS**]———————

Per cup: 63.9 calories; 0.4 g fat; 1.9 g protein; 14.7 g carbs; 4.2 g fiber; 85.7 mg sodium.

HEART-PROTECTIVE CARROT-GINGER SOUP WITH CHIVES

Tangy, tasty, and warming from the inside out, the combination of carrots with ginger will delight not only your taste buds but your entire digestive system. This soup is packed with the antioxidants vitamin A and beta-carotene, together with tons of fiber and B-complex vitamins. It doesn't get better than this for high-energy, nutrient-dense soups.

2 tablespoons (28 ml) extra-virgin olive oil or coconut oil

1 large onion, chopped

6 large carrots, chopped

2 cups (280 g) chopped butternut squash, skin on

5 cups (1.2 L) Digestive Vegetable Stock (page 224)

½ teaspoon salt, Celtic or sea

1 teaspoon chopped fresh ginger, peeled

¼ teaspoon each ground cumin, coriander powder, and garlic powder

1 cup (60 g) chopped fresh parsley

6 tablespoons (90 g) Immune-Boosting Yogurt (page 278)

2 tablespoons (6 g) chopped fresh chives

Melt the oil in a large pot. Add the onions and cook for several minutes over medium heat until they begin to sweat. Add the carrots and butternut squash and cook for about 3 minutes. Add the vegetable stock, salt, ginger, cumin, and coriander and garlic powders. Bring to a boil, reduce the heat, and simmer, about 15 to 20 minutes, or until you can pierce the pieces easily with a fork.

Purée the soup in a blender or food processor with the parsley. Serve with 1 tablespoon of yogurt in each bowl and top with fresh chives.

Yield: 6 servings

Note: Ginger is a stimulating herb that gets the blood flowing and the circulation going. Because of this, it can make you feel warm when nothing else seems to do the trick.

[NUTRITIONAL ANALYSIS]

Per serving: 183.3 calories; 6.3 g fat; 4.5 g protein; 30.6 g carbs; 8.3 g fiber; 256.1 mg sodium.

LOVE-YOUR-HEART RED LENTIL SOUP

Enjoy a warm bowl of this tasty lentil soup with its classic herbs and vegetables reminiscent of Northern Italy. Lentils are one of the healthiest sources of plant-based protein around in addition to their numerous other nutritional benefits. They are packed with heart-healthy soluble fiber, which helps moderate blood sugar levels and promote digestive health.

2 cups (384 g) dried red lentils

2 bay leaves

6 cups (1.4 L) Digestive Vegetable Stock (page 224) or filtered water

3 tablespoons (45 ml) extra-virgin olive oil

2 cups (320 g) diced onions

3 cloves garlic, diced

2 cups (360 g) chopped fresh tomatoes

2 cups (240 g) sliced zucchini

1½ tablespoons (4.5 g) dried oregano

2 tablespoons (5 g) chopped fresh basil

2½ tablespoons (35 ml) apple cider vinegar

2½ teaspoons onion powder

1 tablespoon salt, Celtic or sea

⅓ cup (90 g) canned tomato paste

1 tablespoon (15 ml) balsamic vinegar

½ teaspoon black pepper

Wash and drain the lentils. Place in a large pot with the bay leaves and stock and bring to a boil. Reduce the heat to medium and cook, stirring occasionally, for 30 minutes, or until the lentils are soft.

In a large skillet, heat the oil over medium heat and sauté the onions and garlic for about 10 minutes, or until the onions are golden brown. Stir in the tomatoes, zucchini, oregano, basil, apple cider vinegar, and onion powder and sauté for about 5 minutes. Set aside.

When the lentils are nearly soft, add the salt and reserved tomato, zucchini, and herb mixture. Stir in the tomato paste, balsamic vinegar, and pepper and simmer for 10 minutes. Remove the bay leaves and serve immediately.

Yield: 6 servings

Recipe Variation

To increase the complete protein content, add ¼ or ½ cup (47 to 95 g) of brown rice and decrease the lentils by the same amount.

[NUTRITIONAL ANALYSIS]

Per serving: 413.5 calories; 9.4 g fat; 20.6 g protein; 61.8 g carbs; 15.3 g fiber; 919.8 mg sodium.

IMMUNE-BOOSTING BASQUE BEAN AND CABBAGE SOUP

This delicious, simple soup is a hearty staple of the Basques, an ethnic group of people from France and Spain that primarily inhabits an area tradition-ally known as the Basque Country. The white beans give it body in the form of fiber and protein, while the cabbage provides tons of vitamin C and other heart-healthy nutrients. Like any thick soup or stew, it tastes even better the day after it is made, so make this one a day ahead of consuming it.

1½ cups (312 g) dried white navy beans

2 tablespoons (28 ml) olive oil

1 medium onion, chopped

3 cloves garlic, minced

1 medium carrot, chopped

½ cup (50 g) chopped celery

8 cups (1.9 L) Digestive Vegetable Stock (page 224)

1 tablespoon (7 g) ground paprika

2 tablespoons (13 g) ground flaxseed

¼ cup (15 g) chopped fresh parsley

1 teaspoon dried thyme

1 bay leaf

¾ pound (340 g) redskin potatoes, scrubbed and cut into ¾-inch (2-cm) cubes

6 cups (420 g) firmly packed shredded green cabbage

1 teaspoon salt, Celtic or sea

½ teaspoon black pepper

Soak the beans overnight. Next morning, rinse the beans under cold water and drain. In a large pot, heat the oil over medium-high heat. Add the onion, garlic, carrot, and celery. Cook for about 5 minutes, or until the onions are translucent, stirring frequently. Add the beans, stock, paprika, flaxseed, parsley, thyme, and bay leaf. Bring to a boil over high heat, then reduce the heat to low and simmer the soup, partially covered, for about 45 minutes, or until the beans are almost tender.

Add the potatoes and cabbage and cook for an addi-tional 20 to 25 minutes, or until the vegetables are very tender. Remove and discard the bay leaf, season with salt and pepper, and serve immediately.

Yield: 8 servings as an appetizer or 6 as an entrée

Note: The soup can be prepared up to 2 days in advance and refrigerated, tightly covered. Reheat over low heat, covered, until hot, stirring occasionally.

———————[NUTRITIONAL ANALYSIS]———————
Per serving: 306.9 calories; 5.3 g fat; 14.4 g protein; 54.3 g carbs; 18.5 g fiber; 182.7 mg sodium.

BUILD-ME-UP BUTTERNUT AND MACADAMIA NUT BISQUE

This creamy, delicious dish is rich in antioxidants, fiber, and anti-inflammatory omega-3s that are particularly important for inclusion in your heart-healthy diet. Butternut squash is warming and good for stabilizing blood sugar levels to keep your system balanced for hours. Macadamia nuts contain essential vitamins and minerals including potassium, manganese, thiamine, and fiber, all of which help your body defend against disease and increase overall energy.

- 2 tablespoons (28 ml) extra-virgin olive oil
- 1 cup (160 g) chopped onions
- ¾ cup (101 g) macadamia nuts, roughly chopped
- 2 teaspoons grated fresh ginger, peeled
- 1 clove minced garlic
- 1 teaspoon ground turmeric
- 1 cup (150 g) green apples, peeled, cored, and diced
- 1 medium to large butternut squash, peeled, seeded, and diced
- 1 cup (235 ml) Nutritive Chicken (page 223) or Digestive Vegetable Stock (page 224)
- 4 tablespoons (60 g) Immune-Boosting Yogurt (page 278)
- 4 teaspoons (68 g) macadamia nuts, roughly chopped

Heat the oil in a large pot. Add the onions, macadamia nuts, ginger, and garlic and sauté until lightly browned, about 3 to 5 minutes. Stir in the turmeric. Add the apple and squash. Stir for about 3 minutes, coating them with the other ingredients, and then add the stock. Cover and cook for about 20 minutes, until the squash is quite soft. Pour all the ingredients into a food processor and blend until smooth and creamy. Add a little hot water if the soup is too thick or for a thinner consistency. Serve with a large dollop of yogurt and a teaspoon of macadamia nuts.

Yield: 4 servings

Note: Macadamia nuts are a good source of protein and vitamin E, a powerful antioxidant that not only protects your cells from free-radical damage but reduces your risk of gastrointestinal cancer.

[NUTRITIONAL ANALYSIS]

Per serving: 476 calories; 40.2 g fat; 6.3 g protein; 30.8 g carbs; 7.8 g fiber; 44.2 mg sodium.

LOW-CARB HERBED CHEDDAR CRACKERS

These are moist and delicious, so I like to make a large batch to keep on hand for all occasions. Believe it or not, topping these savory, delectable crackers with sweet spreads is simply scrumptious.

- **2 teaspoons butter**
- **2 cups (230 g) almond flour**
- **2 cups (240 g) grated sharp Cheddar cheese**
- **1 teaspoon fresh thyme, or ½ teaspoon dried**
- **1 teaspoon fresh sage, or ½ teaspoon dried**
- **¼ teaspoon cayenne pepper**
- **1 teaspoon baking soda**
- **6 tablespoons (90 ml) cold filtered water**

Preheat the oven to 300°F (150°C, gas mark 2). Grease 2 baking sheets with butter. In a large bowl, combine the almond flour, Cheddar, thyme, sage, cayenne, and baking soda. Add the cold water, mix, and form into a flat dough. Cover and refrigerate for about 30 minutes.

Remove the dough from the refrigerator. Take 1 teaspoon dough, roll it into a ball, and squeeze down with your fingers onto the prepared baking sheet. Continue this process until all of the dough has been used. Each cracker should be about ⅛-inch (3 mm) thick and at least ¾-inch (2 cm) away from the next cracker. Bake in the oven for 30 minutes, or until the edges start to brown. The crackers should look pale in the center. Turn the oven down to 200F (95°C).

Remove the sheets from the oven and let cool for 5 minutes. Turn each cracker over and return the trays to the oven. Bake for 20 minutes, turn the oven off, and let the crackers sit in the oven until the oven has cooled somewhat, about 10 minutes. Remove the sheets from the oven and cool completely. The crackers should be slightly browned, but still pale. Serve these topped with your favorite condiments. Store the crackers between waxed paper in an airtight container.

Yield: About 50 crackers

Note: Almond flour is not only gluten free, but also low in carbohydrates and sugars and high in protein.

————[**NUTRITIONAL ANALYSIS**]————
Per serving: 38.7 calories; 3.1 g fat; 2 g protein; 0.9 g carbs; 0.4 g fiber; 64 mg sodium.

BLOOD SUGAR–BALANCING BUTTERNUT & LEEK PIES

You'll love the sweet, subtle flavors and smooth texture of these satisfying and delectable pies. The high-fiber and antioxidant-laden butternut squash marries nicely with the sweet, delicate flavor of leeks, all the while adding impressive amounts of the B vitamin folate. Folate supports the cardiovascular system by keeping homocysteine in proper balance. Warning: You may need to eat more than just one.

1 cup (140 g) butternut squash, peeled, seeded, and diced

1½ tablespoons (21 g) butter

¾ cup (78 g) chopped leeks

1 tablespoon (20 g) organic honey

1 clove garlic, minced

10 eggs

⅓ cup (33 g) grated Parmesan cheese

⅓ cup (80 ml) Bone-Building French Cream (page 277)

Dash of cayenne pepper

½ teaspoon salt, Celtic or sea

½ teaspoon black pepper

Preheat the oven to 350°F (180°C). Lightly oil a large, 6-hole muffin tin.

In a medium-size pot, steam the squash in a small amount of water for about 10 minutes, or until it starts to soften. Drain and set aside. Heat the butter in a small skillet and add the leeks. Stir and sauté for about 3 minutes, or until the leeks start to wilt. Add the honey and garlic and cook, stirring, for 3 to 4 minutes. Remove from the heat and set aside.

In a large bowl, combine the eggs, Parmesan, and cream and mix well. Add the squash, leeks, cayenne pepper, salt, and black pepper. Divide the mixture evenly among the muffin tin holes and bake for 30 to 40 minutes, until the tops of the pies feel firm. Remove from the oven and let cool for a few minutes before removing from the molds. Serve at room temperature or cold. Refrigerate in an airtight container, where they will keep for up to 5 days.

Yield: 6 servings

Note: Leeks, like onions and garlic, are part of the sulfur-containing Alliaceae family, which are high in antioxidant flavonoids well known for their anti-inflammatory properties.

———[**NUTRITIONAL ANALYSIS**]———
Per serving: 243.1 calories; 16.8 g fat; 13.7 g protein; 9.6 g carbs; 1.2 g fiber; 361.6 mg sodium.

HIGH-ENERGY CHICKEN & CAULIFLOWER CROQUETTES

Gain more energy when you nosh on these high-protein and fiber-filled goodies. The chicken and cauliflower pair nicely with the fresh herbs and Parmesan cheese to create a creamy and crunchy texture that will explode with flavor in your mouth.

½ cup (80 g) chopped onions

1 tablespoon (15 ml) extra-virgin olive oil

1 pound (455 g) chicken, minced

1 cup (100 g) chopped cauliflower

1 teaspoon fresh thyme

1 tablespoon (4 g) chopped fresh parsley

½ teaspoon salt, Celtic or sea

½ teaspoon pepper

2 eggs, divided

½ cup (50 g) grated Parmesan cheese

1 cup (115 g) almond flour

⅓ cup (80 ml) coconut oil

In a medium to large skillet over medium heat, sauté the onions in olive oil until tender, about 5 minutes. Add the chicken and cook for about 20 minutes on low until all the moisture has evaporated. In a separate pot, steam the cauliflower until just soft, about 8 minutes. Drain and place into a food processor with the chicken and onions and add the thyme, parsley, salt, pepper, and 1 egg and blend until smooth. Refrigerate the mixture for 30 minutes.

Mix the Parmesan cheese with the almond flour and spread onto a large, flat plate. Whip the remaining egg in a bowl until light and fluffy. Remove the chicken mixture from the refrigerator and form into small croquettes, about 1 by 2 inches (2.5 by 5 cm). Dip them into the beaten egg and roll in the almond and cheese flour until well covered. Heat the coconut oil in a nonstick pan and fry the croquettes, turning them frequently, until golden brown. When cooked, place the croquettes onto a double layer of kitchen paper towels to remove excess oil. Serve warm with Antioxidant BBQ Sauce (page 274) or Spice-It-Up Sweet Chili Sauce (page 272).

Yield: About 16 croquettes

Recipe Variation

Change the protein content by swapping the chicken with salmon, shrimp, or any white-meat fish you prefer.

—————[NUTRITIONAL ANALYSIS]—————

Per serving: 151.4 calories; 12.1 g fat; 9.5 g protein; 2.6 g carbs; 1 g fiber; 132.8 mg sodium.

TURKEY, LAMB, OR BEEF KOFTAS WITH A HEART-HEALTHY KICK

Spiced with tasty herbs and spices, these delicious treats will satisfy your palate and keep you well nourished at the same time. Kofta is a type of spicy meatball or kebab made popular in the Middle East, South Asia, and the Balkans. The ground meat in this dish provides texture and all nine essential amino acids. The spices add extra flavor along with exemplary heart-healthy benefits.

1 pound (455 g) turkey, lamb, or beef, minced

½ cup (80 g) finely chopped onion

1 clove garlic, minced

1 teaspoon each dried coriander, cumin, and turmeric

½ teaspoon ground cinnamon

½ teaspoon finely chopped dried chile pepper

1 teaspoon tomato paste

1 tablespoon (6 g) chopped fresh mint

1 tablespoon (1 g) chopped fresh cilantro

3 tablespoons (45 ml) coconut oil

In a large bowl, combine the turkey, lamb, or beef with all the other ingredients except the coconut oil and mix well, using your hands. Form into 12 to 15 small balls, using about a heaped teaspoon per ball. Heat the coconut oil in a large, nonstick frying pan over medium to high heat and cook the koftas until browned all over, about 3 minutes. Layer a bowl with crumpled-up paper towels and place the koftas into the bowl to remove any excess oil. Serve hot or cold with Antioxidant BBQ Sauce (page 274), Spice-It-Up Sweet Chili Sauce (page 272), or another sauce of your choosing.

Yield: 12 to 15 koftas

Recipe Variation

Turn these koftas into a vegetarian dish by removing the meat and using brown rice, bulgur, or beans instead.

─── [NUTRITIONAL ANALYSIS] ───
Per serving: 109.5 calories; 9.2 g fat; 5.5 g protein; 0.8 g carbs; .2 g fiber; 29.8 mg sodium.

SPICED HONEY-GLAZED NUTS

Enjoy a handful or two of these sweet, delicious, and flavorful nuts packed with notable health-benefiting nutrients. Heart-friendly fiber, essential fatty acids, protein, and antioxidant vitamins and minerals are loaded in every bite from the nuts, which are made even better by the addition of honey and herbs to spice things up.

> **1 cup each raw almonds (145 g), walnuts (120 g), pecans (100 g), and cashews (145 g) or macadamia nuts (135 g)**
>
> **¼ cup (85 g) organic honey**
>
> **1 teaspoon ground cinnamon**
>
> **1 pinch ground cloves**
>
> **¼ teaspoon each ground turmeric, coriander, and cumin**
>
> **1 teaspoon coconut oil**

Preheat the oven to 350°F (180°C, gas mark 4). Spread the nuts onto a large baking sheet and bake for 5 to 10 minutes, or until they are crisp and lightly browned, ensuring they do not get overbrowned. Remove from the oven and allow to cool.

Combine the honey and all the spices in a bowl and mix well. Heat a large, nonstick frying pan over medium heat and add the nuts. Sprinkle the spice and honey mixture over the nuts and stir for about 5 minutes, or until the nuts start to turn golden. The honey will heat and become thinner and coat the nuts. Using a wooden spoon, gently separate the nuts if they start to stick together. When the nuts are cooked, remove them from the heat, spread them onto the baking sheet coated with coconut oil, and allow them to cool. Store the nuts in an airtight container.

Yield: 16 servings

Note: Raw honey contains a full spectrum of essential vitamins and minerals and is an excellent source of antioxidants. Whenever possible, purchase locally grown, organic raw honey, as it will be of higher nutrient content. Pasteurizing honey through heating removes some of its best qualities. In recipes that require heating the honey, don't use raw honey but go for plain honey and choose organic whenever you can.

[NUTRITIONAL ANALYSIS]

Per serving: 414 calories; 37.6 g fat; 9.6 g protein; 16.6 g carbs; 5.1 g fiber; 1.8 mg sodium.

CALMING COCONUT-DATE BALLS

These sweet, delicious treats are rich in heart-healthy nutrients such as fiber, potassium, and magnesium, along with numerous antioxidants. The coconut adds a nice, chewy texture plus provides essential fatty acids. A couple of these are enough to satisfy any sweet tooth and keep your appetite satiated for hours.

- **1 cup (160 g) pitted, halved dates**
- **1 cup (130 g) dried apricots**
- **1 cup (145 g) raisins**
- **1 cup walnuts (120 g)**
- **1 tablespoon (15 ml) maple syrup**
- **3 tablespoons (45 ml) fresh orange juice**
- **¼ teaspoon salt, Celtic or sea**
- **1 cup (80 g) shredded coconut, unsweetened, divided**

Place the dates, apricots, raisins, walnuts, maple syrup, orange juice, and salt in a food processor and grind to a paste. Add half the coconut and process again until smooth. Check the consistency: Pinch the dough and make sure that it sticks together. If the dough is too dry, add a teaspoon or two of water until it sticks.

Place some cold water in a bowl and dip your fingers in the bowl. With moist hands, form small balls out of the date paste and roll in the remaining coconut. Refrigerate in an airtight container.

Yield: 30 to 35 balls

Note: Soaking your dates and dried fruits helps release essential vitamins and minerals and makes them easier to digest. The soak water is fortifying for the heart.

———————[NUTRITIONAL ANALYSIS]———————
Per serving: 76.9 calories; 3.9 g fat; 1.1 g protein; 11 g carbs; 1.4 g fiber; 11.3 mg sodium.

DETOXIFYING LIMA BEAN BLINIS WITH ARTICHOKE HERBED DIP

Well known for their meaty texture and mild buttery flavor, lima beans are a good source of protein, providing all nine essential amino acids. These deliciously buttery beans are also an excellent source of both soluble and insoluble dietary fiber that are well known for their digestive benefits. The combination of antioxidant-laden artichokes and herbs adds greatly to the many medicinal benefits of this delicious and satisfying dish.

FOR THE BLINIS:

- **1 cup (156 g) dried lima beans**
- **6 eggs**
- **1 tablespoon (15 ml) Bone-Building French Cream (page 277)**
- **2 cloves garlic, minced**
- **1 tablespoon (1.7 g) chopped fresh rosemary**
- **1 teaspoon salt, Celtic or sea**
- **½ teaspoon black pepper**
- **Dash of cayenne pepper**

FOR THE DIP:

- **1 can (13¾ [390 g] ounces) artichoke hearts in water, drained, rinsed, and coarsely chopped**
- **8 ounces (225 g) cream cheese, diced into small cubes**
- **⅓ cup (75 g) Heart-Healthy Almond Mayonnaise (page 271)**
- **½ cup (50 g) grated fresh Parmesan cheese**
- **¼ cup (15 g) chopped fresh parsley**
- **2 tablespoons (5 g) chopped fresh basil**
- **1 teaspoon grated lemon zest**
- **½ teaspoon black pepper**
- **Dash of cayenne pepper**

———————[NUTRITIONAL ANALYSIS]———————
Per serving: 53.8 calories; 2.9 g fat; 3.1 g protein; 4.5 g carbs; 1.2 g fiber; 109.2 mg sodium.

To make the blinis: Soak the beans overnight. The next day, drain and rinse them under cold water. Place the beans in a medium-size pan, add water to cover the beans, cover the pot, bring to a boil, and reduce to a simmer for 1 hour, until the beans are quite soft. Drain the beans and set aside.

Preheat the oven to 350°F (180°C, gas mark 4).

In another bowl combine the eggs and cream and whip until fluffy. Pour into a food processor along with the beans, garlic, rosemary, salt, pepper, and cayenne. Blend until smooth.

Lightly grease a 12-hole muffin tin with coconut or olive oil. Pour about 1 inch (2.5 cm) of the mixture into each muffin hole and bake for about 10 minutes. The blinis only need to set firmly; they do not need to brown. Repeat this process until all of the blinis are made. Let cool and then refrigerate in an airtight container. These will keep for a few days and are great with any other toppings.

Yield: 30 blinis

To make the dip: Preheat the oven to 425°F (220°C, gas mark 7).

In a medium bowl, mix all the dip ingredients together. Transfer to a lightly oiled ovenproof casserole dish or 9-inch (23-cm) pie pan and bake for about 20 minutes, until hot and bubbly. Serve on top of the blinis and with cut-up raw vegetables such as celery and carrots.

Yield: Approximately 3 cups

Note: Thanks to their high antioxidant content, artichokes have been ranked number seven in a study conducted by the U.S. Department of Agriculture that examined antioxidant levels of one thousand different foods. Among their many powerful antioxidants, artichokes also contain two important components, luteolin and cynarin, which are believed to provide heart-healthy benefits.

· ON THE ·
DINNER MENU

More than a family ritual, your last meal of the day is just as important as your first, because it provides an opportunity to consume nutrients that may have been lacking during the day. A balanced, nutrient-packed dinner also provides your body with essential vitamins and minerals to help it repair, rebuild, and regenerate your cells, organs, and tissues during sleep.

In this section you'll find tantalizing, balanced options that pack in the antioxidants and vitamins while providing a diversity of both nutrition and flavor. From meatless main dishes to poultry, seafood, and beef, all are stocked with nature's most powerful ingredients. There's also a hearty selection of irresistible vegetables, grains, and beans, which by no means should only be reserved for the side of the plate. Experiment a little and have fun with your meals. Perhaps rather than making meat the mainstay of your meal, try filling half your plate with vegetables or building your dishes around the ingredients that offer the greatest nutritional benefits and bang for the bite.

SPICY MOROCCAN TEMPEH WITH LENTILS

Tempeh is more than just a delicious meat substitute for vegetarians. It is made from fermented soybeans, which are a rich source of probiotics, friendly microorganisms that help maintain a healthy digestive system and boost immunity. Tempeh has the added advantage of soaking up the flavors of whatever other items it is cooked with and has a rich, chewy texture that many meat eaters often can't tell apart from meat. Together, the tempeh and lentils in this recipe provide plenty of healthy, plant-based protein, fiber, and an array of heart-healthy vitamins and minerals.

- 1 package (8 ounces [225 g]) tempeh, cut into 1-inch (2.5-cm) cubes
- 1 tablespoon (15 ml) each wheat-free tamari and brown rice vinegar
- 2 tablespoons (28 ml) coconut oil, divided
- 1 small onion, diced
- 2 cloves garlic, minced
- 2 medium celery stalks, diced
- 2 small carrots, diced
- 2 tablespoons (32 g) tomato paste
- ¼ cup (60 ml) red or white wine
- 1 teaspoon each ground cumin and turmeric
- 1 cup (192 g) brown lentils
- 5½ cups (1.3 L) Digestive Vegetable Stock (page 224)
- 1 teaspoon salt, Celtic or sea
- 1 teaspoon capers
- 1 tablespoon (15 ml) extra-virgin olive oil

Preheat the oven to 375°F (190°C, gas mark 5). Toss the tempeh with the tamari and vinegar and let sit for at least 20 minutes. Toss with 1 tablespoon (15 ml) of coconut oil and transfer to a baking sheet. Bake for 15 minutes and set aside.

Heat the remaining tablespoon of coconut oil in a large pan over medium heat. Add the onion, garlic, celery, and carrots and sauté until they are tender and start to brown, about 8 to 10 minutes. Add the tomato paste and sauté a few more minutes, until it starts to brown. Add the wine and stir to release any browned bits from the bottom of the pan. Add the cumin, turmeric, lentils, and stock. Cover and simmer gently until the lentils are soft, about 40 minutes. Add the salt and capers and simmer for 5 to 10 more minutes. Toss in the baked tempeh and cook until warmed. Serve hot, drizzled with the olive oil.

Yield: 4 servings

Note: The fermentation process that soy undergoes to become tempeh makes it more easily digestible and metabolized by the body than traditional soy products, and it is much healthier. One 4-ounce (115-g) serving of tempeh provides more than a third of the average daily protein requirement.

—————[**NUTRITIONAL ANALYSIS**]—————

Per serving: 394.8 calories; 15.3 g fat; 19.7 g protein; 45.4 g carbs; 17.3 g fiber; 836 mg sodium.

HI-FIBE RED BEAN BURGERS

Chock-full of tasty herbs and spices and loaded with heart-healthy nutrients, these delicious meatless burgers can hold their own against any frozen burger you'd buy in a supermarket. They are so easy to make and you'll be pleased to have created such a vegetarian delight.

1 cup (250 g) dried red kidney beans

2½ cups (570 ml) Digestive Vegetable Stock (page 224) or filtered water

½ cup (70 g) sunflower seeds and ½ cup (70 g) pumpkin seeds

½ cup (55 g) peeled, grated carrots

½ cup (80 g) finely chopped onion

½ cup (75 g) finely chopped green bell pepper

1 teaspoon ground cumin

1 tablespoon (4 g) finely chopped fresh parsley

1 tablespoon (1 g) finely chopped cilantro

1 teaspoon salt, Celtic or sea

½ teaspoon black pepper

4 eggs

1 tablespoon (15 ml) fresh lemon or lime juice

2 tablespoons (28 ml) coconut oil

Soak the beans overnight. Drain and wash under cold water until the water runs clear. Place the beans into a pot and cover with stock or water, bring to a boil, reduce the heat to a simmer, and cook for up to 2 hours, or until soft but not mushy. They should still have a slight firmness to them. Grind the sunflower and pumpkin seeds in a food processor or use a coffee grinder until the consistency resembles a cereal meal, about a minute or less.

Place the kidney beans into a food processor and process until coarsely chopped. Combine with the sunflower and pumpkin seed meal, carrots, onion, bell pepper, cumin, parsley, cilantro, salt, pepper, eggs, and lemon or lime juice and knead with your hands until mixed through. Divide into 4 pieces and form into patties.

Add the coconut oil to a large, nonstick skillet over medium heat. Cook each patty for approximately 10 minutes on each side, or until they are slightly browned on the outside. Serve hot or cold with Antioxidant BBQ Sauce (page 224), Spice-It-Up Sweet Chili Sauce (page 272), or another sauce of your choosing.

Yield: 4 burgers

Note: Put a little olive oil on your hands when shaping the patties to prevent sticking.

[NUTRITIONAL ANALYSIS]

Per serving: 555.4 calories; 29.8 g fat; 26 g protein; 51.1 g carbs; 17.3 g fiber; 479.9 mg sodium.

PROTEIN-PACKED VEGETARIAN SHEPHERD'S PIE

Shepherd's pie is pure comfort food, and this vegetarian version will satisfy the taste buds of meat eaters and vegetarians alike. The goat cheese adds a slightly sweet and sometimes salty undertone, plus it's loaded with calcium, vitamin D, protein, and the amino acid tryptophan, which is a feel-good chemical that relaxes you. Numerous other heart-healthy nutrients, such as potassium, B_2, and fiber, are loaded into the mix to help give you energy and contribute to good health.

- **1 cup (208 g) each dried black and navy beans**
- **½ cup each (96 g) green split peas and green lentils**
- **4 cups (946 ml) Digestive Vegetable Stock (page 224), divided**
- **2 ½ cups (250 g) roughly chopped cauliflower**
- **½ teaspoon each salt, Celtic or sea, and black pepper**
- **¼ teaspoon ground nutmeg**
- **⅓ cup (43 g) peeled, chopped carrots**
- **⅓ cup (33 g) chopped celery**
- **1 cup (160 g) chopped onion**
- **1 cup (150 g) chopped green bell pepper**
- **¼ cup (56 g) butter or ghee**
- **¾ cup (135 g) peeled, sliced tomatoes**
- **¼ teaspoon cayenne pepper**
- **¼ teaspoon freshly cracked black pepper**
- **½ cup (75 g) goat cheese**
- **½ cup (50 g) grated Parmesan cheese**

Soak the black and navy beans overnight. Drain and rinse under cold water. Place the black beans into a large pot with the split peas and lentils and add 2½ cups (570 ml) vegetable stock and a little salt. Cover and simmer gently for up to 2 hours, or until the pulses have absorbed the stock and are soft. Remove them from the heat and mash just a little with a fork. At the same time, place the navy beans into another pot and cover with the remaining stock, cover, and cook for up to 2 hours. Remove and drain.

Preheat the oven to 375°F (190°C, gas mark 5). Steam the cauliflower until soft, about 5 minutes. Toss the cauliflower and navy beans into a food processor and blend until smooth, adding the salt, black pepper, and nutmeg. Set aside. Next, take the carrots, celery, onion, and bell pepper and process in the food processor until finely chopped.

Melt the butter or ghee in a large skillet over medium heat and add the vegetables. Cook for about 10 to 15 minutes, or until they are soft and tender. Set aside. Add the cooked vegetables to the pulse mixture and combine well. Pour the mixture into a 10-inch (25-cm) square baking dish and arrange the tomatoes in overlapping slices on the top.

Combine the mashed cauliflower and navy bean mixture with the goat cheese and season with cayenne pepper, and freshly cracked pepper. Spread the mixture over the tomatoes in the baking dish. Top with grated Parmesan cheese and bake on the top shelf in the oven for about 30 minutes, or until the top is lightly browned. Remove from the oven and let sit for 10 minutes. Serve. Store covered in the refrigerator.

Yield: 4 servings

[NUTRITIONAL ANALYSIS]

Per serving: 668.9 calories; 21.3 g fat; 40.7 g protein; 97 g carbs; 37.3 g fiber; 619.7 mg sodium.

NUTRIENT-RICH ROASTED QUINOA WITH MUSHROOMS, CUMIN, AND CORIANDER

Light, fluffy, and easy to prepare, quinoa is chock-full of nutrients such as protein and fiber and an array of essential vitamins and minerals. It's great for ensuring a healthy digestive system because the complex carbohydrates digest slowly to keep you feeling full longer. The spices add extra goodness and flavor.

1 cup (170 g) quinoa, rinsed and drained

1 cup (70 g) diced porcini mushrooms

1½ cups (355 ml) Digestive Vegetable Stock (page 224)

½ teaspoon salt, Celtic or sea

1 tablespoon (7 g) ground cumin

1 tablespoon (6 g) ground coriander

Dash of cayenne pepper

½ cup (8 g) chopped fresh cilantro

1 tablespoon (15 ml) fresh lemon or lime juice

Preheat the oven to 350°F (180°C, gas mark 4). Place the quinoa on a baking sheet and bake for about 10 minutes, or until you get a crispy texture. Transfer to a medium-size pot and add the mushrooms, stock, and salt. Set aside.

Place the cumin and coriander in a dry skillet over medium heat. Toast them, stirring often, about 1 to 2 minutes. Add them to the quinoa mixture. Bring to a boil, reduce the heat, cover with a lid, and simmer for about 10 minutes to allow flavors to meld together. Transfer into a serving dish, fluff with a fork, and stir in the fresh cilantro and lemon or lime juice.

Yield: 2 servings

Recipe Variation

To add more plant protein to dishes that call for rice, use quinoa instead. It cooks quickly and is generally done when the water has been absorbed and the germ has separated from the seed.

───────[NUTRITIONAL ANALYSIS]───────

Per serving: 378 calories; 5.4 g fat; 14.3 g protein; 70.8 g carbs; 9.7 g fiber; 416.3 mg sodium.

HIGH-FIBER BUTTERNUT GNOCCHI WITH HERBED CREAM SAUCE

Sublimely delicious and with all-around goodness, this flavorsome dish transforms butternut squash into something special. With its tangerine hue indicating an abundance of the antioxidants known as carotenoids, butternut squash also delivers an ample dose of dietary fiber, making it an exceptionally heart-friendly choice. The delicious mix of herbs in the cream sauce provides a ton of antioxidants to boost your health and increase the flavor.

FOR THE GNOCCHI:

2 pounds (910 g) fresh butternut squash, unpeeled, seeded, and cut into large chunks

3 eggs

½ teaspoon salt, Celtic or sea

¼ teaspoon ground nutmeg

½ cup (50 g) grated Parmesan cheese

1 cup (115 g) almond flour

FOR THE SAUCE:

⅓ cup (75 g) butter

1 clove garlic, minced

1 tablespoon each fresh basil (2.5 g), parsley (4 g), and tarragon (4 g), all finely chopped

4 sage leaves, finely chopped

1 cup (235 ml) Bone-Building French Cream (page 277)

⅓ cup (33 g) grated Parmesan cheese, divided

½ teaspoon salt, Celtic or sea

¼ teaspoon black pepper

Preheat the oven to 320°F (160°C).

To make the gnocchi: Place the butternut squash in an ovenproof dish and bake for 30 to 40 minutes, or until soft.

Start making the cream sauce while the squash is baking (see directions that follow). When the squash is cooked, remove it from the oven and let it cool a little. Place it into a food processor and process until smooth. Add the eggs, salt, nutmeg, cheese, and almond flour and process to combine. Pour the mixture into a 9- by 13-inch (23- by 33-cm) baking dish lined with parchment paper and bake for 1 hour, or until the gnocchi feels firm. Remove from the oven and let sit for 5 minutes. Cut the gnocchi into squares or triangle shapes and serve hot with the Herbed Cream Sauce.

Yield: Approximately 4 servings (1 cup each)

To make the sauce: Melt the butter in a small skillet on medium heat. Add the garlic, basil, parsley, tarragon, and sage and stir for approximately 1 minute. Add the cream and half the Parmesan. Stir and cook until the Parmesan has melted. Add the salt and pepper. Do not boil the mixture, just sauté on low heat until all ingredients have combined to a creamy consistency, about 2 to 3 minutes. Serve hot over top of the sliced gnocchi and garnish with the remaining Parmesan.

Yield: Approximately 4 servings

[NUTRITIONAL ANALYSIS]

Per serving: 337.8 calories; 20.1 g fat; 17.1 g protein; 29.5 g carbs; 9.3 g fiber; 399.7 mg sodium.

REVITALIZING VEGETABLE BIRYANI

Warming spices combined with basmati rice lend a distinctive Indian aroma and flavor to this high-fiber, heart-healthy dish. The colorful addition of saffron provides a richness of flavor as well as many vital antioxidants and vitamins, including folic acid, niacin, riboflavin, and vitamins A and C. Basmati rice is a good source of soluble fiber as well as the heart-healthy and fat-soluble vitamin E, which is an antioxidant known for preventing blood platelets from clumping and reducing the risk of heart disease. The cashews add healthy fats and give the dish a nice, crunchy texture.

1½ cups (270 g) white basmati rice

2½ cups (570 ml) Digestive Vegetable Stock (page 224) or filtered water

1 teaspoon salt, Celtic or sea

Pinch of saffron threads

2 tablespoons (28 g) ghee or coconut oil

½ cup (80 g) diced onion

1 tablespoon (6 g) minced fresh ginger, peeled

1 teaspoon ground turmeric

1 to 2 cloves garlic, minced

1 small carrot, diced

¾ cup (98 g) frozen peas

½ cup (75 g) raisins

½ cup (72 g) whole raw cashews

1 tablespoon (1 g) chopped fresh cilantro

Rinse and drain the rice. Combine the rice, stock or water, salt, and saffron in a large pot with a fitted lid and bring to a boil over medium-high heat. Reduce the heat to low, cover, and cook until the rice is tender, about 12 to 15 minutes. Turn off the heat and let stand, covered for a few minutes, before fluffing with a fork.

Heat the ghee or oil in a pan over medium-high heat. Add the onion, ginger, turmeric, garlic, and carrot and sauté until softened, about 5 to 8 minutes. Remove from the heat, add the peas and raisins, and set aside.

Uncover the rice and gently fluff with a fork. Add the carrot mixture and cashews and gently combine. Garnish with fresh cilantro and serve hot.

Yield: 4 servings

Note: Basmati rice comes in brown and white colors, and it is generally best to soak it for up to 2 hours prior to cooking with it. Soaking it first separates the grains and allows for a more fluffy, less sticky rice.

――――――[NUTRITIONAL ANALYSIS]――――――

Per serving: 357 calories; 13 g fat; 7.7 g protein; 54 g carbs; 6.4 g fiber; 556 mg sodium.

COMFORTING CHEDDAR AND BROCCOLI QUICHE WITH QUINOA CRUST

You can take comfort in knowing that this dish is superhigh in overall nutrient richness to promote optimum health. Quinoa is especially high in plant protein, folate, magnesium, and tryptophan. Sweet-tasting Swiss chard contains more than 800 percent of your daily intake of vitamin K, which is needed throughout the body for myriad functions from bone health to regulating normal blood clotting. Broccoli contains high amounts of vitamins A, C, folic acid, fiber, and calcium, all of which ensure an efficiently running metabolism. The cheeses add a creamy finish to this tasty dish that will leave you feeling good all over.

1 cup (170 g) quinoa

2 tablespoons (28 ml) extra-virgin olive or coconut oil

1 medium red onion, diced

1 tablespoon (10 g) chopped garlic

2 cups (110 g) Swiss chard, roughly chopped

4 cups (284 g) medium-size broccoli florets

1 cup (120 g) grated Cheddar cheese

12 eggs

2 cups (475 ml) whole milk

2 tablespoons (5 g) fresh thyme leaves

½ teaspoon salt, Celtic or sea

Dash of black pepper

¼ cup (25 g) grated Parmesan cheese

Preheat the oven to 350°F (180°C, gas mark 4).

Rinse the quinoa well and set aside to drain. Heat the oil in a pan over medium heat. Add the onion and garlic and sauté until the onion begins to brown, about 8 minutes. Add the Swiss chard and broccoli and sauté for 1 minute, then turn off the heat. Cool slightly. Transfer the mixture to a lightly greased 9- by 13-inch (23- by 33-cm) casserole dish and spread evenly. Sprinkle the Cheddar cheese evenly over the top of the vegetable mixture. Set aside.

In a large bowl, combine the eggs, milk, thyme, salt, pepper, and rinsed quinoa and whisk until thoroughly combined. Pour immediately over the cheese-topped vegetable mixture. Bake the casserole in the oven until cooked through and the top is just starting to brown, about 40 minutes. Remove the casserole from the oven and sprinkle the Parmesan over the top. Return to the oven and bake until the Parmesan is melted and just starting to brown, about 5 more minutes. Let the casserole sit for at least 10 minutes before serving. Serve with a mixed lettuce or spinach salad.

Yield: 6 to 8 servings

Recipe Variation

You can use kale instead of Swiss chard if you wish. Swiss chard eaten raw makes a nice base for smoothies, too, as it tends to be sweeter than kale.

————————[NUTRITIONAL ANALYSIS]————————

Per serving: 360 calories; 19.6 g fat; 20.8 g protein; 22.5 g carbs; 3.9 g fiber; 480.3 mg sodium.

STRENGTHENING SPINACH, FETA, AND RICE CASSEROLE

The feta and rice in this dish provide ample protein and a delicious, creamy texture that explodes with flavor in every mouthful. Spinach is a nutrition superstar that's loaded with fiber, vitamins, and minerals, some of which are hard to find in other foods. You can be certain of getting all your important and heart-healthy nutrients and then some in this dish.

1 cup (180 g) white basmati rice

¾ cup (175 ml) Digestive Vegetable Stock (page 224)

½ cup (75 g) raisins

2 tablespoons (28 g) ghee or coconut oil

1 small red onion, peeled and medium diced

1 tablespoon (10 g) minced garlic

1 teaspoon chopped fresh dill

½ teaspoon salt, Celtic or sea

¼ teaspoon black pepper

1 tablespoon (15 ml) white wine

1 teaspoon fresh lemon or lime juice

4 chops (120 g) chopped spinach

1½ cups (225 g) crumbled feta cheese

2 medium tomatoes, sliced

Preheat the oven to 350°F (180°C, gas mark 4). Lightly grease a 9- by 13-inch (23- by 33-cm) casserole dish and set aside. Rinse and drain the rice. Place the rice in a large pot with a fitted lid, add the stock, and bring to a boil. Reduce the heat to low, cover, and cook until the rice is tender, about 15 minutes. Fluff with a fork and gently mix in the raisins. Cover and set aside.

Heat the ghee or oil in a pan over medium heat. Add the onion and garlic and sauté until the onion is tender, about 5 minutes. Add the dill, salt, pepper, and wine and sauté a few more minutes. Add the lemon or lime juice and spinach and stir until well combined. Remove from the heat and allow to cool. Toss in the feta cheese.

Cover the bottom of the greased casserole dish with the rice mixture. Layer the spinach mixture over the rice. Cover with the tomato slices. Cover with foil and bake until heated through, about 30 to 40 minutes. Serve hot, garnished with extra feta cheese and a drizzle of extra-virgin olive oil, if desired.

Yield: 6 to 8 servings

Note: Spinach contains oxalic acid, which can block the absorption of calcium and iron. Lightly steaming spinach first reduces oxalic acid and makes the minerals more bioavailable to your body.

[NUTRITIONAL ANALYSIS]

Per serving: 234.2 calories; 8.5 g fat; 7.5 g protein; 33 g carbs; 3.5 g fiber; 451.3 mg sodium.

IMMUNE-BOOSTING THAI TEMPEH CAKES WITH SWEET SPICY DIPPING SAUCE

These delicious tempeh cakes are one of my favorite go-to dishes for taste, flavor, and nourishment. They taste just like the ones you would get in a Thai restaurant, only they are healthier. I also like to serve these delicious treats as an appetizer or snack.

1 tablespoon (4 g) lemongrass, fresh or dried

2 cloves garlic, chopped

⅓ cup (50 g) raisins, chopped

4 spring onions, chopped, divided in half

3 chiles, seeded, finely chopped, divided

1 teaspoon finely chopped fresh ginger, peeled

1 tablespoon (6 g) ground coriander

6 tablespoons (6 g) chopped fresh cilantro, divided

2¼ cups (374 g) tempeh, cut into strips

1 tablespoon (15 ml) fresh lime juice

3 tablespoons (21 g) almond flour

1 large egg, lightly beaten

½ teaspoon salt, Celtic or sea

Freshly ground black pepper, to taste

3 tablespoons (45 ml) each coconut oil, mirin, and white wine vinegar

To make the cakes: Place the lemongrass, garlic, raisins, 2 spring onions, 2 chiles, ginger, coriander, and 2 tablespoons (2 g) cilantro into a food processor. Blend into a coarse paste. Add the tempeh and lime juice and blend until combined. Add the almond flour, egg, salt, and pepper and blend again until the mixture forms a coarse, sticky paste.

Divide the mixture into 8 equal parts. Lightly cover your hands in flour to avoid sticking and form the paste into balls. Press the balls to form small cakes. Heat the coconut oil in a large frying pan over medium heat and cook the tempeh cakes for 5 to 6 minutes, turning once, until golden in color. Drain the cakes on paper towels and serve warm with dipping sauce, garnished with chopped cilantro.

To make the sauce: In a small bowl, mix together the mirin, white wine vinegar, and the remaining spring onions, chile, and the cilantro.

Yield: 8 cakes

Recipe Variation

Mirin is a sweet cooking wine made from rice. It is generally available at most supermarkets. You can use sake or sweet sherry instead of the mirin if you like. This recipe was adapted from one of my other books, Foods That Fight Fibromyalgia.

———[**NUTRITIONAL ANALYSIS**]———
Per serving: 201.5 calories; 12.2 g fat; 10.3 g protein; 13 g carbs; 1.3 g fiber; 177.7 mg sodium.

STRESS-LESS SHIITAKE AND ASPARAGUS RISOTTO

Your immune system will get a big boost from this nourishing, succulent, and tender dish, and so will your heart. Apart from their smoky flavor, shiitake mushrooms are known for their ability to lower blood pressure levels as well as their high levels of selenium, vitamin C, protein, and fiber. The addition of asparagus, a known anti-inflammatory vegetable, makes it a powerful duo.

1 teaspoon saffron threads

4 cups (946 ml) Digestive Vegetable Stock (page 224)

1 tablespoon (15 ml) extra-virgin olive oil or coconut oil

1 small onion, chopped

2 cloves garlic, chopped

1 teaspoon dried basil

1 teaspoon chopped fresh basil

2 sprigs fresh thyme

1 teaspoon salt, Celtic or sea

1½ cups (285 g) brown rice

½ cup (120 ml) dry white or red wine

6 asparagus spears, cut into 1-inch (2.5-cm) lengths

1 cup (70 g) sliced shiitake mushrooms

¼ cup (35 g) fresh or frozen peas

1 teaspoon grated lemon zest

1 tablespoon (2.5 g) chopped fresh basil

½ cup (30 g) chopped fresh parsley

Dash of black pepper

Place the saffron and stock in a medium pot and warm over low heat.

In a large pan, heat the oil over medium to high heat and add the onion and garlic until transparent, about 3 to 4 minutes. Add the dry and fresh basil, thyme sprigs, and salt and sauté for about 1 minute. Add the rice and stir and cook for several minutes. Add the wine and stir for 2 minutes. Add the asparagus, mushrooms, and peas and stir them into mixture. Add the saffron and vegetable stock, 1 cup (235 ml) at a time, and stir continuously. Remove the thyme sprigs and cook uncovered, stirring often, until most of the water is absorbed and the rice is thickened and slightly creamy, about 2 to 3 minutes. Add more stock if the rice is dry and needs it. Stir in the lemon zest, fresh basil, parsley, and black pepper. Serve immediately.

Yield: 4 servings

Note: When shopping for mushrooms, look for ones that are firm, ripe, plump, and clean. Avoid ones with wet, slimy spots. Prior to cooking, cleanse them in water and pat them dry with a paper towel so they do not become soggy. Always store fresh mushrooms in the refrigerator to ensure freshness and use them within a couple days of purchase.

[NUTRITIONAL ANALYSIS]

Per serving: 278.1 calories; 4.9 g fat; 7.1 g protein; 50.6 g carbs; 8.2 g fiber; 434.1 mg sodium.

EASY BEEF SAUTÉ WITH FRESH HERBS

Eating beef occasionally, especially when it's grass fed, gives you from two to six times more omega-3s than factory-farmed beef and is only surpassed by the vegetables you add to the dish. This one has got your heart health covered. Enjoy!

- 2 tablespoons (28 ml) extra-virgin olive oil
- 2 cloves garlic, minced
- 1 medium onion, minced
- 1 small chile pepper, minced
- 4 to 6 ounces (115 to 170 g) lean grass-fed beef, chopped into 1- to 2-inch (2.5- to 5-cm) cubes
- 1 cup (120 g) sliced zucchini
- 3 large carrots, sliced
- 8 cremini or shiitake mushrooms, sliced
- 1 large green bell pepper, chopped
- 2 tablespoons (28 ml) tamari
- ½ teaspoon each salt, Celtic or sea, and black pepper
- 2 tablespoons (8 g) chopped fresh parsley

In a skillet over medium-high heat, add the oil and sauté the garlic, onion, and chile pepper until softened, about 5 minutes. Add the beef and cook until tender, about 3 to 5 minutes. Add the remaining ingredients except the parsley. Cook, stirring often, until the vegetables are crisp and tender, about 2 to 3 minutes. Add the fresh parsley at the end. Serve immediately.

Yield: 2 servings

Note: Grass-fed beef contains conjugated linoleic acid (CLA) and the antioxidant vitamin E, both of which support a healthy cardiovascular system. Factory-farmed beef contains significantly lower amounts of these nutrients.

———[**NUTRITIONAL ANALYSIS**]———
Per serving: 374.8 calories; 60.4 g fat; 25.5 g protein; 29.5 g carbs; 6.8 g fiber; 1098.2 mg sodium.

FAVORITE SWEET, SPICY, AND CRUNCHY MEATLOAF

This dish is one of my favorite heartwarming meals. The vegetables ensure you are getting plenty of essential vitamins and minerals, the raisins add a particularly sweet flavor, and the nuts give this meal a crunchy texture.

- **2 tablespoons (28 g) butter or ghee**
- **1 medium onion, chopped**
- **3 cloves garlic, chopped**
- **1 small zucchini, chopped**
- **1 medium carrot, chopped finely**
- **2 stalks celery, chopped finely**
- **¼ cup (18 g) chopped shiitake mushrooms**
- **1 small chile pepper, chopped finely (optional)**
- **1 teaspoon ground turmeric**
- **1 teaspoon ground cumin**
- **1 teaspoon salt, Celtic or sea, divided**
- **½ teaspoon black pepper, divided**
- **1 pound (455 g) lean ground beef, grass fed and organically raised**
- **1 to 2 eggs, beaten**
- **1 tablespoon (15 ml) tamari**
- **½ cup (60 g) roughly chopped walnuts**
- **½ cup (75 g) raisins**
- **4 tablespoons (64 g) unsweetened tomato paste**

Preheat the oven to 350°F (180°C, gas mark 4). Melt the butter or ghee in a large frying pan, add the onion and garlic, and sauté on medium-high heat until the onion softens, about 4 minutes. Add the zucchini, carrot, celery, mushrooms, and chile and cook until they soften and brown, about 5 minutes. Add the turmeric, cumin, half the salt, and half the pepper, then turn the heat off and allow it to cool down to around room temperature (refrigerate to speed up the process if necessary).

In a large bowl, add the beef, eggs, tamari, walnuts, raisins, tomato paste, and remaining salt and pepper and mix together. Then add the cooked vegetables and herbs and blend together well. Transfer the mixture to a greased loaf pan or casserole dish and bake for 30 minutes. Serve hot or cold topped with Spice-It-Up Sweet Chili Sauce (page 272) or tomato sauce.

Yield: 4 servings

Recipe Variation

To increase the fiber in your meat loaf, add ½ cup (85 g) cooked brown rice, lentils, or quinoa. You may need to add an extra egg when you do this so it's moist enough.

————[**NUTRITIONAL ANALYSIS**]————

Per serving: 506.4 calories; 32.9 g fat; 27.5 g protein; 27.4 g carbs; 4.5 g fiber; 907.9 mg sodium.

NICE AND SPICED BEEF OR CHICKEN STIR-FRY

Enjoy the tender and tangy elements of the meat, ginger, and pineapple that cozy up to the hearty, sweet flavor of snow peas in this dish. This meal is nutritious and surprisingly simple, quick, and easy to prepare.

1 tablespoon (15 ml) extra-virgin olive or coconut oil

1 pound (455 g) sirloin or tenderloin, cut into thin 2-inch (5-cm) strips, or 2 chicken breasts, thinly sliced

½ red bell pepper, thinly sliced

1 teaspoon chopped fresh ginger, peeled

¼ teaspoon cayenne pepper

1 cup (155 g) finely chopped pineapple

½ teaspoon hot chile flakes

3 tablespoons (45 ml) fresh lemon juice

2 tablespoons (28 ml) tamari

1 cup (75 g) snow peas, washed and halved

1 green onion, thinly sliced

In a large, nonstick frying pan, heat the oil over medium-high heat. Add the beef or chicken and cook for 3 to 4 minutes, until lightly cooked through. Add the bell pepper, ginger, cayenne, pineapple, chile flakes, lemon juice, tamari, and snow peas. Cook until tender-crisp, about 2 to 3 more minutes. Sprinkle with green onion and serve over rice or with vegetables.

Yield: 4 servings

Note: Snow peas provide us with good amounts of vitamins C and B complex, particularly the critical cardioprotective B vitamin, choline.

Which Foods to Brown?

For meat such as beef, browning is the initial step to a delicious dish; it's an optional step for poultry and pork, and totally unnecessary for fish and seafood. What browning accomplishes is actually enhancing the foods for better flavor.

———[**NUTRITIONAL ANALYSIS**]———
Per serving: 306.1 calories; 12.9 g fat; 36.5 g protein; 10.1 g carbs; 1.8 g fiber; 507.4 mg sodium.

FISHERMAN'S OMEGA-3 FISH FINGERS

High in omega-3 essential fatty acids, this dish has unexpected ginger and turmeric, making it distinctively healthy and delicious. Any kind of greens, particularly sautéed kale or spinach, or a spinach salad with red onions and vinaigrette, makes a great side.

1 pound (455 g) firm, white, deboned fish (mackerel, halibut, or trout)

1 egg

1 teaspoon minced fresh ginger, peeled

¼ teaspoon ground turmeric

½ teaspoon salt, Celtic or sea

½ teaspoon black pepper

1 cup (115 g) almond flour

2 to 3 tablespoons (28 to 45 ml) coconut oil

1 lemon, cut into wedges

Cut the fish into finger lengths. In a small bowl, combine the egg, ginger, turmeric, salt, and pepper. Place the almond flour onto a flat surface. Dip the fish into the egg mixture and then into the almond flour, turning it to cover on all sides.

Heat the oil in a nonstick frying pan over medium to high heat. Place the floured fish fingers into the frying pan and brown lightly until cooked through, about 3 to 4 minutes per side. Serve with a wedge of lemon.

Yield: 4 servings

Note: Apart from their high content of omega-3 essential fatty acids, cold-water varieties of fish, such as mackerel, tuna, salmon, halibut, sardines, and herring, provide other essential nutrients such as coenzyme Q_{10}, selenium, tryptophan, B vitamins, and potassium. All of these nutrients help to support a healthy heart.

Omega-3s Help More Than the Heart

Omega-3 fats lower both blood pressure and triglycerides. They protect the brain and the heart, support circulation, and boost mood. They've been studied for their effects on depression, cardiovascular health, skin, joints, and diabetes. Many studies of behavioral and mood problems have shown a correlation between these issues and low levels of omega-3s. Omega-3s are being studied at Harvard University for their role in combating depression. And a great deal of research has shown that omega-3s are great for the heart.

————————[**NUTRITIONAL ANALYSIS**]————————

Per serving: 431.5 calories; 29 g fat; 37.9 g protein; 7.4 g carbs; 3 g fiber; 326.2 mg sodium.

MEGA-OMEGA SPICE-CRUSTED SALMON

This meal is crunchy on the outside, melt-in-your-mouth delicious on the inside, and ready in just 10 minutes. Pair this dish with our Anti-Ox Pumpkin and Cauliflower Mash (page 264) and Sumptuous Spinach and Swiss Chard with Pine Nuts (page 267) and you'll create a restaurant-style meal that's heart-friendly, too!

1 tablespoon each coriander seeds (6 g), cumin seeds (6 g), and sesame seeds (8 g)

¼ teaspoon dried thyme

1 teaspoon salt, Celtic or sea

½ teaspoon black pepper

4 salmon fillets with skin on one side (about 3 to 4 ounces [85 to 115 g] each)

1 egg white, whisked

1 to 2 tablespoons (15 to 30 ml) coconut oil

Place a dry skillet over medium heat and toast the coriander seeds and cumin seeds, stirring constantly until they become fragrant, about 1 minute. Remove and place in a bowl. Repeat the process with the sesame seeds, remove from the heat, add to the coriander and cumin seeds, and crush with a pestle and mortar. Add the thyme, salt, and pepper and combine.

Dip the skin side of the salmon fillets into the egg white. Press into the spice mixture. Heat the coconut oil in the skillet over high heat and place the fillets into the pan with the seeded side on the oil. Fry for 2 minutes and then turn the heat to low. Flip the fillets and cook on low for up to 8 minutes, depending on how well done you would like them. Serve immediately.

Yield: 4 servings

Note: Farm-raised salmon is inferior in omega-3 essential fatty acid content when compared with wild-caught salmon. We prefer the Vital Choice brand of salmon because it is very high in omega-3s, and we discovered it to be free of harmful mercury and other toxins via independent lab testing. It truly is the best salmon in the world—wild, from Alaska. You can purchase it directly from their website at www.vitalchoice.com.

─────[NUTRITIONAL ANALYSIS]─────
Per serving: 197.2 calories; 10.7 g fat; 25 g protein; 2 g carbs; 1 g fiber; 482.1 mg sodium.

TANTALIZING THAI FISH CAKES

You'll love this delicious variation from regular grilling or baking, high in protein, rich in omega-3s, and bursting with the flavor of mixed Thai spices. The chiles add plenty of heat, so consider adding more or less depending on your palate. I like to pair this dish with Zesty Broccoli with Garlic and Ginger (page 265) or a mixed green salad with Simply Nourishing Salad Dressing (page 217).

¾ pound (340 g) firm, white, deboned fish (mackerel, halibut, or trout)

1 teaspoon chopped red chile peppers

1 tablespoon (20 g) organic honey

1 tablespoon (15 ml) fish sauce

1 tablespoon (1 g) chopped fresh cilantro

1 tablespoon chopped lemongrass

½ cup (50 g) green beans, finely sliced

½ cup (75 g) finely chopped red bell peppers

1 tablespoon (15 ml) coconut oil

Place the fish, chiles, honey, fish sauce, cilantro, and lemongrass in a food processor and process until smooth. Transfer the mixture to a bowl and add the beans and red bell pepper and mix thoroughly. Divide the mixture into 8 balls and shape into flat patties.

Heat the oil in a large frying pan over medium to high heat and add the patties. Fry evenly on each side for about 4 minutes, until golden and cooked through. Serve with Spice-It-Up Sweet Chili Sauce (page 272).

Yield: 8 cakes

Note: The American Heart Association recommends eating fatty fish, such as salmon, herring, sardines, albacore tuna, mackerel, and trout, at least 2 times per week to prevent heart disease, and 3 times per week if you are already at risk for or have heart disease.

How to Make Stock

Save the bones and head of the fish to make a healthy fish stock. It is quick and easy to make and a great standby to have in the freezer as to use as a base for soups and sauces. Wash any fish heads and bones well to remove any trace of blood, place them into a large saucepan, cover with water, add onion, peppercorns, lemon, and a few bay leaves, and simmer for twenty minutes. Remove from heat, strain out the solids, cool, and freeze until needed.

―――――[NUTRITIONAL ANALYSIS]―――――
Per serving: 89.3 calories; 3 g fat; 11.7 g protein; 3.6 g carbs; 0.4 g fiber; 163.4 mg sodium.

SOUL-WARMING TUNA LASAGNA

This tuna lasagna has become a family favorite ever since I started using tuna instead of beef in my lasagna dishes. You can make this dish several days before consuming it, which makes the flavors meld together for a richer flavor. It's a great dish for a dinner party, and there will be plenty left over for seconds, too! Serve it with a mixed green salad with our Simply Nourishing Salad Dressing (page 217).

1 tablespoon (15 ml) extra-virgin olive oil

1 cup (160 g) chopped onion

3 minced cloves garlic

½ cup (50 g) chopped celery

1 cup (130 g) chopped carrots

1 teaspoon fresh or ½ teaspoon dried thyme

1 tablespoon (2.5 g) chopped fresh basil

½ teaspoon salt, Celtic or sea

1 cup (248 g) tomato purée

1 cup (235 ml) Digestive Vegetable Stock (page 224)

1½ cups (270 g) chopped fresh tomatoes

2 cans tuna (7 ounces [195 g] each), in spring water

2 cups (240 g) chopped zucchini, sliced lengthwise

1 teaspoon ground nutmeg

1½ cups (150 g) grated Parmesan cheese, divided in half

Preheat the oven to 350°F (180°C, gas mark 4). Heat the olive oil in a large saucepan over medium to high heat. Add the onion and garlic and cook until tender, about 5 minutes. Add the celery, carrot, thyme, basil, and salt. In a small bowl, combine the tomato puree with the stock and gently add it to the pot, stirring constantly until evenly distributed. Add the tomatoes and tuna and mix in thoroughly.

After a few minutes, add the nutmeg. Pour a small amount of the sauce to cover the bottom of a 9- by 13-inch (23- by 33-cm) baking dish. Add a layer of zucchini slices, pour half of the sauce onto the zucchini layer, and top with half of the Parmesan. Add another layer of zucchini and top with sauce and the remaining cheese. Bake in the oven for about 40 minutes. Remove when cooked and serve immediately. This dish can be frozen and reheated in the oven at a later date.

Yield: 4 to 6 servings

Note: Because tuna fish is high on the food chain, it can contain higher mercury levels than smaller fish. That's why we prefer the canned albacore tuna that Vital Choice sells on its website, which uses only the younger, smaller albacore tuna (14 pounds [6.4 kg] or less) and contains optimal purity, flavor, and omega-3 levels.

—————[NUTRITIONAL ANALYSIS]—————
Per serving: 250.3 calories; 10.8 g fat; 23.6 g protein; 14.8 g carbs; 3.6 g fiber; 811.4 mg sodium.

HEALING BAKED HALIBUT OR SALMON AND SHIITAKE

This dish is simple and easy to prepare and loaded with immune-boosting, heart-healthy nutrients. In addition to adding a pungent, woodsy flavor and meaty texture, shiitake mushrooms provide an impressive array of vitamins and minerals that includes fiber, potassium, magnesium, selenium, zinc, and B complex. You'll love the textures and flavors in this satisfying dish.

1 tablespoon (14 g) butter

1 cup (70 g) chopped shiitake mushrooms

4 fillets salmon or halibut (4 ounces [115 g] each)

2 tablespoons (28 ml) fresh lemon or lime juice

1 tablespoon (14 g) butter, melted

1 tablespoon (7 g) almond flour

1 teaspoon ground paprika

1 teaspoon salt, Celtic or sea

½ teaspoon black pepper

1 tablespoon (4 g) chopped fresh parsley

Preheat the oven to 350°F (180°C, gas mark 4). In a small to medium pan, melt 1 tablespoon (14 g) butter over medium heat and toss in the shiitake mushrooms. Cook until just softened, about 2 to 3 minutes.

Place the fish fillets in a buttered baking dish. Pour the lemon or lime juice over them and brush with the melted butter. Pour the shiitake mushrooms over the top, sprinkle on the almond flour, and coat evenly. Sprinkle on the paprika, salt, and pepper and bake for 15 to 20 minutes, or until the fish is almost cooked.

Turn the heat to broil. Place under the broiler for about 1 minute until the flour browns. Sprinkle with fresh parsley and serve immediately.

Yield: 4 servings

Note: Dry-heat methods such as baking, broiling, and grilling work well for fattier fish such as halibut and salmon.

———————[NUTRITIONAL ANALYSIS]———————

Per serving: 291.2 calories; 18.6 g fat; 24 g protein; 5.5 g carbs; 1.1 g fiber; 402.2 mg sodium.

SPICY SHRIMP AND TOMATO KEBABS WITH HERBED LIMA BEANS

These shrimp kebabs are easy to make and bursting with flavor and goodness. Shrimp is an excellent source of protein and contains a variety of heart-healthy nutrients that include omega-3s, magnesium, selenium, tryptophan, choline, zinc, and B-complex vitamins. The herbed lima beans complement the flavorful kebabs nicely with added fiber and minerals.

1½ pounds (670 g) large, raw, uncooked shrimp, peeled, deveined, and cut in half

2 cups (300 g) cherry tomatoes

8 small cloves garlic, unpeeled

1 lemon, cut into 8 pieces

4 tablespoons (50 ml) extra-virgin olive oil, divided

1 teaspoon salt, Celtic or sea, divided

½ teaspoon black pepper, divided

1 can (15 ounces [425 g]) lima beans, rinsed

1 teaspoon chopped fresh sage

1 teaspoon chopped fresh basil

1 tablespoon (4 g) chopped fresh parsley

Soak 8 wooden skewers in water for about 15 minutes. In a medium bowl, combine the shrimp, tomatoes, garlic, lemon, 2 tablespoons (28 ml) of the oil, ³/₄ teaspoon of the salt, and ¼ teaspoon of the pepper.

Turn the broiler on. Thread the shrimp, tomatoes, garlic, and lemon pieces on the skewers and broil, turning occasionally, until the shrimp is cooked through and the lemon wedges are lightly charred, about 5 to 7 minutes.

Meanwhile, heat the remaining 2 tablespoons (28 ml) oil in a small saucepan over medium heat. Add the lima beans, sage, basil, and parsley, and the remaining salt and pepper. Cook, tossing occasionally, until the beans are warm and covered with the herbs, about 2 to 3 minutes. Serve with the kebabs.

Yield: 4 servings

Note: These kebabs can be assembled ahead of time and stored for up to 12 hours in the refrigerator. Simply reheat them in the oven for about 15 to 20 minutes at 275°F (140°C, gas mark 1) before serving.

[NUTRITIONAL ANALYSIS]

Per serving: 462.5 calories; 17.7 g fat; 43.6 g protein; 33.4 g carbs; 9.7 g fiber; 718.7 mg sodium.

MIGHTY MOROCCAN CHICKEN TAGINE

This healthy and traditional North African favorite requires minimal work and features braised chicken seasoned with fragrant spices and dried fruits. Its flavorsome, sweet sauce combines nicely and tenderizes the chicken, which just melts in your mouth. Feel free to add other vegetables such as cauliflower, carrots, tomatoes, or broccoli to increase its goodness.

1 tablespoon (15 ml) coconut oil

1 clove garlic, minced

1½ cups (240 g) diced onion

1 cup (150 g) chopped red bell pepper

1 teaspoon minced fresh ginger, peeled

2 pounds (910 g) chicken pieces, skin and bones removed

1 teaspoon each ground turmeric, coriander, cumin, and black pepper

2 cups (475 ml) Nutritive Chicken Stock (page 223)

⅔ cup (87 g) chopped dried apricots

½ cup (75 g) raisins

⅔ cup (117 g) prunes, pits removed

1 tablespoon (7 g) ground cinnamon

1½ tablespoons (10 g) almond flour

½ cup (55 g) slivered almonds

Melt the oil in a large pot over high heat and sauté the garlic and onion until soft, about 4 minutes. Add the bell pepper and ginger and sauté for about 2 more minutes, until soft. Add the chicken, turmeric, coriander, cumin, and black pepper and pour in the chicken stock. Half cover with a lid, turn the heat down, and cook for about 30 minutes. Add the apricots, raisins, prunes, cinnamon, and almond flour and cook for a further 15 minutes. In a small, dry pan, toast the slivered almonds. Serve decorated with the toasted almonds. This dish is delicious served with Luscious Lima Bean Mash or Anti-Ox Pumpkin and Cauliflower Mash.

Yield: 4 servings

Note: Tagine, which is often served with couscous, is traditionally cooked in an earthenware pot, also called a tagine, but you can use a heavy lidded pan or slow cooker if you don't have a tagine.

———[**NUTRITIONAL ANALYSIS**]———

Per serving: 655.2 calories; 16.9 g fat; 66.4 g protein; 61 g carbs; 8.9 g fiber; 890.5 mg sodium.

METABOLISM-BOOSTING CHICKEN CURRY FEAST

Because of its combination of spices, this traditional Indian dish has numerous health benefits, including the ability to stimulate your metabolism to feel full quicker, so you eat less and lose weight. Turmeric is one of the main spices used in curry, which also gives it the yellow pigment that brightens up most curry dishes. Coriander, small red or green chiles, cumin, ginger, and onion are also common ingredients in curry and burst with vital nutrients to keep your metabolism running efficiently.

3 tablespoons (45 ml) coconut oil or ghee

2 cups (320 g) finely chopped onion

4 cloves garlic, minced

2 teaspoons minced fresh ginger, peeled

1 teaspoon ground turmeric

1 small red or green chile pepper, minced

1 tablespoon (6 g) ground coriander

1 teaspoon ground cumin

½ teaspoon ground fennel

2 teaspoons ground paprika

1 teaspoon salt, Celtic or sea

2 tablespoons (28 ml) apple cider vinegar

2½ pounds (1.1 kg) chicken thighs, deboned, cut into chunks

2 medium tomatoes, peeled and chopped

5 cardamom pods

1 stick cinnamon

1 stalk lemongrass, minced

1 cup (235 ml) coconut milk

Heat the oil or ghee in a large frying pan or wok over medium heat. Add the onions, garlic, and ginger and cook until the onions are golden and tender, about 5 minutes. Add the turmeric, chile, coriander, cumin, fennel, paprika, salt, and vinegar and stir until well combined. Add the chicken and stir until it is thoroughly coated with the spices. Add the tomatoes, cardamom, cinnamon, and lemongrass and cover. Cook over medium heat for 45 minutes. Remove the lid and add the coconut milk. Stir and cook uncovered for 2 minutes.

Serve with Balancing Basmati Almond Rice (page 266), Antioxidant Ginger, Date, and Orange Chutney (page 275), and Restorative Cucumber-Yogurt Raita (page 277).

Yield: 4 servings

Note: Studies have shown that turmeric, one of the main spices in curry, almost completely prevented joint swelling in rats with arthritis.

———————[**NUTRITIONAL ANALYSIS**]———————
Per serving: 232.6 calories; 16.7 g fat; 7.7 g protein; 13.2 g carbs; 2.2 g fiber; 390.5 mg sodium.

TANTALIZING CHICKEN SATAY WITH POWERFUL PEANUT-COCONUT SAUCE

Succulent and full of flavor, this Thai-style chicken satay is marinated in a tasty, nutrient-dense peanut-coconut sauce, which is the perfect complement to chicken. Even more, this is simple and easy to make and will explode with flavor in your mouth.

1 pound (455 g) chicken breast

½ cup (120 ml) coconut milk

1 tablespoon (15 ml) fish sauce

2 teaspoons red curry paste

1 teaspoon ground turmeric

1 teaspoon organic honey

2 tablespoons (2 g) chopped fresh cilantro

½ teaspoon salt, Celtic or sea

¼ teaspoon black pepper

1 tablespoon (15 ml) coconut oil

Chop the chicken into 2-inch (5-cm) strips. Place the coconut milk, fish sauce, curry paste, turmeric, honey, cilantro, salt, and pepper in a large bowl and combine well. Add the chicken, cover, and let marinate in the refrigerator for at least 1 hour.

Thread the chicken strips onto 8 skewers. Heat the oil in a large frying pan over medium to high heat and cook the chicken for about 7 minutes, turning them halfway through. They should be lightly browned and cooked through. Top them with Punchy Peanut-Coconut Sauce (page 272) and serve over Balancing Basmati Almond Rice (page 266).

Yield: 4 servings

Note: These satays also make a great starter for your meal or may be served as finger food when you are expecting guests. You can make them a day in advance and reheat them in the oven for several minutes before serving.

———————[NUTRITIONAL ANALYSIS]———————

Per serving: 280.2 calories; 13.7 g fat; 34.9 g protein; 4.7 g carbs; 0.5 g fiber; 567.6 mg sodium.

SUPERCHARGED CHICKEN OR TURKEY MEATLOAF

This dish is a family favorite and supereasy to prepare. It provides plenty of protein and vitamin- and mineral-rich veggies. The turmeric and cumin give it a decidedly bold flavor and marry nicely with the raisins. The walnuts are loaded with omega-3s and add a delicious, crunchy texture. This meat loaf pairs nicely with steamed asparagus, broccoli, or cauliflower and tastes great with Spice-It-Up Sweet Chili Sauce (page 272) or Antioxidant BBQ Sauce (page 274) on top.

1 tablespoon (14 g) butter or coconut oil

1 pound (455 g) minced or ground chicken or turkey

2 cloves garlic, minced

1 teaspoon grated fresh ginger, peeled

1 teaspoon ground turmeric

1 teaspoon ground cumin

2 eggs

¾ cup (83 g) grated peeled carrots

1 cup (150 g) finely chopped red bell pepper

½ cup (75 g) raisins

½ cup (60 g) walnuts, roughly chopped

Preheat the oven to 350°F (180°C, gas mark 4). Grease a 4- by 8-inch (10- by 20-cm) loaf pan or casserole dish with butter or coconut oil.

Place the chicken or turkey, garlic, ginger, turmeric, cumin, and eggs in a large bowl and blend together using your hands or a large wooden spoon. Mix in the carrots and bell pepper. Add the raisins and walnuts and mix together. Pack the ingredients into the greased oven dish and bake in the oven for 40 minutes, until the loaf is cooked through and golden on top. Remove from the oven and let stand for 10 minutes. Cut into slices and serve.

Yield: 4 servings

Note: It's always best to choose certified organic ground turkey and chicken, as these are a source of other important nutrients, such as vitamin C, iron, magnesium, and phosphorus, based on the organic diet that was fed to the animals.

―――――[NUTRITIONAL ANALYSIS]―――――
Per serving: 506 calories; 30.4 g fat; 38 g protein; 21.5 g carbs; 3.4 g fiber; 197 mg sodium.

ANTI-INFLAMMATORY TURMERIC TURKEY BURGERS

Enjoy the delicious combination of herbs and spices in these flavorful burgers that pack a punch of powerful, nutrient-dense compounds. Turmeric has more positive qualities than any other spice, particularly when it comes to anti-inflammatory antioxidants. The active compound in turmeric is curcumin, which has been shown to prevent the oxidation of cholesterol and plaque buildup in the body that can lead to cardiovascular disease. Turmeric reduces fat in the liver, which in turn helps the liver metabolize other fats that have accumulated there, perhaps from excess sugars and refined carbohydrates.

1 pound (455 g) ground turkey, preferably organic

1 small onion, chopped

2 eggs, beaten

½ cup (75 g) raisins (optional)

2 tablespoons (14 g) ground turmeric

1 or 2 cloves garlic, minced

1 teaspoon chopped fresh ginger, peeled

1 teaspoon ground cumin

½ teaspoon salt, Celtic or sea

Pinch of black pepper

Dash of cayenne pepper (optional)

1 tablespoon (15 ml) extra-virgin olive or coconut oil

2 teaspoons tamari

These burgers can be grilled or baked. If baking, preheat the oven to 350°F (180°C, gas mark 4). Combine all the ingredients in a large bowl and mix well. Divide the mixture into 6 pieces, shape into burger patties, and place on an oiled baking sheet. Bake for 20 minutes, or until cooked through. The burgers should reach an internal temperature of 165°F. If grilling, place on the heat and cook for about 4 minutes, until browned on one side, then flip over and cook for about 2 to 3 minutes, or until cooked through.

Serve the burgers on buns or alone and with toppings of your choice. The Antioxidant BBQ Sauce (page 274) goes well and tastes delicious with these burgers!

Yield: 6 burgers

Note: Turmeric is the powder of a rhizome. It looks like yellow ginger and is part of curry powder, but it is not curry. For the most curcumin, use turmeric rather than curry powder. Try to select organically grown turmeric to ensure against irradiation. Store turmeric powder in a tightly sealed container in a cool, dark, and dry place.

[NUTRITIONAL ANALYSIS]

Per serving: 265.8 calories; 14 g fat; 23.7 g protein; 11.2 g carbs; 0.7 g fiber; 328.5 mg sodium.

GET-UP-AND-GO INDIAN CHICKPEA DELIGHT

Enjoy the buttery, nutlike taste of chickpeas (aka garbanzo beans) along with an aromatic blend of heart-healthy spices in this nourishing Middle Eastern dish. Chickpeas are an excellent source of fiber, manganese, and folate as well as providing ample amounts of protein. I often make this dish to nosh on as a snack or to accompany my raw salad at lunchtime.

- **1 tablespoon (14 g) ghee or coconut oil**
- **½ medium red onion, chopped**
- **2 cloves garlic, minced**
- **2 teaspoons minced fresh ginger, peeled**
- **1½ teaspoons each coriander, cumin, and chili powder**
- **½ teaspoon each ground cardamom, cloves, and nutmeg**
- **1 teaspoon ground cinnamon**
- **1 teaspoon ground turmeric**
- **2 cups (480 g) crushed tomatoes**
- **½ teaspoon each salt, Celtic or sea, and black pepper**
- **2 cups (328 g) cooked chickpeas, or use canned**
- **1½ cups (355 ml) coconut milk**
- **2 tablespoons (2 g) chopped fresh cilantro**

Heat the ghee or oil in a sauté pan over medium-high heat. Add the onion, garlic, and ginger and cook until softened, about 5 minutes. Add the coriander, cumin, chili powder, cardamom, cloves, nutmeg, cinnamon, and turmeric and sauté for 1 minute. Reduce the heat to medium-low, add the tomatoes, salt, and pepper, and simmer gently for about 25 minutes.

Transfer the mixture to a blender and purée until smooth. Return the purée to the pan, add the chickpeas and coconut milk, and simmer until heated through, about 5 to 8 minutes. Garnish with cilantro. Serve immediately.

Yield: 4 servings

Note: Unlike most other canned vegetables, chickpeas lose very little nutrients when canned. Just be sure to rinse them well with filtered water after removing them from the can.

[NUTRITIONAL ANALYSIS]

Per serving: 400 calories; 19.3 g fat; 9.7 g protein; 44.6 g carbs; 7.9 g fiber; 887.7 mg sodium.

FRAGRANT CAULIFLOWER-QUINOA RISOTTO

This combination of nutritional superstars is a balanced meal all in itself. Quinoa contains all nine essential amino acids that are the building blocks of protein, fiber, and the minerals manganese and magnesium. Cauliflower is loaded with antioxidant nutrients C, K, and B complex to boost detoxification and support a healthy heart. The spices add a rich, pungent flavor and nutritional kick.

1 tablespoon (15 ml) coconut oil

1 medium leek, diced

1 clove garlic, minced

1 teaspoon minced fresh ginger, peeled

½ teaspoon ground cumin

¼ teaspoon ground nutmeg

4 cups (400 g) cauliflower, cut into small florets

1½ tablespoons (22 g) Bone-Strengthening Lemon Tahini (page 271)

1½ cups (355 ml) Digestive Vegetable Stock (page 104)

1½ cups (255 g) cooked quinoa

1 teaspoon lemon juice

½ teaspoon salt, Celtic or sea

Dash of black pepper

2 tablespoons (2 g) chopped fresh cilantro

Heat the oil in a large frying pan over medium heat. Add the leek and garlic and sauté for about 2 minutes, until they wilt. Add the ginger, cumin, and nutmeg and mix for about 1 minute. Stir in the cauliflower, then cook the mixture for about 5 minutes to remove some of the moisture and soften, stirring occasionally. While the cauliflower is cooking, whisk together the tahini and vegetable stock in a medium bowl.

When the cauliflower is cooked, add the quinoa to the pan and pour in the whisked vegetable broth mixture. Mix together well. Bring the risotto to a simmer and cook until all the excess liquid has evaporated, about 5 minutes. Remove from the heat and stir in the lemon juice, salt, and pepper. Sprinkle with cilantro and serve immediately.

Yield: 4 servings

Note: One cup of dry quinoa yields about 3 cups of cooked quinoa. Rinse quinoa well in a mesh strainer before cooking, as this removes the natural bitterness of its outer coating.

———————[**NUTRITIONAL ANALYSIS**]———————

Per serving: 239.7 calories; 8.1 g fat; 8.3 g protein; 37 g carbs; 7.6 g fiber; 241.9 mg sodium.

LUSCIOUS LIMA BEAN MASH

Make the most of the delicate, buttery flavor of fresh lima beans in this mellow, mouthwatering mash. Better than traditional mashed potatoes, this preparation provides more nutrients such as protein, fiber, magnesium, iron, and folate and works wonders on the digestive system. You'll love the flavorful spices in it and probably come back for seconds.

1 cup (156 g) dried lima beans

1 cup (235 ml) Digestive Vegetable Stock (page 224)

½ cup (120 ml) filtered water

1 clove garlic, minced

½ teaspoon salt, Celtic or sea

½ teaspoon black pepper

2 tablespoons (28 ml) extra-virgin olive oil

1½ tablespoons (9 g) fennel seeds

2 tablespoons (8 g) chopped fresh parsley

½ lemon, juiced

1 tablespoon grated lemon rind

Soak the lima beans overnight in filtered water. Next morning, discard the water and rinse the beans well. Place the beans in a medium-size pot and cover with vegetable stock and filtered water. Bring to a boil and simmer for up to 2 hours, until the beans have softened. Drain and place into a food processor, adding the garlic, salt, pepper, oil, fennel, parsley, and lemon juice. Process until smooth. Serve with grated lemon zest sprinkled on top.

Yield: 4 servings

Note: Lima beans are excellent for energy and keeping blood sugar levels balanced. This is due mainly to their high fiber content, which prevents blood sugar levels from rising too fast and provides slow-burning energy.

Recipe Substitution

You can use fava beans, also known as broad beans, in place of the lima beans in this recipe. Fava beans provide adequate amounts of folate, selenium, manganese, potassium, and vitamin K, all of which support heart health.

—————[**NUTRITIONAL ANALYSIS**]—————

Per serving: 200.8 calories; 7.5 g fat; 10 g protein; 30.2 g carbs; 10.6 g fiber; 194 mg sodium.

VEGETABLES, GRAINS & BEANS ON THE SIDE

ANTI-OX PUMPKIN AND CAULIFLOWER MASH

Smooth, sweet, and rich in phytonutrients and antioxidants, this succulent combination is the perfect addition to any meal. Butternut squash and pumpkins are abundant in nutrients known as carotenoids, which are amazingly beneficial for overall cardiovascular health. Cauliflower has a mild flavor and is an excellent source of vitamin C, K, folate, and fiber.

3 cups (420 g) diced butternut squash, peeled

2 cups (200 g) cauliflower, cut into large florets

3 tablespoons (42 g) butter or ghee

¼ cup (30 g) grated Cheddar cheese

1 teaspoon salt, Celtic or sea

1 teaspoon black pepper

2 tablespoons (18 g) pumpkin seeds

2 tablespoons (8 g) chopped fresh parsley

Place the butternut squash in a large saucepan, cover with water, and bring to a boil. Add the cauliflower and let simmer for about 5 minutes, or until both vegetables are soft. Transfer to a food processor, add the butter or ghee, cheese, salt, pepper, and pumpkin seeds and process until smooth. Garnish with fresh parsley and serve immediately.

Yield: 4 servings

Note: Add an Italian taste to this dish by using Parmesan cheese instead of Cheddar. You can also sprinkle a little over the top and place under the broiler for a minute or two to brown on top.

Pumpkin—the Potassium Heavyweight

Pumpkin is a nutritious but overlooked vegetable that is ridiculously low in calories while very high in potassium and vitamin A. Pumpkin is actually a potassium heavyweight, more so than even bananas. One 49-calorie cup of mashed pumpkin contains a whopping 564 mg of the stuff.

Why should you care? Let us count the ways! Several large epidemiological studies suggest that increased potassium intake is associated with a decreased risk of stroke. Four large studies have reported significant associations between dietary potassium and bone mineral density. And a number of studies have shown that people who eat a lot of potassium have lower blood pressure than people who don't.

---————[**NUTRITIONAL ANALYSIS**]————

Per serving: 284.8 calories; 11.1 g fat; 2.9 g protein; 15.8 g carbs; 4.3 g fiber; 350.8 mg sodium.

SAUTÉED SHIITAKE MUSHROOMS WITH A KALE KICK

The rich, buttery, meaty flavor and chewy texture of shiitake mushrooms pair nicely with the earthy-flavored kale. Shiitakes are high in B-complex vitamins, protein, fiber, and numerous minerals, and are well known for their effective immune-strengthening qualities. Kale is considered to be one of the healthiest vegetables around because of its antioxidants and high mineral content. This is medicinal food at its best.

- 2 tablespoons (28 g) butter
- 2 cloves garlic, minced
- 2 cups (140 g) shiitake mushrooms, sliced
- 1 teaspoon salt, Celtic or sea
- ½ teaspoon black pepper
- 2 cups (110 g) kale, chopped
- ¼ cup (60 ml) dry red wine

Melt the butter in a medium saucepan over medium heat. Add the garlic and cook for about 1 minute, or until soft. Add the mushrooms, salt, and pepper and sauté for about 5 minutes. Add the kale and red wine and cook for about 3 minutes longer. Serve immediately.

Yield: 4 servings

Note: This recipe can be served as a side dish or as a topping over chicken, fish, venison, or beef.

ZESTY BROCCOLI WITH GARLIC AND GINGER

Delicious, tender broccoli florets flavored with orange zest and garlic, served as a side dish and ready in a snap. High in antioxidant vitamins and minerals, broccoli is one vegetable you'll want to include in your diet on a regular basis.

- 2 tablespoons (28 g) butter or ghee
- 1 clove garlic, minced
- 1 teaspoon chopped fresh ginger, peeled
- 3 cups (213 g) broccoli, cut into small florets
- ½ teaspoon salt, Celtic or sea
- ½ teaspoon black pepper
- 1 teaspoon grated orange zest

Melt the butter or ghee in a medium saucepan over medium heat. Add the garlic and ginger and cook for about 1 minute, or until soft. Add the broccoli, salt, and pepper and sauté for about 5 minutes, until the broccoli is softened. Add the orange zest at the end and mix in. Serve immediately.

Yield: 4 servings

Note: Broccoli is a good source of minerals such as manganese, magnesium, calcium, selenium, zinc, iron, and phosphorus.

———[NUTRITIONAL ANALYSIS]———
Per serving: 115.7 calories; 6.1 g fat; 2 g protein; 13.2 g carbs; 2.1 g fiber; 343.2 mg sodium.

———[NUTRITIONAL ANALYSIS]———
Per serving: 70.9 calories; 6 g fat; 2.1 g protein; 3.8 g carbs; 2 g fiber; 183.8 mg sodium.

BALANCING BASMATI ALMOND RICE

This fragrant and savory Indian-style rice dish flavored with spices and fresh vegetables is almost a meal in itself. It's easy to digest and is chock-full of fiber, B vitamins, and iron. It goes well with Indian curry or dal (lentils).

- **1 cup (180 g) brown basmati rice**
- **¼ cup (48 g) brown rice**
- **1 cup (235 ml) Digestive Vegetable Stock (page 224)**
- **1 cup (235 ml) filtered water**
- **½ cup each carrots (65 g), zucchini (62 g), and green bell peppers (75 g), all chopped**
- **½ teaspoon salt, Celtic or sea**
- **2 tablespoons (28 ml) extra-virgin olive oil**
- **½ teaspoon cumin seeds**
- **¼ teaspoon black pepper**
- **Pinch each of ground nutmeg and cinnamon**
- **½ cup (72 g) roasted almonds, chopped**
- **¾ cup (45 g) chopped fresh parsley**
- **Dash of cayenne pepper (optional)**

Wash and drain the rice. In a medium-size pot, combine the rice, stock, water, carrots, zucchini, bell peppers, and salt and bring to a boil. Reduce to low heat and simmer, covered, for 20 minutes, or until the rice is soft and the liquids are absorbed.

In a small skillet, melt the olive oil over medium heat and sauté the cumin seeds for 30 seconds. Stir in the pepper, nutmeg, and cinnamon. Add the spice mixture to the cooked rice and vegetables and mix together with a fork. Stir in the almonds, parsley, and cayenne, if using. Serve immediately.

Yield: 4 servings

Note: Because basmati is refined white rice that has been stripped of its bran layer, mixing basmati rice with brown rice ensures that you get the benefits of more fiber in your diet.

——————[**NUTRITIONAL ANALYSIS**]——————
Per serving: 327.5 calories; 13.9 g fat; 8.5 g protein; 45.1 g carbs; 4.6 g fiber; 206.1 mg sodium.

SUMPTUOUS SPINACH AND SWISS CHARD WITH PINE NUTS

A staple of the Mediterranean diet, Swiss chard and spinach are about as good as it gets when it comes to heart-healthy nutrients. They are loaded with antioxidants for strengthening your heart, nourishing your cells, and even reversing aging. The pine nuts add a nice crunch and help bring out the vegetable flavors. You'll enjoy every bite of this tasty dish that's oh-so easy to make!

2 tablespoons (28 ml) extra-virgin olive oil, coconut oil, or ghee

2 small shallots or 2 cloves garlic, minced

4 cups (210 g) Swiss chard, chopped

8 cups (240 g) baby spinach

¼ cup (35 g) toasted pine nuts

Dash salt, Celtic or sea

Heat the oil or ghee in a large frying pan over medium heat. Add the shallots or garlic and sauté for a minute or two, until translucent. Add the Swiss chard and sauté for 2 more minutes. Add the spinach and stir until wilted. Stir in the toasted pine nuts and salt. Serve immediately.

Yield: 4 servings

Note: Pine nuts are a great source of monounsaturated fats, as well as ample amounts of vitamins E and K and the minerals iron, copper, and manganese, all of which help support the cardiovascular system.

Swiss Chard: Low-Cal Superfood

Chard is a member of the goosefoot family of plants. It's a relative of beets, and it comes in both red and white varieties. The red kind is a standout in supermarkets. It's very quick cooking—like spinach—so for goodness sake don't overcook it, or you'll compromise its nutritional value.

Speaking of nutritional value, this vegetable is nothing short of a powerhouse. A cup of cooked chard gives you almost 4 grams of fiber (!), more than 100 mg of calcium, an almost unbelievable 961 mg of potassium, and more than 10,000 IUs of vitamin A. And all this for about 35 calories. Talk about a superfood!

—————[**NUTRITIONAL ANALYSIS**]—————

Per serving: 174.4 calories; 13 g fat; 6.5 g protein; 11.8 g carbs; 6 g fiber; 437 mg sodium.

CARDIOPROTECTIVE GREEN BEANS

These are crunchy, buttery, and lightly steamed to bring out their peak flavor. Green beans are loaded with heart-healthy minerals, potassium, and calcium.

4 cups (400 g) green beans, cut into 1-inch (2.5-cm) pieces

1 teaspoon finely chopped fresh ginger, peeled

½ teaspoon salt, Celtic or sea

1 teaspoon butter or extra-virgin olive oil

1 tablespoon (15 ml) fresh lemon or lime juice

3 tablespoons (21 g) slivered, roasted almonds

4 tablespoons finely chopped fresh parsley (16 g) or cilantro (4 g)

Place the beans in a medium bowl, add the ginger and salt, and mix lightly. Place the beans in a steamer on medium to high heat and cook for 7 to 10 minutes, until bright green and still crisp. Remove from the heat and place in a serving dish. Add the butter or oil and let it melt into the beans. Toss with lemon or lime juice and sprinkle with almonds and parsley or cilantro.

Yield: 4 servings

Note: If you are unable to obtain fresh green beans, use frozen, because they will still retain at least 90 percent of their B vitamins.

SUSTAINING GINGER-SESAME CARROTS

Carrots are loaded with beta-carotene and vitamin C, both antioxidants that strengthen arterial walls and contribute to heart health. Sesame seeds are a good source of calcium to build strong bones and of B vitamins, which are essential to the health of red blood cells and support your body's ability to derive energy from food. The ginger adds not only a special flavor and zest, it also helps improve digestion.

1 tablespoon (15 ml) sesame oil

4 medium carrots, peeled and cut diagonally

1 tablespoon (6 g) finely chopped fresh ginger, peeled

1½ teaspoons salt, Celtic or sea

1 tablespoon (8 g) sesame seeds

Heat the sesame oil in a medium pan, add the carrots, and sauté for 3 minutes. Add the ginger and salt and cook for about 15 minutes on low heat, or until tender. Transfer to a serving dish and sprinkle with sesame seeds.

Yield: 4 servings

Note: To add more variety and nutrition to this dish, include green beans along with carrots.

───────[NUTRITIONAL ANALYSIS]───────

Per serving: 84 calories; 4 g fat; 3.3 g protein; 9.7 g carbs; 4.8 g fiber; 205.1 mg sodium.

───────[NUTRITIONAL ANALYSIS]───────

Per serving: 69.3 calories; 4.5 g fat; 1.1 g protein; 6.6 g carbs; 2 g fiber; 207.4 mg sodium.

· NOURISHING · ACCOMPANIMENTS
AND MENU ENHANCEMENTS

Your heart-healthy menu would not be complete without a set of team-player foods and dishes that contribute a complementary blend of nutritional attributes and synergy in the form of condiments, sauces, preserves, and fermented foods. I included these dishes as much for their flavor as their nutrient-dense beneficial qualities. The recipes in this section comprise an extraordinary collection of culinary superstars you'll want to keep on hand to enhance your flavorful and nutritive experience. Enjoy the condiments alongside your favorite vegetables, smeared over crackers, wraps, and sandwiches, or added to salads, meats, and fish. Fermented foods provide a healthy dose of friendly bacteria known as probiotics to strengthen both your immunity and digestion. You'll find a pleasing array of antioxidant-laden sauces to enjoy with many of the other dishes in this book. Last but not least, I've included several of my favorite preserves that are simply scrumptious, irresistibly good for your health, and easy to make.

MEDITERRANEAN BLACK OLIVE TAPENADE

This bold, zesty, Mediterranean-inspired, and nutritious dip is loaded with essential fatty acids, vitamins E and C, as well as amino acids and protein, all of which support a healthy heart. It can be enjoyed as a delicious pasta sauce, too.

1 cup (100 g) pitted black kalamata olives

1 clove garlic, minced

1 teaspoon Dijon mustard

1 teaspoon fresh lemon or lime juice

2 tablespoons (6 g) dulse flakes

1 tablespoon (15 ml) extra-virgin olive oil

¼ cup (60 ml) filtered water

1 tablespoon (8 g) walnuts

½ teaspoon grated lemon zest

Place all the ingredients in a food processor and puree. Transfer to a small bowl and let stand for at least 20 minutes to allow the flavors to meld together and develop. Spread over Low-Carb Herbed Cheddar Crackers (page 229) and vegetables or use in sandwiches and wraps.

Yield: ⅔ cup

Note: Black olives help stimulate the production of hydrochloric acid in the stomach, which is vital for digestion and breaking down food.

SUPER-HEALTHFUL HUMMUS

This creamy, fiber-filled dip goes especially well with crackers and raw vegetables or can be used as a spread in sandwiches or wraps. Garbanzo beans, affectionately known as chickpeas, are high in folate, tryptophan, iron, and antioxidants and are a good source of plant protein.

2 cups (328 g) cooked garbanzo beans

2 cloves garlic, minced

2 tablespoons (18 g) sunflower seeds

2 tablespoons (30 g) Bone-Strengthening Lemon Tahini (page 271)

⅓ cup (80 ml) fresh lemon or lime juice

1 small celery stalk, chopped

½ teaspoon ground paprika

¾ teaspoon salt, Celtic or sea

1 tablespoon (15 ml) extra-virgin olive oil

Dash of cayenne pepper

Place all the ingredients in a food processor and blend until smooth and creamy. Transfer to a bowl and serve. This will keep in the refrigerator for up to 1 week.

Yield: About 2 cups

Note: Use a dollop of healthy hummus in place of mayonnaise—it will add more protein and fiber and keep you feeling satisfied longer, which can aid in weight loss.

────[NUTRITIONAL ANALYSIS]────

Per tablespoon: 13.8 calories; 1.2 g fat; 0.1 g protein; 0.2 g carbs; 0.1 g fiber; 34.2 mg sodium.

────[NUTRITIONAL ANALYSIS]────

Per tablespoon: 40.6 calories; 1.7 g fat; 1.3 g protein; 5.3 g carbs; 1.1 g fiber; 123.3 mg sodium.

BONE-STRENGTHENING LEMON TAHINI

As far as health foods go, there aren't many that are as versatile or that pack the same nutritional punch as this tasty tahini. It is loaded with heart-healthy nutrients such as calcium and almost a full profile of B-complex vitamins for helping you strengthen bones and reduce stress.

- **1 cup (240 g) raw tahini**
- **¼ cup (60 ml) lemon juice**
- **¼ cup (60 ml) extra-virgin olive oil**
- **½ cup (120 ml) filtered water**
- **½ teaspoon salt, Celtic or sea**
- **1 clove garlic, minced**
- **1 teaspoon chopped cilantro**
- **Dash of cayenne pepper (optional)**
- **½ cup (72 g) sesame seeds**

in a quart-size jar, combine the tahini, lemon juice, olive oil, and water and thoroughly stir together. Stir in the salt, garlic, cilantro, and cayenne, if using. In a medium skillet over medium heat, toast the sesame seeds for 5 minutes, or until golden brown. Do not let them burn. Transfer the sesame seeds to a food processor and blend until coarsely ground. Stir the sesame seeds into the tahini mixture. Serve as a dip for veggies or with Low-Carb Herbed Cheddar Crackers (page 229). Store in the refrigerator.

Yield: About 2 cups (480 g)

Note: Turn this dip into a salad dressing by adding more water until you reach the desired consistency.

HEART-HEALTHY ALMOND MAYONNAISE

A healthy, delicious homemade mayonnaise recipe is something for every health-conscious person to have up their sleeve, or in their refrigerator! This one is loaded with vitamin E for your healthy heart, and numerous essential minerals. Plus, you won't believe how much better it tastes than the store-bought kind.

- **2 egg yolks**
- **2 tablespoons (28 ml) fresh lemon juice**
- **2 tablespoons (28 ml) filtered water**
- **1 teaspoon raw organic honey**
- **1 teaspoon mustard powder**
- **½ teaspoon salt, Celtic or sea**
- **½ teaspoon white pepper**
- **1 cup (235 ml) grapeseed oil**
- **2 tablespoons (12 g) ground almonds**

Place 1 cup (235 ml) of water into a small pot and bring it to a simmer. Place a heatproof bowl in the pot. Add the egg yolks, lemon juice, water, honey, mustard, salt, and pepper and whisk until the mixture thickens. Remove from the heat and pour into a food processor. Add a small amount of oil to the mixture and blend together. Add the almonds and blend into the mixture. While blending, continue pouring small amounts of oil until it is all gone and the mixture has thickened. Pour the mayonnaise into a sealed jar and refrigerate. It will keep for up to 4 weeks in the refrigerator.

Yield: 1½ cups (340 g)

Note: Use this mayonnaise in egg and chicken salads and open-faced tuna sandwiches and wraps.

[NUTRITIONAL ANALYSIS]

Per tablespoon: 72.9 calories; 6.3 g fat; 1.8 g protein; 2.6 g carbs; 0.9 g fiber; 26.2g; sodium.

[NUTRITIONAL ANALYSIS]

Per tablespoon: 89 calories; 9.5 g fat; 0.2 g protein; 0.4 g carbs; 0 g fiber; 0.7 mg sodium.

PUNCHY PEANUT-COCONUT SAUCE

This spicy sauce has a delicious Thai taste and is perfect with chicken, shrimp, or beef dishes. Peanuts are rich in vitamins, minerals, and fiber that provide energy and contain monounsaturated fatty acids, especially oleic acid, which has been shown to be beneficial for heart health. Apart from its creamy, rich flavor, coconut milk contains magnesium, potassium, phosphorus, and iron, all of which support a healthy metabolism.

- 1 cup (235 ml) coconut milk
- 1 tablespoon (15 g) red curry paste
- ½ cup (130 g) crunchy, sugar-free peanut butter
- ½ cup (120 ml) Nutritive Chicken Stock (page 223)
- 2 tablespoons (40 g) organic honey
- 2 tablespoons (28 ml) fresh lime juice
- ½ teaspoon salt, Celtic or sea

Pour the coconut milk into a small saucepan and bring to a boil. Whisk in the curry paste until dissolved. Add the peanut butter, stock, and honey. Reduce the heat and simmer until smooth, stirring constantly, about 5 minutes. Remove from the heat and add the lime juice and salt. Let cool to room temperature before refrigerating in an airtight container, where it will keep for up to 1 week.

Yield: About 2 cups

Note: Peanuts belong to the legume or bean family, which are the best sources of plant protein because of their high percentages of essential amino acids.

SPICE-IT-UP SWEET CHILI SAUCE

This sweet chili sauce is simple to make and makes a superb condiment that goes with many dishes. It's great as a dip with finger foods and shrimp or as a glaze over chicken, beef, pork, and even grilled vegetables. Chiles are a good source of antioxidants, such as vitamins C and A, and contain a beneficial amount of heart-healthy minerals such as potassium, magnesium, manganese, calcium, and iron.

- 1 tablespoon (15 ml) coconut oil
- ½ cup (80 g) chopped red onion
- 8 cloves garlic, minced
- 4 large red chile peppers, seeds removed, finely chopped
- 2 red bell peppers, chopped
- 3 tablespoons (24 g) grated fresh ginger, peeled
- 6 kaffir lime leaves
- 3 lemongrass stems, chopped
- 1 bunch cilantro, chopped
- 1 cup (340 g) organic honey
- 4 tablespoons (60 ml) filtered water
- 2 tablespoons (28 ml) apple cider vinegar
- 1 tablespoon (16 g) tomato paste
- 1 teaspoon fish sauce
- 1 teaspoon salt, Celtic or sea

Heat the oil in a medium saucepan over medium heat, add the onion and garlic, and cook until they turn a light golden brown and become slightly crispy. Remove from the pan and set aside.

In a food processor, combine the chiles, bell pepper, ginger, lime leaves, lemongrass, and cilantro and blend until finely chopped. Set aside.

[NUTRITIONAL ANALYSIS]

Per tablespoon: 59.9 calories; 4.5 g fat; 1.9 g protein; 2.8 g carbs; .2 g fiber; 76.4 mg sodium.

[NUTRITIONAL ANALYSIS]

Per tablespoon: 26.2 calories; .3 g fat; .2 g protein; 6.8 g carbs; .2 g fiber; 46.9 mg sodium.

In the same saucepan, place the honey and water and heat until the honey starts to simmer. Add the chile paste mixture, vinegar, tomato paste, fish sauce, and salt and simmer for about 2 minutes. Return the onions and garlic to the pot and for cook an additional 1 minute. Adjust the taste, adding more fish sauce if you like it saltier, or more honey if you'd like it sweeter. Transfer the contents to an airtight jar and store in the refrigerator, where it will keep for up to 2 months.

Yield: About 3 cups (825 ml)

Note: Chile peppers are available year-round in either fresh, dried, or powdered form. Whenever possible, buy fresh chiles instead of powder, as these may contain adulterated spicy mixtures. Kaffir lime leaves and lemongrass are available in most Asian supermarkets.

HEALTH-GIVING HOLLANDAISE SAUCE

There's nothing better than homemade healthy hollandaise that's not only supersimple to make but packed full of goodness and fantastic flavor. This one is loaded with protein and healthy fats that most store-bought brands are devoid of and that usually contain inferior, genetically modified oils such as soybean or vegetable oil.

3 egg yolks
2 tablespoons (28 ml) filtered water
¾ cup (165 g) unsalted butter, cubed
2 tablespoons (28 ml) fresh lemon juice
¼ teaspoon salt, Celtic or sea
Dash of black pepper

Place a heatproof bowl over a medium-size saucepan filled a quarter of the way with hot, but not boiling, water and maintain the temperature at a simmer. Put the egg yolks and water into the bowl and whisk for about 3 minutes, or until the mixture thickens and has doubled in volume. Add the butter, one cube at a time, ensuring each cube has fully melted before adding the next one. This will take approximately 10 minutes. Whisk constantly until the sauce thickens and then remove from heat. Whisk in the lemon juice, salt, and pepper. Feel free to use an electric whisk to speed up the process and reduce time. Serve immediately. This sauce is best used soon after making it and does not keep well in the refrigerator.

Yield: About 1 cup

Note: Include this hollandaise over your favorite egg dishes, such eggs Benedict, or over fresh, steamed asparagus, spinach, kale, broccoli, or cauliflower.

———[NUTRITIONAL ANALYSIS]———
Per tablespoon: 87 calories; 9.5 g fat; .6 g protein; .2 g carbs; 0 g fiber; 31.8 mg sodium.

ANTIOXIDANT BBQ SAUCE

If you're a lover of livening up certain dishes with barbecue sauce like I am, then you'll love this healthy, homemade version that's overflowing with antioxidant nutrients and flavor. Most store-bought versions of barbecue sauce contain high-fructose corn syrup and lots of sugar. This one is naturally sweetened with raisins and honey, plus it's packed with antioxidant vitamins and minerals. You'll never go back to store-bought brands once you've tasted this delicious blend, which will give your body a healthy boost.

10 large tomatoes

3 tablespoons (45 ml) extra-virgin olive oil

1½ cups (240 g) diced onions

5 cloves garlic, minced

1 teaspoon minced fresh ginger, peeled, optional

1½ cups (180 g) diced celery

1 medium green bell pepper, diced

½ cup (75 g) raisins

½ cup (170 g) organic honey

¾ cup (175 ml) apple cider vinegar

2 teaspoons each dried mustard powder, ground paprika, and salt, Celtic or sea

1 teaspoon black pepper

½ teaspoon dried, whole chile pepper

½ teaspoon cayenne pepper

Place the whole tomatoes into a pot of boiling water for 1 to 2 minutes to loosen their skins and make them easier to remove. Remove and rinse under cold water. Set aside to cool and drain. Once the tomatoes are cool enough to handle, remove their skins and then dice them.

Add the oil to a large pot over medium heat. Add the onions and garlic and sauté until soft, about 3 to 5 minutes. Add the ginger, celery, and bell pepper and cook until soft, about 3 to 4 minutes. Add the raisins, honey, vinegar, mustard powder, paprika, salt, black pepper, chile, and cayenne and bring to a boil, stirring constantly. Turn the heat down and let simmer, stirring often, for about 1 hour, or until thickened to your liking. Remove from the heat and let cool. Pour into a food processor and process until smooth. Transfer to sealed glass containers and refrigerate for 2 or more hours to allow the flavors to meld. This can be frozen for later use.

Yield: 1 quart (946 ml)

Note: Liberally spread this sauce over your favorite meats, poultry, beans, grains, and other dishes that are sure to be enhanced by its superb taste and nutritional goodness.

[NUTRITIONAL ANALYSIS]

Per tablespoon: 25.3 calories; .8 g fat; .3 g protein; 5 g carbs; .5 g fiber; 62.9 mg sodium.

ANTIOXIDANT GINGER, DATE, AND ORANGE CHUTNEY

Who doesn't love the hot, sour, and sweet taste of tangy chutney, especially one that's loaded with antioxidant goodness to provide multiple health benefits? This condiment goes well with rice, quinoa, vegetables, and meats, and believe it or not, it's wonderfully delicious smeared over toast, sandwiches, and wraps accompanied with other fillings.

2 oranges, peeled, seeded, and chopped

1½ cups (240 g) chopped dates

1 tablespoon (8 g) grated fresh ginger, peeled

¼ cup (60 ml) fresh orange juice

1 tablespoon (6 g) finely grated orange zest

3 tablespoons (45 ml) apple cider vinegar

2 tablespoons (40 g) organic honey

3 tablespoons (45 ml) lemon or lime juice

1 teaspoon mustard seeds

1 tablespoon (7 g) ground cinnamon

¼ teaspoon salt, Celtic or sea

Dash of cayenne pepper

Place all the ingredients in a nonstick saucepan and cook, covered, over medium-low heat for 30 minutes, stirring occasionally. Add more liquids if needed. Let cool before transferring the mixture to an airtight jar and store in the refrigerator. The chutney will keep for up to 3 or 4 weeks refrigerated.

Yield: 2 cups

Note: Experiment with the flavors of fruit and spices by switching some out for other favorites, such as mango, tamarind, tomatoes, peaches, or whatever is in season.

BERRY-BUZZ JELLY

This delectable, sugar-free berry jam is simple to make and loaded with heart-healthy antioxidant nutrients. It contains vitamins C and E, minerals such as potassium and magnesium, and lots of fiber, too. It's a great choice for spreading over muffins, breads, bagels, scones, pancakes, yogurt, or ice cream.

1 cup (145 g) blueberries

1 cup (125 g) raspberries

½ cup (170 g) organic honey

3 tablespoons (45 ml) fresh orange juice

½ teaspoon salt, Celtic or sea

Place all the ingredients in a saucepan, cover, and bring to a boil over medium heat. Simmer for 1 hour, stirring occasionally. The jam should thicken with a small amount of juice left. Remove from the stove and let cool. Transfer to an airtight container and refrigerate for at least 3 hours before serving.

Yield: About 1 cup (320 g)

Note: Berries have been found to contain some of the highest antioxidant power of any fresh fruits, consistently scoring high on the ORAC test, which has been used by the U.S. Department of Agriculture and other agencies to measure the antioxidant power of foods. Antioxidants inhibit oxidation, which prevents damaging effects to cells and promotes longevity.

————[NUTRITIONAL ANALYSIS]————
Per tablespoon: 33.8 calories; 0.1 g fat; 0.3 g protein; 8.9 g carbs; 1 g fiber; 14.7 mg sodium.

————[NUTRITIONAL ANALYSIS]————
Per tablespoon: 42.3 calories; 0.1 g fat; 0.2 g protein; 11.2 g carbs; 0.8 g fiber; 42.2 mg sodium.

IMMUNE-BUILDING LEMON-GINGER BUTTER

Enjoy the creamy texture and deliciously sweet and sour flavors of this healthy spread, which is super-quick and easy to make. The addition of ginger not only provides antioxidants and improves digestion, it adds pungent flavor. Lemons are an excellent source of vitamin C, which is well known for boosting the immune system and cleansing the liver by helping to produce more bile. In doing so, this speeds up the process of digestion.

½ cup (112 g) butter, melted

½ cup (170 g) organic honey

½ cup (115 g) Immune-Boosting Yogurt (page 278)

½ cup (120 ml) lemon juice

2 tablespoons grated lemon rind

½ teaspoon minced fresh ginger, peeled

¼ teaspoon salt, Celtic or sea

½ teaspoon vanilla extract

Place the butter and honey in a food processor and blend until fluffy. Add the yogurt, lemon juice, lemon rind, ginger, salt, and vanilla extract and whip until the butter becomes fluffy. Transfer the contents to an airtight container and refrigerate for at least 3 hours before using.

Yield: 2 cups

Note: Ginger has been used for centuries both for its culinary offerings and powerful medicinal benefits. Several health compounds in ginger, including gingerols and zingerone, are effective anti-inflammatory agents and have gastrointestinal soothing effects. Some research has shown ginger to be more effective against bacterial infections than antibiotics.

Sweet and Savory Sensations

Use Immune-Building Lemon and Ginger Butter as a creamy, delicious base for cakes and muffins. Or, for a tantalizing taste sensation, add a dollop over cooked pasta and seafood dishes such as seared or roasted salmon or grilled clams.

[NUTRITIONAL ANALYSIS]

Per tablespoon: 47.6 calories; 3.1 g fat; 0.3 g protein; 5.1 g carbs; 0 g fiber; 37.4 mg sodium.

BONE-BUILDING FRENCH CREAM

This highly versatile, European-style, sour-tasting cream is loaded with beneficial bacteria called probiotics that provide a wide array of health benefits. This will become an indispensable ingredient in your kitchen, and you'll probably never go back to store-bought sour cream again after trying this one.

2½ cups (570 ml) heavy whipping cream, preferably organic

½ cup (115 g) Immune-Boosting Yogurt (page 278), or use plain yogurt, preferably organic

Pour the cream into a saucepan over medium heat and bring to just before boiling. Do not let boil. Remove from the heat and transfer to a glass jar with a screw-top lid. Mix in the yogurt, let cool to room temperature, secure with the lid, and place inside a cupboard at room temperature for 24 hours. After 24 hours remove the jar gently from the cupboard and refrigerate for at least 8 hours. It will keep in the refrigerator for up to 2 weeks.

Yield: 3 cups

Note: Studies have shown that fermented dairy products alleviate symptoms of lactose intolerance and improve calcium absorption.

RESTORATIVE CUCUMBER-YOGURT RAITA

Raita is a very versatile and cooling side dish that goes well with curry and over the top of spicy foods or hot dishes such as beans or rice. Cucumbers are loaded with antioxidant nutrients, such as vitamin C, and contain the heart-healthy minerals potassium and magnesium. Increase the sweetness of this dish by adding a few grapes or some diced pineapple.

2 cups (460 g) Immune-Boosting Yogurt (page 278), or use unsweetened natural yogurt

1 cucumber, peeled and coarsely grated

2 fresh scallions, finely chopped

1 small green chile pepper, finely chopped

1 clove garlic, minced

1 teaspoon grated fresh ginger, peeled

Juice of 1 lemon or lime

1 tablespoon (6 g) chopped fresh mint

¼ teaspoon black peppercorns

1 teaspoon cumin seeds

Pour the yogurt and cucumber into a small bowl and combine well. Add the scallions, chile, garlic, ginger, lemon or lime juice, mint, and peppercorns and blend together. Heat the cumin seeds over medium heat in a dry pan until they smoke, about 30 seconds, then add to the raita. Leave at least 1 hour in the refrigerator before serving so that flavors meld.

Yield: 2 ½ cups

Note: Yogurt is a good source of bioavailable calcium and protein because of its live cultures.

———————[NUTRITIONAL ANALYSIS]———————
Per tablespoon: 46 calories; 4.8 g fat; 0.4 g protein; 0.6 g carbs; 0 g fiber; 7.3 mg sodium.

———————[NUTRITIONAL ANALYSIS]———————
Per tablespoon: 10.4 calories; 0.5 g fat; 0.5 g protein; 0.9 g carbs; 0.2 g fiber; 6.7 mg sodium.

IMMUNE-BOOSTING YOGURT

No healthy kitchen is complete without fermented foods such as yogurt, which are laden with enzymes and friendly bacteria that balance your "inner eco-system." The probiotics in yogurt have a powerful, beneficial effect on your gut's immune system, your first line of defense against pathogens. Flavor your yogurt using 3 tablespoons of a natural, all-fruit jam, such as our Berry-Buzz Jelly (page 275).

1 quart (946 ml) milk, preferably organic

¼ cup (60 g) natural yogurt or 1 package powdered yogurt starter such as Greek or Bulgarian

Scald the milk by bringing it to just below boiling in a medium pan. Do not boil. Allow it to cool to around 110°F (43°C). Whisk in the yogurt or starter culture and pour into a screw-top jar and attach lid. Store for 24 hours in a dark place at room temperature. Yogurt is finished culturing when the milk solids gently separate from the walls of the jar when tipped gently to one side. When the yogurt is finished culturing, reserve ¼ cup to be used to culture your next batch. Refrigerate in an airtight jar for up to 2 weeks.

Yield: 2 cups

Note: To make coconut milk yogurt, use 1 quart (946 ml) of coconut milk in place of the dairy milk. Coconut milk yogurts are not typically able to be recultured time and time again as are dairy-based yogurts.

PROBIOTIC FRUIT CHUTNEY

Pineapple is rich in food enzymes, particularly bromelain, which helps to break down protein. It is also a good source of manganese. The fresh cilantro and serrano chiles give a nice kick to this dish, which goes well with grilled fish or meats or with a salad.

1 small, ripe pineapple, peeled, cored, and chopped

2 ripe pears, peeled, cored, and chopped

1 cup (16 g) finely minced cilantro leaves

1 tablespoon (10 g) finely minced ginger, peeled

2 serrano chile peppers, seeded if desired, and minced

½ teaspoon ground cloves

1 teaspoon ground cinnamon

¼ cup whey starter culture plus 2 additional tablespoons

In a food processor, place all the ingredients except the starter culture and process until finely chopped. Stir in ¼ cup of the starter culture. Spoon the chutney mixture in batches into a mason jar and mash with a wooden spoon until the pineapple and pear release their juices. Continue spooning the mixture into the jar and mashing it until the liquid covers the pineapple and pear solids. Spoon the additional 2 tablespoons starter culture over the chutney and cover it loosely, leaving 1 inch (2.5 cm) of headspace to allow for expansion. Place the chutney in a dark spot in your kitchen at room temperature and allow to ferment for 2 to 3 days before removing to cold storage. Secure the lid before refrigerating. It should keep for 6 to 8 weeks if refrigerated.

Yield: 1 quart

─────[NUTRITIONAL ANALYSIS]─────
Per tablespoon: 19.4 calories; 1 g fat; 1 g protein; 1.5 g carbs; 0 g fiber; 15.6 mg sodium.

─────[NUTRITIONAL ANALYSIS]─────
Per tablespoon: 9.3 calories; 0.1 g fat; 0.2 g protein; 2.2 g carbs; 0.3 g fiber; 8.8 mg sodium.

SWEET ENDINGS
DESSERTS
AND OTHER DELIGHTS

Few things are more rewarding in life than treating yourself to the occasional sweet treat, especially one that is packed with antioxidants, minerals, phytonutrients, and more! These simple and delectable pleasures are made entirely from nature's finest sweets, utilizing natural, high-quality ingredients and smart substitutions for notoriously no-no ingredients. Dried and fresh fruits, fruit juice and fruit juice concentrate, honey, molasses, and maple syrup are healthier choices compared to sugar and artificial sweeteners. I've also included whole grains, nuts, and even a few vegetables that come from whole food sources. They are nutrient dense to provide plenty of essential vitamins and minerals, and will not only satisfy your desire to indulge those sweet cravings, but actually enhance the flavors and improve the desserts. These are sweets to celebrate.

HEARTY HAZELNUT ROUNDS

Enjoy the sweet, nutty burst of flavor with these crispy cookies made from a combination of nut flours. Hazelnuts, also known as filberts, are packed full of heart-healthy nutrients, such as magnesium, calcium, protein, fiber, and vitamins E and B complex. Hazelnut is quite often added to coffee for a rich, delicious flavor, so enjoy one or two of these with your morning or afternoon brew.

2½ cups (338 g) hazelnuts

⅓ cup (75 g) butter, softened

⅔ cup (230 g) organic honey

3 eggs

2½ cups (288 g) almond flour

¼ teaspoon ground cardamom

¼ teaspoon ground cloves

½ teaspoon ground ginger

1 teaspoon ground cinnamon

1 teaspoon vanilla extract

1 teaspoon grated orange or lemon rind

Dash of salt, Celtic or sea

Preheat the oven to 300°F (150°C, gas mark 2). Line a baking sheet with parchment paper or grease with butter.

Place the hazelnuts in a food processor and grind into a meal. In a medium bowl, combine the butter, honey, and eggs until creamy. In another bowl, combine the almond flour, hazelnut meal, spices, vanilla extract, and lemon rind and mix together until smooth. Spread the dough onto the baking sheet about ¼ inch (6 mm) thick. Bake for 20 minutes. Remove from the oven and let cool for about 10 minutes. Using a round cookie cutter, cut out as many shapes as possible. Store them in an airtight container.

Yield: About 20 cookies

Note: Hazelnuts are one of the best sources of the antioxidant vitamin E, which is supportive of the heart muscle and all other muscles in the body.

---[NUTRITIONAL ANALYSIS]---

Per serving: 188 calories; 14.1 g fat; 4.7 g protein; 13.5 g carbs; 2.1 g fiber; 48 mg sodium.

LUSCIOUS LEMON-PINEAPPLE YOGURT CAKE

With its combination of sweet and sour tastes, this deliciously light and moist yogurt cake is a perfect after-dinner treat or something to enjoy with your morning tea on those special occasions. Pineapple and lemons are both rich in antioxidants, particularly vitamin C, to support a healthy heart, and are known for their anti-inflammatory qualities. This one is sure to be a hit with the whole family and your guests.

1 teaspoon butter or coconut oil

4 eggs, separated

½ cup (170 g) organic honey

2 teaspoons vanilla extract

½ teaspoon almond extract

2 cups (460 g) Immune-Building Yogurt (page 278)

Juice of 1 lemon

Rind of 1 lemon, finely grated

1 cup (155 g) pineapple, finely chopped

2 cups (230 g) almond flour

2 teaspoons baking soda

1 cup (125 g) raspberries

Preheat the oven to 350°F (180°C, gas mark 4). Grease an 8-inch (20-cm) square baking tin with the butter or coconut oil.

In a large mixing bowl, combine the egg yolks with the honey, vanilla and almond extracts, yogurt, lemon juice, and rind and mix well. Add the pineapple. In a separate bowl, combine the almond flour with the baking soda and add to the egg yolk mixture. Beat the egg whites until stiff, about 3 or 4 minutes, and gently fold into the mixture. Pour the mixture into the prepared cake tin and bake for 1 hour, or until the cake feels spongy. Let cool before removing from the tin. Serve with fresh raspberries and Bone-Building French Cream (page 277).

Yield: 8 servings

Note: Pineapple contains the enzyme bromelain, which helps regulate the secretions of the pancreas to aid in digestion.

————[**NUTRITIONAL ANALYSIS**]————

Per serving: 363.7 calories; 21 g fat; 13.5 g protein; 34.5 g carbs; 4.3 g fiber; 417.1 mg sodium.

HEALTH-GRATIFYING GRAPEFRUIT AND ORANGE CAKE

This lusciously light and fluffy cake is a family favorite that doesn't last long whenever I make it. It has just the right amount of tang and sweetness, which is enhanced when served with the sour taste of Bone-Building French Cream (page 277). Oranges and grapefruits are loaded with antioxidant nutrients that protect against heart disease and are effective in preventing and treating many others.

FOR THE CAKE:

1 tablespoon (14 g) coconut butter

2 medium oranges

1 lemon

1 teaspoon minced fresh ginger, peeled

¾ cup (255 g) organic honey

6 eggs

½ cup (58 g) coconut flour

1 ½ cups (173 g) almond flour

1 teaspoon baking soda

½ teaspoon salt, Celtic or sea

FOR THE SYRUP:

¾ cup (255 g) organic honey

½ cup (120 ml) fresh grapefruit juice

½ cup (120 ml) fresh orange juice

Rind from half of orange, thinly sliced

Rind from half of grapefruit, thinly sliced

To make the cake: Preheat the oven to 350°F (180°C, gas mark 4). Grease a 9-inch (23-cm) round cake pan with the coconut butter. Wash the orange and lemon and place them whole in a saucepan covered with cold water. Bring to a boil and simmer for 1 hour, or until the fruit becomes soft. Check the water level and add more if needed. Slice the fruit open, remove the seeds, place in a food processor, and puree. Add the ginger, honey, eggs, flours, baking soda, and salt and blend well. Add a tablespoon of filtered water if the mixture is too dry. Pour the mixture into the greased cake pan and bake for 1 hour, until a toothpick stuck in the center comes out clean. Cool in the pan for 2 hours before removing.

To make the syrup: Place the honey, grapefruit and orange juices, and rinds in a small saucepan. Bring to a boil. Simmer for about 10 minutes, until the rinds look translucent. Remove the rinds and decorate the top of the cake with them. Pour the syrup over the top and serve with Bone-Building French Cream.

Yield: 6 to 8 servings

Note: Grapefruit contains compounds that are known to increase circulating levels of certain drugs, including statins. If this is an issue for you, then you may want to eliminate the grapefruit and add more orange instead. In general, it's recommended that you avoid consuming grapefruit if you take any pharmaceutical medications.

————[NUTRITIONAL ANALYSIS]————

Per serving: 109.6 calories; 0.1 g fat; 0.3 g protein; 29.2 g carbs; 0.1 g fiber; 1.6 mg sodium.

ALMIGHTY ALMOND AND WALNUT PUMPERNICKEL BREAD

This dense, high-fiber bread has a wonderful flavor that goes well with sweet or savory toppings. The nuts and seeds give it extra nutrients, while the almond flour allows you to consume baked bread without any gluten.

1 cup (120 g) walnuts

¼ cup (36 g) sunflower seeds

¼ cup (35 g) pumpkin seeds

3 cups (345 g) almond flour

1 teaspoon baking soda

½ teaspoon ground nutmeg

1 teaspoon anise or caraway seeds (optional)

½ teaspoon salt, Celtic or sea

3 eggs

⅓ cup (75 g) butter or ghee

1 tablespoon (20 g) unsulphured molasses

1 teaspoon vanilla extract

Preheat the oven to 350°F (180°C, gas mark 4). Grease a 4- by 8-inch (10- by 20-cm) loaf pan. Place the walnuts, sunflower seeds, and pumpkin seeds into a food processor and blend for about 10 seconds. Remove the sharp blade from the processor and insert the mixing blade. Add the flour, baking soda, nutmeg, anise or caraway seeds, and salt and pulse the ingredients together. Add the eggs, butter or ghee, molasses, and vanilla extract and blend into the mixture. Pour the batter into the greased loaf pan and bake for 45 minutes, or until the top is browned and cracked. Remove from the oven and let cool before removing from the pan. Transfer to an airtight container and refrigerate. It will keep for up to 1 week.

Yield: 10 silces

Recipe Variation

You can add a banana, or 1 cup (145 g) of raisins or dates (160 g), to this bread to increase sweetness or add more flavor.

---[**NUTRITIONAL ANALYSIS**]---

Per serving: 382.5 calories; 34.6 g fat; 11.9 g protein; 12.3 g carbs; 4.8 g fiber; 59.1 mg sodium.

POWERHOUSE PUMPKIN, SPICE, AND ALMOND BREAD

This mouthwatering, nutritious pumpkin bread is a good source of dietary fiber and helps in regulating blood sugar levels. The combination of almond flour and coconut flour creates a more breadlike texture than using either one alone. This tastes great as is or with a smearing of butter or fruit jelly.

1 tablespoon (15 ml) coconut oil

3 cups (345 g) almond flour

½ cup (58 g) coconut flour

½ teaspoon salt, Celtic or sea

1 teaspoon baking soda

3 large eggs

¼ cup (55 g) butter or ghee

1 tablespoon (15 ml) apple cider vinegar

1 cup (240 g) pumpkin, peeled, cooked, and mashed

1 teaspoon minced fresh ginger, peeled

½ teaspoon cinnamon

½ teaspoon ground cloves (optional)

1 tablespoon (6 g) grated orange zest

1 cup (120 g) walnuts, chopped

½ cup (75 g) raisins (optional)

Preheat the oven to 350°F (180°C, gas mark 4). Grease an 8-inch (20-cm) loaf tin with the coconut oil. In a food processor, pulse the almond flour, coconut flour, salt, and baking soda together. Add the eggs, butter, and vinegar and mix together. Add the pumpkin, ginger, cinnamon, cloves, if using, and orange zest and blend together. Toss in the walnuts and raisins, if using. Transfer the contents to the prepared loaf tin and bake for 35 to 45 minutes, until the top of the loaf feels firm. Cool the bread in the pan for 2 hours before removing. Serve immediately or store in an airtight container in the refrigerator.

Yield: 10 slices

Note: This bread freezes well. Thaw at room temperature for 2 hours and reheat by placing in the oven for 10 minutes.

————[**NUTRITIONAL ANALYSIS**]————
Per serving: 368.6 calories; 30.1 g fat; 11.4 g protein; 17.6 g carbs; 5 g fiber; 215 mg sodium.

NOURISHING CRUSTY ONION AND PARMESAN ROLLS

These scrumptious rolls are always a hit and are snapped up quickly whenever I make them. I sometimes spice them up with a clove of fresh garlic, which goes nicely with Italian dishes, such as lasagna. The almond flour not only gives them a delicious, nutty taste compared with wheat flour but contains heart-healthy micronutrients such as vitamin E, potassium, and calcium.

- **4 tablespoons (56 g) butter or ghee, divided**
- **1 large onion, finely chopped**
- **2 tablespoons (40 g) organic honey**
- **1 teaspoon finely chopped rosemary**
- **1 teaspoon salt, Celtic or sea**
- **1 teaspoon black pepper**
- **2 large eggs**
- **3 cups (345 g) almond flour**
- **1 teaspoon baking soda**
- **¾ cup (75 g) grated Parmesan or Cheddar cheese**
- **1 tablespoon (4 g) finely chopped parsley**
- **1 tablespoon (15 ml) olive oil**

Preheat the oven to 350°F (180°C, gas mark 4). Grease a 9- by 13-inch (23- by 33-cm) baking sheet with 1 tablespoon (14 g) butter or ghee. Heat 1 tablespoon butter or ghee in a large skillet over medium-high heat. Add the onions, honey, rosemary, salt, and pepper and cook for about 5 to 7 minutes, until golden brown.

In a large bowl, whisk together the eggs and 2 tablespoons (28 g) butter or ghee, then add the flour, baking soda, cheese, and parsley and blend together. Add the cooked onion mixture and knead together until a sticky dough forms. Moisten your hands with water, form the dough into 8 balls, and place them onto the greased baking sheet, spacing evenly. With a sharp knife, trace a cross over the top of the buns and brush the tops with the olive oil. Bake until the rolls are golden, about 15 to 20 minutes. The rolls should feel firm. Remove from the oven and let cool for several minutes before serving.

Yield: 8 rolls

Note: The rolls can be made into biscuits by increasing the onion and cheese to 1 cup each. Form into drop biscuits on a parchment-lined sheet, and bake for 15 to 20 minutes, or until lightly browned on top and cooked through.

———————[NUTRITIONAL ANALYSIS]———————
Per serving: 390.5 calories; 32.5 g fat; 14.8 g protein; 15.5 g carbs; 4.9 g fiber; 440 mg sodium.

FORTIFYING FIG AND MINTY BLUEBERRY BRÛLÉE

Enjoy the creamy, sweet taste of these delicious fresh fruit and custard treats. Figs are loaded with potassium, a mineral that helps to control blood pressure. Blueberries contain a ton of antioxidants, especially vitamin C, and a tangy flavor that comes to life in this dish.

½ cup (85 g) ripe fresh figs, sliced

1 cup (145 g) fresh blueberries

1 tablespoon (6 g) finely chopped fresh mint

3 cups (705 ml) Bone-Building French Cream (page 277)

5 egg yolks

¼ cup (85 g) organic honey

1 teaspoon vanilla extract

3 fresh strawberries, halved

Preheat the oven to 350°F (180°C, gas mark 4). Set aside 6 small ramekins. Combine the figs, blueberries, and mint in a bowl. In a medium saucepan over medium heat, pour the cream, egg yolks, honey, and vanilla extract and whisk until well combined, about 1 minute. Do not boil. Remove from the heat and set aside.

Place the fruit into the bottom of the ramekins. Add the cream mixture over the top of the fruit. Place the ramekins into a deep baking dish with water that reaches halfway up the ramekins and bake for 35 minutes, until the custard has set but is still slightly jiggly. Remove from the water bath and let cool at room temperature before refrigerating. Refrigerate for at least 3 hours before serving. Garnish with half a strawberry on top.

Yield: 6 servings

Note: Switch up the flavors by changing the fruits you use. For example, add 1 tablespoon of orange zest when heating the cream and eggs, and line the bottom of the ramekins with fresh orange pieces.

[NUTRITIONAL ANALYSIS]

Per serving: 485.4 calories; 42.2 g fat; 5.8 g protein; 23.6 g carbs; 1.2 g fiber; 67.3 mg sodium.

ENERGY-GIVING COCONUT, ALMOND, AND RAISIN CUSTARD

This refreshing nondairy custard is delicious served for dessert or enjoyed at breakfast over granola. The coconut and almond milks contain more nutrients than dairy milk and provide your body with protein and hea lthy fats to boost your metabolism. Feel free to add a few dates with the raisins for added sweetness.

½ cup (75 g) raisins

1 cup (235 ml) almond milk

1 cup (235 ml) coconut milk

5 egg yolks, whisked

1 teaspoon vanilla extract

½ teaspoon ground nutmeg

1 teaspoon cinnamon

1 cup (145 g) strawberries, halved

Preheat the oven to 300°F (150°C, gas mark 2). Evenly sprinkle the raisins over the bottom of an 8-inch (20-cm) square oven dish. Have a larger-size oven dish at the ready that will house the smaller dish.

In a medium saucepan, combine the almond milk, coconut milk, and egg yolks over medium heat. Do not boil. Remove from the heat and stir in the vanilla extract. Pour the mixture over the raisins and sprinkle with nutmeg and cinnamon. Place the dish inside of the larger oven dish and fill the larger dish with hot water until it reaches halfway up the smaller dish. Gently place in the oven for 35 minutes, or until the top starts to feel firm but is still slightly jiggly.

Remove from the oven and water bath and let stand for 5 or 10 minutes before serving or refrigerating. Decorate with slices of strawberry before serving.

Yield: 6 servings

Note: Almond milk is high in heart-healthy vitamin E and is a good source of calcium.

------[NUTRITIONAL ANALYSIS]------

Per serving: 186.3 calories; 11 g fat; 3.7 g protein; 16.9 g carbs; 1.4 g fiber; 42.7 mg sodium.

BLUEBERRY AND APPLE CRUMBLE GONE NUTS

Blueberries and apples are a great combination for a wonderful, warm crisp that can be made in a snap. They are loaded with antioxidant vitamins C, A, and E and minerals such as selenium and zinc, all of which boost your immune system. Walnuts add a crunchy texture and are rich in essential ALA, the plant-based form of omega-3 fatty acids.

FOR THE FILLING:

4 large green apples, peeled, cored, and cut into thin wedges

Juice of ½ lemon (about 1 tablespoon [15 ml])

¼ cup (60 ml) filtered water

1 teaspoon grated lemon rind

2 tablespoons (40 g) organic honey, divided

2 cups (290 g) blueberries, fresh or frozen

½ teaspoon cinnamon

¼ teaspoon mace (optional)

FOR THE TOPPING:

⅔ cup (76 g) almond flour

½ cup (40 g) rolled oats

¼ cup (55 g) butter

1 teaspoon organic honey

1 cup (120 g) walnuts

Preheat the oven to 350°F (180°C, gas mark 4). Grease an 8-inch (20-cm) square baking dish with butter.

To make the filling: Toss the apples, lemon juice, water, lemon zest, and 1 tablespoon of the honey into a medium saucepan and cook, covered, for 5 minutes, over low heat. Remove the lid and simmer on high for another 5 minutes. Remove from the heat, add the blueberries, cinnamon, and mace to the pot, and let sit for about 10 minutes, until the blueberries soften and flavors meld. Drain the fruit of its juices in a sieve and set the fruit aside in a small bowl. Pour the juice back into the saucepan, adding the remaining tablespoon of honey, and simmer until reduced down by half. Retain this syrup for later. Cool the fruit in the refrigerator.

To make the topping: In a food processor, add the almond flour, rolled oats, butter, honey, and walnuts and blend until chunky crumbs are formed. Refrigerate the crumble for 10 minutes. When the fruit has cooled, place the fruit into a baking dish and top it with the crumble. Bake for 20 minutes. Serve warm topped with Bone-Building French Cream (page 277) or Immune-Boosting Yogurt (page 278).

Yield: 4 servings

Note: This nutritionally loaded dish is great served at breakfast or as an afternoon snack.

[NUTRITIONAL ANALYSIS]

Per serving: 659 calories; 41.7 g fat; 11.9 g protein; 69.1 g carbs; 12.1 g fiber; 87.3 mg sodium.

BERRY-BENEFICIAL BLUEBERRY AND PECAN PIE

This pecans in this classic pie are an excellent source of the antioxidant vitamin E, which is well known for improving heart health. Blueberries are packed with the antioxidant vitamin C and add a tangy flavor that comes to life when you add a hint of lemon.

FOR THE CRUST:

2½ cups (250 g) pecans

2 tablespoons (28 ml) coconut oil

¼ cup (85 g) organic honey

1 teaspoon vanilla extract

½ cup (58 g) coconut flour

1 egg

¼ teaspoon salt, Celtic or sea

½ teaspoon baking soda

FOR THE FILLING:

3 cups (465 g) frozen blueberries

2 green apples, peeled, cored, and cut into thin wedges

⅓ cup (80 ml) fresh lemon juice

1 teaspoon grated fresh lemon zest

¾ cup (255 g) organic honey

To make the crust: Soak the pecans in filtered water for 1 hour and then drain and dry with a paper towel. When dried, spread the nuts evenly over a baking sheet and place in an oven heated to 150°F for about 5 hours, or until crispy. Remove from the oven, transfer the crispy nuts to a food processor, and grind to a nut butter. Transfer to a large bowl. Turn the oven temperature up to 300°F (150°C, gas mark 2). Add the oil, honey, and vanilla extract to the processed nuts and blend. Add the coconut flour, egg, salt, and baking soda and blend together. If the batter is too soft, add more coconut flour, 1 teaspoon at a time, until it thickens into a ball. Press the crust batter into a greased 9-inch (23-cm) round pie dish and bake for 30 minutes, until the crust is golden brown. If the crust is getting too dark, cover with a piece of foil. Remove from the oven and let cool completely at room temperature.

To make the filling: Place the blueberries, apples, lemon juice, zest, and honey in a large pot and bring to a boil. Reduce to a simmer and cook uncovered for about 15 to 20 minutes, until the liquid has thickened. Remove from the heat, place in a covered bowl, and refrigerate for at least 3 to 4 hours, or overnight. Once set, fill the piecrust with the mixture. Serve warm or cold with Bone-Building French Cream (page 277).

Yield: 6 to 8 servings

Note: Research has shown that adding just a small handful of pecans to your diet each day can inhibit unwanted oxidation of blood lipids, thus helping prevent the oxidation of LDL cholesterol.

———[NUTRITIONAL ANALYSIS]———
Per serving: 589.3 calories; 33 g fat; 7.4 g protein; 75.9 g carbs; 11.9 g fiber; 169.3 mg sodium.

ANTI-OX ORANGE MOUSSE

Enjoy the tangy, sweet taste of oranges in this super-simple mousse. Oranges contain a high amount of antioxidants and more than 170 phytonutrients and 60 flavonoids, all of which have been shown to have anti-inflammatory, anticancer, and heart-healthy benefits and to promote optimum health. It's deliciously smooth and creamy.

½ cup (170 g) organic honey, divided

Grated rind from 1 orange

¼ cup (60 ml) + 2 tablespoons (28 ml) cold filtered water, divided

1 teaspoon gelatin

1½ cups (355 ml) Bone-Building French Cream (page 277)

⅔ cup (160 ml) fresh orange juice

2 tablespoons (28 ml) lemon juice

1 teaspoon vanilla extract

½ teaspoon ground nutmeg

1 teaspoon cinnamon

4 orange slices

In a small, nonstick saucepan, combine the honey, orange zest, and ¼ cup (60 ml) water and simmer for 1 minute. Turn the heat off. Soak the gelatin in 2 tablespoons (28 ml) cold water and add to the hot honey, stirring well. Transfer the contents to a ceramic bowl, refrigerate for about 20 minutes, and then remove.

In a medium bowl, whip the cream until quite thick. Add the orange and lemon juices, vanilla extract, and the thickened honey. Pour equal amounts of the mixture into 6 individual ramekins and refrigerate for at least 3 to 4 hours, until the mousse sets. Remove from the refrigerator and dip the ramekins into hot water for about 10 seconds. Using a knife, separate the edges of the mousse away from the ramekins and place upside down onto the center of a dessert plate. Decorate with nutmeg, cinnamon, and a slice of orange and serve.

Yield: 4 servings

Note: Apart from their delightful taste, oranges also contain vitamins A and B_1. One medium-size orange contains nearly 100 percent of the daily intake of vitamin C.

[NUTRITIONAL ANALYSIS]

Per serving: 472 calories; 29 g fat; 3.4 g protein; 53.5 g carbs; 0.3 g fiber; 47.2 mg sodium.

SOOTHING PEAR, DATE, AND ALMOND PUDDING WITH GRAPEFRUIT CREAM SAUCE

The soft, sweet, buttery flesh of pears studded with sticky dates makes for a comforting dessert fit for any occasion. Pears are packed with heart-healthy fiber, potassium, and vitamin C. Dates are loaded with essential minerals such as calcium, iron, potassium, magnesium, and phosphorus. Serve it with whipped cream or as-is—it's simply divine!

FOR THE PUDDING:

3 tablespoons (42 g) butter, room temperature

2 tablespoons (40 g) organic honey, divided

1½ cups (173 g) almond flour

½ teaspoon salt, Celtic or sea

1 teaspoon vanilla extract

1 teaspoon almond extract or 2 tablespoons (28 ml) amaretto liqueur

1 whole egg

3 eggs, separated

7 to 8 large dates, pitted and finely chopped

2 large pears, peeled, cored, and finely chopped

FOR THE SAUCE:

3 egg yolks

4 tablespoons (80 g) organic honey

1 teaspoon vanilla extract

1 cup (235 ml) Bone-Building French Cream (page 277)

½ cup (120 ml) fresh grapefruit juice

1 teaspoon grated orange zest

Preheat the oven to 370°F. Lightly butter 6 small ramekins.

To make the pudding: In a large bowl, add the butter and 1 tablespoon (20 g) honey and beat until creamy. Blend in the almond flour, salt, vanilla extract, almond extract or amaretto, whole egg, and 3 egg yolks. Fold the dates and pears into the mixture.

In a separate bowl, whisk the egg whites until they stiffen, about 2 to 3 minutes with a handheld whisk or 1 minute with an electric beater. Add the rest of the honey and whisk until thick and creamy. Fold this into the almond flour mixture. Spoon the mixture into the prepared ramekins and bake for 25 to 30 minutes, or until the puddings feel spongy. Remove from the oven and let cool for 10 minutes before turning them onto serving plates. Top with grapefruit cream sauce. Sprinkle with orange zest.

To make the sauce: In a small bowl, combine the egg yolks, honey, and vanilla extract and place in a pot of hot water that reaches a quarter of the way up the bowl. Simmer the water gently and do not let it boil. Remove from the heat after 2 minutes as it begins to thicken. Add the cream, grapefruit juice, and orange zest and whisk until smooth. Let cool and serve with the puddings.

Yield: 6 servings

Note: For a different taste sensation, try swapping the pears for pineapple or apple or a combination of these with the pears.

———[**NUTRITIONAL ANALYSIS**]———
Per serving: 531.8 calories; 36.7 g fat; 12.8 g protein; 44.3 g carbs; 5.1 g fiber; 232 mg sodium.

SWEET BROWN RICE PUDDING WITH AN ANTIOXIDANT TWIST

Because of its high fiber content, this delicious pudding is especially helpful in maintaining a healthy digestive system. The eggs and cream combine well to give a fluffy texture, and the nuts provide crunch as well as nutrient density. Enjoy this tasty, hearty dish for dessert, breakfast, or as an anytime snack.

3 eggs

1 cup (235 ml) Bone-Building French Cream (page 277) or use heavy cream, preferably organic

⅓ cup (80 ml) maple syrup

1 teaspoon vanilla extract

1 teaspoon ground cinnamon

½ teaspoon ground nutmeg

1 cup (160 g) whole grain brown rice, rinsed, drained, and cooked

1 tablespoon (8 g) finely grated fresh ginger, peeled

1 cup (145 g) raisins

1 cup (110 g) pecans or walnuts (120 g), chopped

1 mashed banana (optional)

Preheat the oven to 325°F (170°C, gas mark 3). Beat the eggs with the cream, maple syrup, vanilla extract, cinnamon, and nutmeg. Stir in the rice, ginger, raisins, nuts, and banana. Pour the contents into a 9-inch (23-cm) baking dish and bake for approximately 45 minutes, or until the eggs have set. Remove from the oven and let cool or serve hot with Bone-Building French Cream (page 277). This will stay fresh refrigerated for up to 1 week.

Yield: 4 servings

Note: Ginger contains several medicinal compounds, including gingerol, which is especially effective for supporting heart health.

—————[**NUTRITIONAL ANALYSIS**]—————
Per serving: 531.5 calories; 29.7 g fat; 10.9 g protein; 62.8 g carbs; 4 g fiber; 60.3 mg sodium.

NO-BAKE SUPERFOOD FUDGE BROWNIES

Enjoy the fruity, nutty, and chocolate flavor of this nutritionally superb dessert that lies somewhere between a brownie and fudge square. Cacao is a well-known superfood because of its high content of antioxidants and other important nutrients such as protein, healthy fat, magnesium, calcium, zinc, fiber, and iron. And best of all, you can make these in about 5 minutes!

1 cup (100 g) raw walnut pieces

1 cup (160 g) packed, soft Medjool dates, (about 10 or 11), pits removed

½ cup (50 g) cacao powder

¾ cup (60 g) shredded coconut, divided

½ teaspoon salt, Celtic or sea

1 to 2 tablespoons (15 to 28 ml) filtered water

½ cup (85 g) cacao nibs

Place the walnuts in a food processor and pulse for a few seconds to form a coarse meal. While the machine is still running, add the dates, cacao powder, ½ cup shredded coconut, salt, and 1 tablespoon (15 ml) of the filtered water, processing until a moist, crumblike dough forms. Depending on the natural moisture of the dates, you may need to add a touch more water to get the crumbs to stick when pinched together.

Spread the mixture into an 8- by 8-inch (20- by 20-cm) pan and sprinkle with the cacao nibs and remaining shredded coconut. Press the mixture firmly into a solid brownie layer. Refrigerate for about 2 hours. Cut into bite-size squares and serve.

Yield: 24 small squares

Note: Cacao is a type of tropical tree that produces the world's chocolate in raw form, before sugar, fat, and other ingredients are added. Several hundred years ago, cacao beans were so valuable that they were used as a form of currency.

---[**NUTRITIONAL ANALYSIS**]---

Per serving: 85.7 calories; 5.8 g fat; 1.7 g protein; 9.1 g carbs; 2 g fiber; 29.7 mg sodium.

A MONTH OF
• MENU PLANS •
FOR HEART HEALTH

WEEK 1 EATING PLAN SUGGESTIONS

Sunday

BREAKFAST

Brain-Boosting Salmon Eggs Benedict (page 205), or Hearty Mediterranean Frittata (page 207)

LUNCH

Feel-Good Turkey or Salmon Tomato Panini (page 222), or Energizing Thai Spice Chicken Salad (page 215) with Energizing Thai Spice Salad Dressing (page 218)

SNACK (OPTIONAL)

Spiced Honey-Glazed Nuts (page 233), or Blood Sugar–Balancing Butternut and Leek Pies (page 230)

DINNER

Protein-Packed Vegetarian Shepherd's Pie (page 239), or Soul-Warming Tuna Lasagna (page 253) with Cardioprotective Green Beans (page 268)

Monday

BREAKFAST

Get-Up-and-Go Banana Berry Quinoa Porridge (page 201), or Melt-in-Your Mouth Baked Granola (page 202)

LUNCH

Cardioprotective Salmon Caesar Salad (page 214) with Cardioprotective Caesar Salad Dressing (page 217), or Stress-Less Turkey, Avocado, and Veggie Nori Wrap (page 219)

SNACK (OPTIONAL)

2 to 3 Low-Carb Herbed Cheddar Crackers (page 229), or High-Energy Chicken and Cauliflower Croquettes (page 231)

DINNER

Revitalizing Vegetable Biryani (page 242), or Anti-Inflammatory Turmeric Turkey Burgers (page 260) with Anti-Ox Pumpkin and Cauliflower Mash (page 264)

Tuesday

BREAKFAST

Regenerating Herb Scrambled Eggs (page 203), or Melt-in-Your Mouth Baked Granola (page 202)

LUNCH

Almighty Avocado and Black Bean Salad (page 211), or Feel-Good Turkey or Salmon Tomato Panini (page 222)

SNACK (OPTIONAL)

High-Energy Chicken and Cauliflower Croquettes (page 231), or Spiced Honey-Glazed Nuts (page 233)

DINNER

Spicy Moroccan Tempeh with Lentils (page 237), or Favorite Sweet, Spicy, and Crunchy Meatloaf (page 248) with Zesty Broccoli with Garlic and Ginger (page 265)

DESSERT

Blueberry and Apple Crumble Gone Nuts (page 288), or Soothing Pear, Date, and Almond Pudding with Grapefruit Cream Sauce (page 291)

Wednesday

BREAKFAST

Protein-Powered Muesli with Coconut and Raisins (page 203), or Melt-in-Your Mouth Baked Granola (page 202)

LUNCH

Pumping Jumping Bean Salad (page 216), or Feel-Good Turkey or Salmon Tomato Panini (page 222)

SNACK (OPTIONAL)

Spiced Honey-Glazed Nuts (page 233), or Calming Coconut-Date Balls (page 234)

DINNER

Strengthening Spinach, Feta, and Rice Casserole (page 244), or Metabolism-Boosting Chicken Curry Feast (page 257) with Sustaining Ginger-Sesame Carrots (page 268)

Thursday

BREAKFAST

Melt-in-Your Mouth Baked Granola (page 202), or Protein-Powered Muesli with Coconut and Raisins (page 203)

LUNCH

Energizing Thai Spice Chicken Salad (page 215) with Energizing Thai Spice Salad Dressing (page 218), or Feel-Good Turkey or Salmon Tomato Panini (page 222)

SNACK (OPTIONAL)

High-Energy Chicken and Cauliflower Croquettes (page 231), or Spiced Honey-Glazed Nuts (page 233)

DINNER

Nutrient-Rich Roasted Quinoa with Mushrooms, Cumin, and Coriander (page 240), or Healing Baked Halibut or Salmon and Shiitake (page 254) with Luscious Lima Bean Mash (page 263)

Friday

BREAKFAST

Fortifying Flourless Chicken Flapjacks (page 204), or Regenerating Herb Scrambled Eggs (page 203)

LUNCH

2 slices of Gluten-Free Mediterranean Veggie Pizza (page 219) or Feel-Good Turkey or Salmon Tomato Panini (page 222)

SNACK (OPTIONAL)

Turkey, Lamb, or Beef Koftas with a Heart-Healthy Kick (page 232), or Spiced Honey-Glazed Nuts (page 233)

DINNER

Stress-Less Shiitake and Asparagus Risotto (page 246), or Supercharged Chicken or Turkey Meat Loaf (page 259) with Sautéed Shiitake Mushrooms with a Kale Kick (page 265)

DESSERT

Blueberry and Apple Crumble Gone Nuts (page 288), or Berry-Beneficial Blueberry and Pecan Pie (page 289)

Saturday

BREAKFAST

Super-Energizing Baked Beans (page 208), or Strengthening Sun-Dried Tomato and Feta-Chive Omelet (page 206)

LUNCH

Build-Me-Up Butternut and Macadamia Nut Bisque (page 228), or 2 slices of Gluten-Free Mediterranean Veggie Pizza (pages 219)

SNACK (OPTIONAL)

High-Energy Chicken and Cauliflower Croquettes (page 231), or Detoxifying Lima Bean Blinis with Artichoke Herbed Dip (page 234)

DINNER

Immune-Boosting Thai Tempeh Cakes with Sweet Spicy Dipping Sauce (page 245), or Nice and Spiced Beef or Chicken Stir-Fry (page 249) with Balancing Basmati Almond Rice (page 266)

DESSERT

Energy-Giving Coconut, Almond, and Raisin Custard (page 287), or Blueberry and Apple Crumble Gone Nuts (page 288)

WEEK 2 EATING PLAN SUGGESTIONS

Sunday

BREAKFAST

Get-Up-and-Go Banana Berry Quinoa Porridge (page 201), or Melt-in-Your Mouth Baked Granola (page 202)

LUNCH

Almighty Avocado and Black Bean Salad (page 211), or Love-Your-Heart Red Lentil Soup (page 226)

SNACK (OPTIONAL)

Blood-Sugar-Balancing Butternut and Leek Pies (page 220), or High-Energy Chicken and Cauliflower Croquettes (page 221)

DINNER

High-Fiber Butternut Gnocchi with Herbed Cream Sauce (page 241), or Metabolism-Boosting Chicken Curry Feast (page 257) with Sumptuous Spinach and Swiss Chard with Pine Nuts (page 267)

Monday

BREAKFAST

Regenerating Herb Scrambled Eggs (page 203), or Fortifying Flourless Chicken Flapjacks (page 204)

LUNCH

Vitalizing Broccoli and Cauliflower Salad (page 213) with Simply Nourishing Salad Dressing (page 217), or Stress-Less Turkey, Avocado, and Veggie Nori Wrap (page 219)

SNACK (OPTIONAL)

Detoxifying Lima Bean Blinis with Artichoke Herbed Dip (page 234), or Spiced Honey-Glazed Nuts (page 233)

DINNER

Protein-Packed Vegetarian Shepherd's Pie (page 239), or Favorite Sweet, Spicy, and Crunchy Meat Loaf (page 258) with Zesty Broccoli with Garlic and Ginger (page 265)

Tuesday

BREAKFAST

Melt-in-Your Mouth Baked Granola (page 202), or Protein-Powered Nut Muesli with Coconut and Raisins (page 203)

LUNCH

Mood-Boosting Chicken and Pineapple Coleslaw with Coconut-Lime Dressing (page 212), or Pumping Jumping Bean Salad (page 216)

SNACK (OPTIONAL)

Turkey, Lamb, or Beef Koftas with a Heart-Healthy Kick (page 232), or Spiced Honey-Glazed Nuts (page 233)

DINNER

Hi-Fibe Red Bean Burgers (page 238), or Nice and Spiced Beef or Chicken Stir-Fry (page 249) with Cardioprotective Green Beans (page 268)

DESSERT

Sweet Brown Rice Pudding with an Antioxidant Twist (page 292), or Fortifying Fig and Minty Blueberry Brûlée (page 286)

Wednesday

BREAKFAST

Regenerating Herb Scrambled Eggs (page 203), or Fortifying Flourless Chicken Flapjacks (page 204)

LUNCH

Feel-Good Turkey or Salmon Tomato Panini (page 222), or Vibrant Avocado and Veggie Salsa Collard Wrap (page 221)

SNACK (OPTIONAL)

1 slice of Almighty Almond and Walnut Pumpernickel Bread (page 283) with Immune-Building Lemon-Ginger Butter (page 276), or Spiced Honey-Glazed Nuts (page 233)

DINNER

Stress-Less Shiitake and Asparagus Risotto (page 246), or Fisherman's Omega-3 Fish Fingers (page 250) with Fragrant Cauliflower-Quinoa Risotto (page 262)

Thursday

BREAKFAST

Get-Up-and-Go Banana Berry Quinoa Porridge (page 201), or Melt-in-Your Mouth Baked Granola (page 202)

LUNCH

Love-Your-Heart Red Lentil Soup (page 226), or Cardioprotective Salmon Caesar Salad (page 214) with Cardioprotective Caesar Salad Dressing (page 217) and 1 Nourishing Crusty Onion and Parmesan Roll (page 285)

SNACK (OPTIONAL)

1 slice of Almighty Almond and Walnut Pumpernickel Bread (page 283) with Super-Healthful Hummus (page 270)

DINNER

Revitalizing Vegetable Biryani (page 242), or Healing Baked Halibut or Salmon and Shiitake (page 259) with Cardioprotective Green Beans (page 268)

Friday

BREAKFAST

Melt-in-Your Mouth Baked Granola (page 202), or Protein-Powered Muesli with Coconut and Raisins (page 203)

LUNCH

2 slices Gluten-Free Mediterranean Veggie Pizza (pages 219), or Feel-Good Turkey or Salmon Tomato Panini (page 222)

SNACK (OPTIONAL)

Blood-Sugar-Balancing Butternut and Leek Pies (page 220), or 2 Calming Coconut-Date Balls (page 224)

DINNER

Spicy Moroccan Tempeh with Lentils (page 237), or Mega-Omega Spice Crusted Salmon (page 251) with Sumptuous Spinach and Swiss Chard with Pine Nuts (page 267)

DESSERT

Hearty Hazelnut Rounds (page 280), or Luscious Lemon-Pineapple Yogurt Cake (page 281)

Saturday

BREAKFAST

Super-Energizing Baked Beans (page 208), or Strengthening Sun-Dried Tomato and Feta-Chive Omelet (page 206) with 1 Zesty Digestive Herb and Cheddar Breakfast Muffin (page 209)

LUNCH

Almighty Avocado and Black Bean Salad (page 211), or Immune-Boosting Basque Bean and Cabbage Soup (page 227)

SNACK (OPTIONAL)

Detoxifying Lima Bean Blinis with Artichoke Herbed Dip (page 234) with 2 to 3 Low-Carb Herbed Cheddar Crackers (page 229), or High-Energy Chicken and Cauliflower Croquettes (page 231)

DINNER

Comforting Cheddar and Broccoli Quiche with Quinoa Crust (page 243), or Spicy Shrimp and Tomato Kebabs with Herbed Lima Beans (page 255) with Sustaining Ginger-Sesame Carrots (page 269)

DESSERT

Berry-Beneficial Blueberry and Pecan Pie (page 289), or Sweet Brown Rice Pudding with an Antioxidant Twist (page 292)

WEEK 3 EATING PLAN SUGGESTIONS

Sunday

BREAKFAST

Strengthening Sun-Dried Tomato and Feta-Chive Omelet (page 206)

LUNCH

1 cup Build-Me-Up Butternut and Macadamia Nut Bisque (page 1228) with 2 Low-Carb Herbed Cheddar Crackers (page 229), or 1 Feel-Good Turkey or Salmon Tomato Panini (page 222)

SNACK (OPTIONAL)

1 to 2 Blood-Sugar-Balancing Butternut and Leek Pies (page 230), or a handful of Spiced Honey-Glazed Nuts (page 233)

DINNER

Protein-Packed Vegetarian Shepherd's Pie (page 239), or Soul-Warming Tuna Lasagna (page 253) with Cardioprotective Green Beans (page 268)

Monday

BREAKFAST

Protein-Powered Muesli with Coconut and Raisins (page 203), or Regenerating Herb Scrambled Eggs (page 203)

LUNCH

Energizing Thai Spice Chicken Salad (page 215), or Vibrant Avocado and Veggie Salsa Collard Wrap (page 221)

SNACK (OPTIONAL)

1 to 2 High-Energy Chicken and Cauliflower Croquettes (page 231), or 1 to 2 Turkey, Lamb, or Beef Koftas with a Heart-Healthy Kick (page 232)

DINNER

Strengthening Spinach, Feta, and Rice Casserole (page 244), or Mega-Omega Spice-Crusted Salmon (page 251) with Zesty Broccoli with Garlic and Ginger (page 265)

Tuesday

BREAKFAST

Fortifying Flourless Chicken Flapjacks (page 204), or Melt-in-Your Mouth Baked Granola (page 202)

LUNCH

Stress-Less Turkey, Avocado, and Veggie Nori Wrap (page 219), or Cardioprotective Salmon Caesar Salad (page 214) with Cardioprotective Caesar Salad Dressing (page 217)

SNACK (OPTIONAL)

1 to 2 slices of Powerhouse Pumpkin, Spice, and Almond Bread (page 284), or handful of Spiced Honey-Glazed Nuts (page 223)

DINNER

Revitalizing Vegetable Biryani (page 242), or Spicy Shrimp and Tomato Kebabs with Herbed Lima Beans (page 255) with Luscious Lima Bean Mash (page 263)

DESSERT

Sweet Brown Rice Pudding with an Antioxidant Twist (page 292), or 1 to 2 Hearty Hazelnut Rounds (page 280)

Wednesday

BREAKFAST

Regenerating Herb Scrambled Eggs (page 203), or Get-Up-and-Go Banana Berry Quinoa Porridge (page 221)

LUNCH

Mood-Boosting Chicken and Pineapple Coleslaw with Coconut-Lime Dressing (page 202), or Pumping Jumping Bean Salad (page 206)

SNACK (OPTIONAL)

1 to 2 Calming Coconut-Date Balls (page 234), or a handful of Spiced Honey-Glazed Nuts (page 233)

DINNER

Favorite Sweet, Spicy, and Crunchy Meat Loaf (page 248) with Anti-Ox Pumpkin and Cauliflower Mash (page 264), or High-Fiber Butternut Gnocchi with Herbed Cream Sauce (page 241)

Thursday

BREAKFAST

Protein-Powered Muesli with Coconut and Raisins (page 203), or Regenerating Herb Scrambled Eggs (page 203)

LUNCH

Stress-Less Turkey, Avocado, and Veggie Nori Wrap (page 219), or Love-Your-Heart Red Lentil Soup (page 226)

SNACK (OPTIONAL)

A handful of Spiced Honey-Glazed Nuts (page 233), or 1 to 2 Calming Coconut-Date Balls (page 234)

DINNER

Stress-Less Shiitake and Asparagus Risotto (page 246), or Mighty Moroccan Chicken Tagine (page 256) with Sustaining Ginger-Sesame Carrots (page 269)

Friday

BREAKFAST

Regenerating Herb Scrambled Eggs page 203), or Fortifying Flourless Chicken Flapjacks (page 204)

LUNCH

Almighty Avocado and Black Bean Salad (page 211), or Mood-Boosting Chicken and Pineapple Coleslaw with Coconut-Lime Dressing (page 212)

SNACK (OPTIONAL)

1 to 2 Turkey, Lamb, or Beef Koftas with a Heart-Healthy Kick (page 232), or a handful of Spiced Honey-Glazed Nuts (page 233)

DINNER

Protein-Packed Vegetarian Shepherd's Pie (page 239), or Nice and Spiced Beef or Chicken Stir-Fry (page 249) with Zesty Broccoli with Garlic and Ginger (page 265)

DESSERT

Blueberry and Apple Crumble Gone Nuts (page 288), or Berry-Beneficial Blueberry and Pecan Pie (page 289)

Saturday

BREAKFAST

Super-Energizing Baked Beans (page 208), or Strengthening Sun-Dried Tomato and Feta-Chive Omelet (page 206)

LUNCH

Pumping Jumping Bean Salad (page 216), or Feel-Good Turkey or Salmon Tomato Panini (page 222)

SNACK (OPTIONAL)

Cup of Build-Me-Up Butternut and Macadamia Nut Bisque (page 228), or 1 to 2 Detoxifying Lima Bean Blinis with Artichoke Herbed Dip (page 234)

DINNER

Comforting Cheddar and Broccoli Quiche with Quinoa Crust (page 243), or Metabolism-Boosting Chicken Curry Feast (page 257) with Cardioprotective Green Beans (page 268)

DESSERT

Slice of Health-Gratifying Grapefruit and Orange Cake (page 282), or 1 to 2 Hearty Hazelnut Rounds (page 280)

WEEK 4 EATING PLAN SUGGESTIONS

Sunday

BREAKFAST

Brain-Boosting Salmon Eggs Benedict (page 205), or Strengthening Sun-Dried Tomato and Feta Chive Omelet (page 206)

LUNCH

Almighty Avocado and Black Bean Salad (page 211), or Stress-Less Turkey, Avocado, and Veggie Nori Wrap (page 219)

SNACK (OPTIONAL)

Blood-Sugar-Balancing Butternut and Leek Pies (page 230), or Detoxifying Lima Bean Blinis with Artichoke Herbed Dip (page 234)

DINNER

Immune-Boosting Thai Tempeh Cakes with Sweet Spicy Dipping Sauce (page 245), or Soul-Warming Tuna Lasagna (page 253) with Vitalizing Broccoli and Cauliflower Salad (page 203)

Monday

BREAKFAST

Melt-in-Your Mouth Baked Granola (page 202), or Sweet Brown Rice Pudding with an Antioxidant Twist (page 292)

LUNCH

Love-Your-Heart Red Lentil Soup (page 226), or Feel-Good Turkey or Salmon Tomato Panini (page 222)

SNACK (OPTIONAL)

Spiced Honey-Glazed Nuts (page 233), or Calming Coconut-Date Balls (page 234)

DINNER

Strengthening Spinach, Feta and Rice Casserole (page 244), or Fisherman's Omega-3 Fish Fingers (page 250) with Zesty Broccoli with Garlic and Ginger (page 265)

Tuesday

BREAKFAST

Melt-in-Your Mouth Baked Granola (page 202), or Protein-Powered Muesli with Coconut and Raisins (page 203)

LUNCH

Cardioprotective Salmon Caesar Salad (page 214) with Cardioprotective Caesar Salad Dressing (page 217), or Vibrant Avocado and Veggie Salsa Collard Wrap (page 221)

SNACK (OPTIONAL)

Spiced Honey-Glazed Nuts (page 233), or Calming Coconut-Date Balls (page 234)

DINNER

Strengthening Spinach, Feta, and Rice Casserole (page 244), or Anti-Inflammatory Turmeric Turkey Burgers (page 260) with Sustaining Ginger-Sesame Carrots (page 269)

DESSERT

No-Bake Superfood Fudge Brownies (page 293), or Fortifying Fig and Minty Blueberry Brûlée (page 286)

Wednesday

BREAKFAST

Regenerating Herb Scrambled Eggs (page 203), or Fortifying Flourless Chicken Flapjacks (page 204)

LUNCH

Pumping Jumping Bean Salad (page 216), or Feel-Good Turkey or Salmon Tomato Panini (page 222)

SNACK (OPTIONAL)

Slice of Almighty Almond and Walnut Pumpernickel Bread (page 283), or a handful of Spiced Honey-Glazed Nuts (page 233)

DINNER

Stress-Less Shiitake and Asparagus Risotto (page 246), or Favorite Sweet, Spicy, and Crunchy Meat Loaf (page 248) and Zesty Broccoli with Garlic and Ginger (page 265)

Thursday

BREAKFAST

Fortifying Flourless Chicken Flapjacks (page 204), or Regenerating Herb Scrambled Eggs (page 203)

LUNCH

Pumping Jumping Bean Salad (page 216), or Feel-Good Turkey or Salmon Tomato Panini (page 222)

SNACK (OPTIONAL)

Super-Healthful Hummus (page 270) with 2 Low-Carb Herbed Cheddar Crackers (page 229)

DINNER

Comforting Cheddar and Broccoli Quiche with Quinoa Crust (page 243), or Tantalizing Thai Fish Cakes (page 252) with Anti-Ox Pumpkin and Cauliflower Mash (page 234)

Friday

BREAKFAST

Regenerating Herb Scrambled Eggs (page 203), or Protein-Powered Muesli with Coconut and Raisins (page 203)

LUNCH

Vitalizing Broccoli and Cauliflower Salad (page 213), or Gluten-Free Mediterranean Veggie Pizza (page 219)

SNACK (OPTIONAL)

Bone-Strengthening Lemon Tahini (page 271) with 2 Low-Carb Herbed Cheddar Crackers (page 229), or a handful of Spiced Honey-Glazed Nuts (page 233)

DINNER

Nutrient-Rich Roasted Quinoa with Mushrooms, Cumin, and Coriander (page 240), or Mighty Moroccan Chicken Tagine (page 256) with Balancing Basmati Almond Rice (page 266) and Zesty Broccoli with Garlic and Ginger (page 265)

DESSERT

Sweet Brown Rice Pudding with an Antioxidant Twist (page 292)

Saturday

BREAKFAST

Strengthening Sun-Dried Tomato and Feta-Chive Omelet (page 206), or Hearty Mediterranean Frittata (page 207)

LUNCH

Cardioprotective Salmon Caesar Salad (page 214) with Cardioprotective Caeser Salad Dressing (page 217), or Vibrant Avocado and Veggie Salsa Collard Wrap (page 221)

SNACK (OPTIONAL)

Blood-Sugar-Balancing Butternut and Leek Pies (page 230), or a handful of Spiced Honey-Glazed Nuts (page 233)

DINNER

Spicy Moroccan Tempeh with Lentils (page 237), or Soul-Warming Tuna Lasagna (page 253) with Sumptuous Spinach and Swiss Chard with Pine Nuts (page 267)

DESSERT

Berry-Beneficial Blueberry and Pecan Pie (page 289)

GLOSSARY

Adenosine triphosphate (ATP)—the body's energy molecule.

Adrenal glands—endocrine glands that sit on top of the kidneys. They secrete stress hormones such as cortisol and adrenaline.

Adrenaline (also known as epinephrine)—a hormone secreted by the adrenal glands that increases heart rate, constricts blood vessels, and participates in the "fight or flight" response.

Advanced glycation end products (AGEs)—the end products of a reaction in which a sugar molecule bonds to a protein molecule. AGEs are implicated in many chronic diseases such as diabetes and heart disease.

All-cause mortality—death from any cause whatsoever.

Allicin—the major biologically active component of garlic, responsible for its broad spectrum of anti-bacterial activity.

Alpha-linolenic acid (ALA)—a plant-based omega-3 fatty acid that helps reduce inflammation and is found in flaxseed, chia seeds, hemp, and walnuts.

Amino acids—molecules that link together to form proteins.

Angina—chest pain or discomfort produced when the heart doesn't get enough blood.

Anthocyanins—compounds found in plants, especially berries, that have powerful antioxidant properties. Anthocyanins provide the pigments responsible for the rich colors of berries.

Arteriosclerosis—general term for any kind of hardening or stiffening of the arteries.

Artery—a blood vessel that carries blood away from the heart.

Astaxanthin—a powerful antioxidant found primarily in wild salmon and krill. It's responsible for salmon's pink-red color.

Atherogenic—capable of producing plaque in the arteries.

Atherosclerosis—a condition in which the arteries thicken, the walls become inflamed, material builds up, and plaque is formed. Commonly referred to as "hardening of the arteries."

Atom–the smallest component of an element having the chemical properties of the element.

Beta blocker–a class of drugs used for various indications such as cardiac arrhythmias and hypertension. It diminishes the effects of stress hormones such as adrenaline.

Bifurcation–to separate into two parts or branches, as when the main stem of a blood vessel divides to become two smaller vessels.

Bile acids–a complex fluid found in the bile of mammals that aids in fat absorption. Bile acids are produced from cholesterol in the liver and stored in the gallbladder.

Blood clot (also known as a thrombus)–blood clots form when there is damage to the lining of a blood vessel. Normal clotting is an important mechanism in helping the body repair injured blood vessels. When unneeded blood clots form, however, this can have potentially serious consequences.

Blood pressure–the pressure exerted against the walls of the blood vessels by circulating blood.

Calcification (as in the arteries)–the process by which calcium builds up in soft tissue, including arteries and heart valves, causing it to harden.

Carbohydrates–one of the three "macronutrients" or classes of food (the others are protein and fat). Carbohydrates include sugars and starch.

Cardiac ischemia (also known as myocardial ischemia)–a decrease in blood flow that reduces your heart's oxygen supply. It can damage your heart muscle.

Cholesterol (includes serum cholesterol)–a waxy sterol that is an essential component of cell membranes. (A sterol is a particular type of fat.) It's the principal sterol synthesized by animals and is important for the manufacture of sex hormones, vitamin D, and bile acids.

Coenzyme Q$_{10}$ (CoQ$_{10}$)–a vitamin-like substance found in every cell in the body; essential for the manufacture of the body's energy molecule, ATP; a powerful antioxidant; approved since 1974 in Japan, where it is used for heart failure. It is significantly depleted by statin drugs.

Conjugated linoleic acid (CLA)–a "good" trans fat found in the meat and milk of grass-fed animals. Much research has shown that it has anticancer properties and may also help with body composition (reduction in body fat).

Control group–a group in a scientific experiment that is treated identically to the experimental group in every way except that it's not given the drug or treatment being tested. In drug tests, the control group gets a placebo. The effects of the drug or treatment are measured in the experimental group, which is then compared to the control group.

Cortisol–a steroid hormone produced by the adrenal gland. It is the primary "stress hormone" in the body

COX-2 inhibitors–a class of compounds (often drugs) that inhibit enzymes in the body called COX (cyclooxygenase). COX-1 maintains the normal lining of the stomach while COX-2 increases in response to inflammation. COX-2 inhibitors reduce inflammation while leaving COX-1 alone.

C-reactive protein–protein in the blood used as a systemic measure of inflammation.

Cytokines–inflammatory chemicals produced by a variety of cells in the body, including those in the adipose (fat) tissue.

D-alpha tocopherol–one of eight forms of vitamin E.

Diabetes, type 1–an autoimmune disease that results in the destruction of the insulin-producing cells in the pancreas. Type 1 diabetics don't produce enough insulin, and the disease is typically fatal unless treated with exogenous insulin (either by injection, inhalation, or insulin pumps).

Diabetes, type 2–a chronic condition in which the cells "ignore" insulin (see *insulin resistance*), usually resulting in dangerously high blood sugar and insulin levels. Ninety to 95 percent of diabetics have this type of diabetes, which is a lifestyle-related disease.

Diet-heart hypothesis–the idea that saturated fat and dietary cholesterol cause or contribute to heart disease.

DL-alpha tocopherol–a synthetic form of vitamin E.

Docosahexaenoic acid (DHA)–an omega-3 fatty acid found primarily in fish. It is particularly important for the brain.

Dolichols–important for the synthesis of glycoproteins, which in turn are important for emotions, cell identification, cell messaging, and immune defense. Statin drugs reduce them, because dolichols are produced by the same pathway that produces cholesterol and is interrupted by statin drugs. Reduced bioavailability of dolichols can affect every cellular process in the body.

Double-blind study–a study in which neither the subjects nor the experimenters know which subjects are getting an active drug and which subjects are getting a placebo. Double-blind studies are believed to minimize the effect of experimenter and patient expectations.

D-ribose–molecule made in the body's cells and used for cellular function.

Eicosanoids–mini hormones that control metabolic processes in the body; also called prostaglandins.

Eicosapentaenoic acid (EPA)–an important omega-3 fatty acid found primarily in fish. It is particularly important for the heart.

Electrons–tiny subatomic particles that carry a negative electric charge and surround the nuclei of atoms.

Ellagic acid–a natural antioxidant found in many vegetables and fruits, particularly raspberries, strawberries, and pomegranates. It is being investigated for its anticancer properties.

Endocrinology–the study of hormones and what they do.

Endothelial dysfunction (ED)—dysfunction of the cells that line the inner surface of all blood vessels. A major feature of endothelial dysfunction is the inability of the arteries to dilate (open) fully. ED contributes to several diseases, including diabetes, and it is always associated with heart disease.

Endothelium—the thin layer of cells that lines the inner surface of blood vessels.

Enzyme—a complex protein that speeds the rate at which certain chemical processes take place.

Epinephrine (also known as adrenaline)—an important stress hormone released by the adrenal glands.

Estrogen—family of hormones that perform about four hundred functions in the human body; produced primarily in the ovaries and adrenal glands; known as the "female hormone" but present in both women and men.

Farnesyl-PP—an intermediate in the HMG-CoA pathway.

Fat—one of the three major classes of nutrients known as "macronutrients" (the others being protein and carbohydrates). It is made up of smaller units called fatty acids.

Fatty acids—the building blocks of fat.

Fiber—indigestible component of food; associated with lower risks of heart disease, diabetes, obesity, and cancer.

Fibrates—a class of drugs used for lowering cholesterol. They also lower triglycerides.

Fibrin—a protein essential for the clotting of blood.

Fibrinogen—a protein that is converted to fibrin during the blood-clotting process.

Flavanols—a group of plant pigments, including the anthocyanins, that are beneficial to health.

Flavonoids—plant compounds that have antioxidant and anti-inflammatory activity.

Folic acid—a water-soluble B vitamin needed for proper development of the human body and to help the body make healthy new cells. Folic acid is the synthetic (man-made) form of folate, found naturally in some foods.

Free radicals—destructive molecules in the body; can harm cells and DNA by producing "oxidative damage."

Fructose—fruit sugar, found naturally in honey, berries, fruits, and most root vegetables. Table sugar is half glucose, half fructose. The most damaging of the sugars when taken in concentrated forms such as sugar, high-fructose corn syrup, or agave nectar. Causes insulin resistance, fatty liver, and elevated triglycerides.

Geranyl-PP—a product of the condensation of dimethallyl-pp and isopentyl-pp.

Glucagon—the "sister" hormone of insulin, made in the pancreas. Increases when blood sugar levels are low. Helps counteract the effects of insulin.

Glucocorticoids—a class of steroid hormones produced by the adrenal glands. Cortisol is the most important glucocorticoid.

Glucose—a simple sugar and component of most carbohydrates. Table sugar is 50 percent glucose. It is measured in the blood as blood glucose.

Glycation–the result of the bonding of a protein molecule with a sugar molecule. It is also known as nonenzymatic glycosylation.

Glycemic Index–measure of how much a portion, specifically 50g, of a given food raises blood sugar.

Hemochromatosis–a disorder that results in too much iron being absorbed from the gastrointestinal tract.

High-density lipoprotein (HDL)–a complex of lipids and proteins that transports cholesterol in the blood and is often thought of as the "good" cholesterol.

High-fructose corn syrup–a sweetener made by processing corn syrup to increase the level of fructose.

HMG-CoA reductase–an enzyme that plays a central role in the production of cholesterol in the liver.

Homeostasis–derived from the Greek, meaning "remaining stable" or "remaining the same." A relatively stable state of equilibrium.

Homocysteine–an amino acid found in the blood, high levels of which increase the chance of heart disease, stroke, osteoporosis, and Alzheimer's. Homocysteine can be lowered with folic acid, vitamin B_6, and vitamin B_{12}.

Hormones–chemical messengers that travel in the bloodstream and affect sexual function, growth, development, mood, and many different metabolic processes.

Hydrogenated or partially hydrogenated oil–the process of adding hydrogen to vegetable oil is called hydrogenation. It makes the oil less likely to spoil but also creates trans fat, the most damaging of all the fatty acids.

Hypertension–high blood pressure.

Hyperviscosity–increased thickness of the blood.

Inflammation, acute–a tissue response to injury, usually of a sudden onset. Examples include injuries to the knee or back, abscesses, and skin outbreaks. Classical signs include pain, heat, redness, and swelling.

Inflammation, chronic–prolonged and persistent inflammation that often flies beneath the pain radar. It is a critical component of nearly all degenerative diseases. Chronic, persistent inflammation of the vascular walls is a major cause of heart disease.

Insulin–fat-storing hormone that, if raised high enough, long enough, and frequently enough, contributes to diabetes, heart disease, and aging.

Insulin resistance–the condition in which the cells stop "listening" to insulin, resulting in high blood sugar and high insulin. Insulin resistance is associated with metabolic syndrome and type 2 diabetes.

Intermediate-density lipoprotein (IDL)–one of five major groups of lipoproteins that transport different types of molecules, including cholesterol, through the bloodstream.

Isopentyl pyrophosphate (IPP)–an intermediate in the HMG-CoA pathway.

Keys, Ancel (1904-2004)–an American researcher and scientist whose Seven Countries Study appeared to show that serum cholesterol was strongly related to coronary heart disease. He persuaded many Americans—and mainstream health organizations—to adopt and endorse a low-fat diet.

L-carnitine–a vitamin-like compound that escorts fatty acids into the mitochondria of the cells, where it can be "burned" for energy.

Left ventricular hypertrophy–enlargement (hypertrophy) of the muscle tissue that makes up the wall of the heart's main pumping chamber (the left ventricle).

Lipid core–an important component of "vulnerable plaque" (plaque prone to rupture). Approximately 40 percent of vulnerable plaque is composed of the lipid core.

Lipid rafts–regions of cell membranes that are involved in intracellular signaling pathways. They are particularly rich in cholesterol.

Lipoproteins–structures that transport fats, especially cholesterol and triglycerides, from place to place within the bloodstream.

Low-density lipoprotein (LDL)–one of five major groups of lipoproteins that transport different types of molecules, including cholesterol, through the bloodstream. It's popularly known as the "bad" cholesterol.

Lumbrokinase (also known as *Boluoke*)–an extract from earthworms that lowers blood viscosity (thickness), helps thin the blood, and helps prevent clots by breaking down fibrinogen.

Macrophages–white blood cells that devour foreign invaders such as fungi and bacteria.

Magnesium–a mineral that helps lower high blood pressure.

Maladaptation–faulty or inadequate adaptation; a trait that has become more harmful than helpful.

Mediterranean diet–the general name given to diets from the Mediterranean Sea areas that emphasize fruits, vegetables, whole grains, olive oil, beans, nuts, fish, and small amounts of red meat.

Meta-analysis–a "study of studies" that combines data from several studies that address a set of related research hypotheses; a statistical procedure for combining data from multiple studies.

Metabolic syndrome–the name for a group of risk factors that occur together and increase the risk for coronary artery disease, stroke, and type 2 diabetes. It's also known as prediabetes, and it's characterized by insulin resistance, high triglycerides, abdominal fat, high blood pressure, low HDL cholesterol, and high blood sugar.

Mevalonate pathway (HMG-CoA reductase pathway)–the biochemical pathway that produces cholesterol as well as coenzyme Q_{10} and other important compounds such as dolichols.

Mitochondria–the power stations in every cell where energy is produced.

Monocytes–a type of white blood cell that attacks bacteria or viruses.

Monounsaturated fatty acids–fats central to the Mediterranean diet; associated with lower rates of heart disease; found in nuts and olive oil; also called omega-9s.

Myocardial infarction–a heart attack.

Nattokinase–an enzyme extracted from the Japanese food called natto (fermented soybeans). A natural blood thinner and clot buster (similar in effect to lumbrokinase).

Neurotransmitters–chemicals produced mainly in the brain that transmit information; examples are serotonin, dopamine, and epinephrine.

Niacin (nicotinic acid, vitamin B$_3$)–often used to lower LDL cholesterol and/or raise HDL.

Nuclear factor kappa B (NF-kB)–a "smoke sensor" that detects dangerous threats, such as free radicals and infectious agents, and responds by unleashing inflammatory responses in chronic diseases. It is produced by the mevalonate pathway and inhibited by statin drugs.

Nutraceutical–combination of the word "nutrition" and "pharmaceutical"; a supplement that provides health benefits.

Omega-3 fatty acids–a class of polyunsaturated fatty acids that have strong anti-inflammatory properties and are important for the brain and the heart.

Omega-6 fatty acids–a class of polyunsaturated fats found in vegetable oils. They are pro-inflammatory, especially when not balanced with enough omega-3s.

Oxidation (also known as *oxidative damage*)–the damage to skin, organs, and arteries caused by free radicals; along with inflammation, one of the initiators of heart disease; implicated in many other diseases as well.

Oxidative stress–the damage done to cells by free radicals of oxygen molecules; another term for oxidation or oxidative damage.

Oxytocin–a chemical often called the "bonding" hormone that is released during breastfeeding and sex. It can elicit the urge to connect to others.

Pantethine–biologically active form of vitamin B$_5$; often used for lowering cholesterol.

Pattern A–desirable distribution of LDL particles in which the big, fluffy, innocuous particles predominate.

Pattern B–undesirable distribution of LDL particles in which the small, atherogenic particles predominate.

Placebo-controlled study–a way of testing in a scientific experiment in which one group (or more) gets the treatment or the drug and another group (the control group) gets an inert substance (placebo).

Plaque (atherosclerotic plaque)–a deposit of fat and other substances that accumulate in the lining of arterial walls.

Platelet–a cell-like particle in the blood that is an important part of blood clotting.

Polyphenols–large class of plant chemicals, many of which have significant health benefits.

Polyunsaturated fatty acids–large class of fatty acids with many members, including both the omega-3s and the omega-6s; found in vegetable oils, nuts, and fish.

Prenylated proteins–proteins anchored to membranes.

Primary prevention–treatment to prevent a first heart attack.

Progesterone–an important hormone secreted by the female reproductive system.

Protein–one of the three "macronutrients" or classes of food (the others are carbohydrates and fat).

Pterostilbene–a chemical related to resveratrol and found in blueberries and grapes; may have significant health benefits.

Randomized study–a study in which subjects are randomly assigned to either treatment or control groups.

Risk reduction, absolute–the actual amount of risk reduction from taking a certain drug or eating a certain diet. For example, if 3 percent of all subjects could be expected to die over the course of a decade but only 2 percent of subjects taking a drug *actually* died over the course of the same decade, the absolute risk reduction is 1 percent.

Risk reduction, relative–risk reduction expressed as the percent difference between expected and observed. In the above example, the difference between 3 percent expected death and 2 percent observed death would be expressed as a 33 percent reduction in *relative risk*, a much more impressive number but very misleading.

Saturated fatty acids–a fatty acid in which there are no double bonds. Saturated fats are found primarily in animal foods and are solid at room temperature.

Secondary prevention–treatment to prevent a subsequent heart attack in patients who have already suffered one or more heart attacks.

Selenoproteins–a class of proteins that contain the essential mineral selenium.

Seven Countries Study–a study by Ancel Keys purporting to show that cholesterol and fat in the diet are the prime causes of heart disease. It was later criticized for bias and poor methodology.

Squalene–a metabolic precursor of sterols.

Statins–a class of drugs used to lower cholesterol. Also known as HMG-reductase inhibitors.

Stress, acute–a kind of stress that is usually short-term; it can be thrilling and exciting, like a run down a challenging ski slope, or it can be unpleasant, like anger or a headache.

Stress, chronic–the grinding stress that wears people down day after day, year after year. It is considered a contributing factor in heart disease.

Sugar–a sweet crystalline substance obtained from various plants, especially sugar beet and sugar cane.

Testosterone–the major male sexual hormone belonging to the steroid family; produced in the testes of males but also produced (in smaller amounts) by females in the ovaries.

Thrombus–a blood clot formed within the vascular system, impeding blood flow.

Tocopherols–a class of four closely related chemical compounds that are part of the vitamin E family.

Tocotrienols–a class of four potent antioxidants and heart-healthy nutrients that are part of the vitamin E family.

Total cholesterol–the sum total of all "types" of cholesterol measured in the blood. Includes LDL and HDL cholesterol, as well as lesser known VLDL and IDL; given as one number on a blood test.

Trans fatty acids–a special kind of fat formed when liquid fats are made into solid fats by the addition of hydrogen atoms; partially hydrogenated or hydrogenated vegetable oils.

Triglycerides–main form of fat found in the body and in the diet and nearly always measured on a standard blood test; high levels increase the risk for heart disease and are a feature of metabolic syndrome.

Vasodilate–the dilation (widening) of blood vessels from the relaxation of the muscular wall of the vessels, resulting in lowered blood pressure.

Very low-density lipoprotein (VLDL)–one of five types of lipoproteins, packages that transport substances such as cholesterol and triglycerides throughout the bloodstream.

Voodoo death–term coined by physiologist Walter Cannon, M.D., that refers to the phenomenon of sudden death brought on by strong emotional shock, stress, or fear.

Yudkin, John (1910-1995)–British physiologist and scientist; pioneer researcher examining the link between sugar and degenerative disease; became internationally known for his book on sugar, *Pure, White and Deadly*.

ENDNOTES

CHAPTER 1

1. M. de Lorgeril et al. "Mediterranean Diet, Traditional Risk Factors, and the Rate of Cardiovascular Complications after Myocardial Infarction: Final Report of the Lyon Diet Heart Study," *Circulation* 99, no. 6 (1999): 779-85.

2. Channing Laboratory, "History," *The Nurses' Health Study*, www.channing.harvard.edu/nhs/?page_id=70.

3. Ibid.

4. M. de Lorgeril et al., "Mediterranean Alpha-Linolenic Acid-Rich Diet in Secondary Prevention of Coronary Heart Disease." *The Lancet*, no. 143 (1994): 1454-59.

5. J. Kastelein et al., "Simvastatin with or without Ezetimibe in Familial Hypercholesterolemia," *New England Journal of Medicine* 358, no. 14 (2008): 1431-43.

6. F. B. Hu et al., "Primary Prevention of Coronary Heart Disease in Women through Diet and Lifestyle," *New England Journal of Medicine* 343, no. 1 (2000): 16-12.

7. Ibid.

CHAPTER 2

1. M. Herper, "America's Most Popular Drugs," *Forbes*, April 19, 2011, www.forbes.com/sites/matthewherper/2011/04/19/americas-most-popular-drugs.

2. D. J. DeNoon, "The 10 Most Prescribed Drugs," *WebMD Health News*, April 20, 2011, www.webmd.com/news/20110420/the-10-most-prescribed-drugs.

3. University of Minnesota, School of Public Health, *Health Revolutionary: The Life and Work of Ancel Keys*, PDF transcript of a video documentary, 2002, www.asph.org/movies/keys.pdf.

4. A. Keys, ed., *Seven Countries: A Multivariate Analysis of Death and Coronary Heart Disease* (Cambridge, MA: Harvard University Press, 1980); A. Keys, "Coronary Heart Disease in Seven Countries," *Circulation* 41, no. 1 (1970): 1-211.

5. M. Kendrick, *About Cavemen's Diet*, online discussion board comments posted to the website of the International Network of Cholesterol Skeptics, February 12, 2002, www.thincs.org/discuss.cavemen.htm.

6. M. Kendrick, *The Great Cholesterol Con* (London: John Blake, 2007), 53.

7. U. Ravnskov, *Ignore the Awkward* (Seattle: CreateSpace, 2010).

8. I.H. Page et al., "Dietary Fat and Its Relation to Heart Attacks and Strokes," *Circulation* 23 (1961): 133-36.

9. G. Taubes, "The Soft Science of Dietary Fat," *Science* 291, no. 5513 (2001): 2536-45.

10. Ibid.

11. University of Maryland, "Trans Fats 101," University of Maryland Medical Center, last modified November 3, 2010, www.umm.edu/features/transfats.htm.

12. Multiple Risk Factor Intervention Trial Research Group, "Multiple Risk Factor Intervention Trial," *Journal of the American Medical Association* 248, no. 12 (1982): 1465-77.

13. Ibid.

14. M. Madjid et al., "Thermal Detection of Vulnerable Plaque," *American Journal of Cardiology* 90, no. 10 (2002): L36-L39.

15. W. Castelli, "Concerning the Possibility of a Nut . . ." *Archives of Internal Medicine* 152, no. 7 (1992): 1371-72.

16. "The Lipid Research Clinics Coronary Primary Prevention Trial Results," *Journal of the American Medical Association* 251, no. 3 (1984): 351-74.

17. G. V. Mann, "Coronary Heart Disease–'Doing the Wrong Things,'" *Nutrition Today* 20, no. 4 (1985): 12-14.

18. Ibid.

19. M. F. Oliver, "Consensus or Nonsensus Conferences on Coronary Heart Disease," *The Lancet* 325, no. 8437 (1985): 1087-89.

20. National Institutes of Health Consensus Development Conference Statement, December 10-12, 1984.

21. National Institutes of Health, "News from the Women's Health Initiative: Reducing Total Fat Intake May Have Small Effect on Risk of Breast Cancer, No Effect on Risk of Colorectal Cancer, Heart Disease, or Stroke," *NIH News*, last modified February 7, 2006, www.nih.gov/news/pr/feb2006/nhlbi-07.htm.

22. A. Ottoboni and F. Ottoboni, "Low-Fat Diet and Chronic Disease Prevention: The Women's Health Initiative and Its Reception," *Journal of American Physicians and Surgeons* 12, no. 1 (2007): 10-13.

23. G. Kolata, "Low-Fat Diet Does Not Cut Health Risks, Study Finds," *New York Times*, February 8, 2006.

24. D. Lundell, *The Cure for Heart Disease* (Scottsdale: Publishing Intellect, 2012).

25. M. de Lorgeril, *A Near-Perfect Sexual Crime: Statins Against Cholesterol* (France: A4Set, 2011).

CHAPTER 3

1. J. M. Gaziano et al., "Fasting Triglycerides, High-Density Lipoprotein, and Risk of Myocardial Infarction," *Circulation* 96, no. 8 (1997): 2520-25.

2. D. Harman, "Aging: A Theory Based on Free Radical and Radiation Chemistry," *Journal of Gerontology* 11, no. 3 (1956): 298-300; D. Harman, "Free Radical Theory of Aging," in *Free Radicals and Aging*, eds. I. Emerit and B. Chance (Basel, Switzerland: Birkhäuser, 1992).

3. "Some Good Cholesterol Is Actually Bad, Study Shows," *Science Daily*, accessed September 12, 2011, www.sciencedaily.com/releases/2008/12/081201081713.htm.

4. Ibid.

5. D. Lundell, *The Cure for Heart Disease* (Scottsdale: Publishing Intellect, 2012).

CHAPTER 4

1. M. Houston, M.D., M.S., director of the Hypertension Institute in Tennessee, May 2, 2012, telephone communication.

2. D. C. Goff et al., "Insulin Sensitivity and the Rise of Incident Hypertension," *Diabetes* Care 26, no. 3 (2003): 805-9, doi.

3. "Too Much Insulin a Bad Thing for the Heart?" *Science Daily*, last modified April 19, 2010, www.sciencedaily.com/releases/2010/04/100419233109.htm.

4. V. Marigliano et al., "Normal Values in Extreme Old Age," *Annals of the New York Academy of Sciences* 673 (1992): 23-28.

5. J. O'Connell, *Sugar Nation: The Hidden Truth Behind America's Deadliest Habit and the Simple Way to Beat It* (New York: Hyperion Books, 2011), 78.

6. Ibid.

7. G. Taubes, "Is Sugar Toxic?" *New York Times Magazine*, April 13, 2011.

8. "Findings and Recommendations on the Insulin Resistance Syndrome," American Association of Clinical Endocrinologists, Washington, D.C., August 25-26, 2002.

9. Ibid.

10. M. Miller, "What Is the Association Between the Triglyceride to High-density Lipoprotein Cholesterol Ratio and Insulin Resistance?" *Medscape Education*, www.medscape.org/viewarticle/588474; T. McLaughlin et al., "Use of Metabolic Markers to Identify Overweight Individuals Who Are Insulin Resistant," *Annals of Internal Medicine* 138, no. 10 (2003): 802-9.

11. Johns Hopkins Medicine, "The New Blood Lipid Tests—Sizing Up LDL Cholesterol," *Johns Hopkins Health Alerts*, last modified on June 13, 2008, www.johnshopkinshealthalerts.com/reports/heart_health/1886-1.html.

12. Taubes, "Is Sugar Toxic?"

13. G. V. Mann, *Coronary Heart Disease: The Dietary Sense and Nonsense* (London: Janus, 1993).

14. G. V. Mann et al., "Atherosclerosis in the Masai," *American Journal of Epidemiology* 95, no. 1 (1972): 26-37.

15. J. Yudkin, *Sweet and Dangerous* (New York: Wyden, 1972).

16. A. Keys, "Letter: Normal Plasma Cholesterol in a Man Who Eats 25 Eggs a Day," *New England Journal of Medicine* 325, no. 8 (1991): 584.

17. National Institutes of Health. "National Cholesterol Education Program," *National Heart, Lung, and Blood Institute*, last modified in October 2011, www.nhlbi.nih.gov/about/ncep.

18. www.who.int/dietphysicalactivity/publications.

19. J. Eilperin, "U.S. Sugar Industry Targets New Study," *Washington Post*, April 23, 2003, www.washingtonpost.com/ac2/wp-dyn/A17583-2003Apr22?language=printer.

20. J. Casey, "The Hidden Ingredient That Can Sabotage Your Diet," *MedicineNet*, last modified January 3, 2005, www.medicinenet.com/script/main/art.asp?articlekey=56589.

21. Taubes, "Is Sugar Toxic?"

22. L. Tappy et al., "Metabolic Effects of Fructose and the Worldwide Increase in Obesity," *Physiological Reviews* 90, no. 1 (2010): 23-46; M. Dirlewanger et al., "Effects of Fructose on Hepatic Glucose Metabolism in Humans," *American Journal of Physiology, Endocrinology, and Metabolism* 279, no. 4 (2000): E907-11.

23. S. S. Elliott et al., "Fructose, Weight Gain, and the Insulin Resistance Syndrome," *American Journal of Clinical Nutrition* 76, no. 5 (2002): 911-22; K.A. Lê and L. Tappy, "Metabolic Effects of Fructose," *Current Opinion in Clinical Nutrition and Metabolic Care* 9, no. 4 (2006): 469-75; Y. Rayssiguier et al., "High Fructose Consumption Combined with Low Dietary Magnesium Intake May Increase the Incidence of the Metabolic Syndrome by Inducing Inflammation," *Magnesium Research Journal* 19, no. 4 (2006): 237-43.

24. K. Adeli and A. C. Rutledge, "Fructose and the Metabolic Syndrome: Pathophysiology and Molecular Mechanisms," *Nutrition Reviews* 65, no. 6 (2007): S13-S23; K.A. Lê and L. Tappy, "Metabolic Effects of Fructose."

25. "Fructose Metabolism by the Brain Increases Food Intake and Obesity, Study Suggests," *Science Daily*, www.sciencedaily.com/releases/2009/03/090325091811.htm.

CHAPTER 5

1. F. B. Hu et al., "Meta-analysis of Prospective Cohort Studies Evaluating the Association of Saturated Fat with Cardiovascular Disease," *American Journal of Clinical Nutrition* 91, no. 3 (2010): 502-9.

2. R. S. Kuipers et al., "Saturated Fat, Carbohydrates, and Cardiovascular Disease," *Netherlands Journal of Medicine* 69, no. 9 (2011): 372-78.

3. F. de Meester and A. P. Simopoulos, eds., "A Balanced Omega-6/Omega-3 Fatty Acid Ratio, Cholesterol and Coronary Heart Disease," *World Review of Nutrition and Dietetics* 100 (2009): 1-21; T. Hamazaki, Y. Kirihara, and Y. Ogushi, "Blood Cholesterol as a Good Marker of Health in Japan," *World Review of Nutrition and Dietetics* 100 (2009): 63-70.

4. Japan Atherosclerosis Society, "Japan Atherosclerosis Society (JAS) Guidelines for Prevention of Atherosclerotic Cardiovascular Diseases," *Journal of Atherosclerosis and Thrombosis* 14, no. 2 (2007): 5-57; de Meester and Simopoulos, "A Balanced Omega-6/Omega-3 Fatty Acid Ratio, Cholesterol and Coronary Heart Disease."

5. T. Hamazaki, et al., "Blood Cholesterol as a Good Marker of Health in Japan," *World Review of Nutrition and Dietetics* 100 (2009): 63–70; de Meester and Simopoulos, "A Balanced Omega-6/Omega-3 Fatty Acid Ratio."

6. D. M. Dreon et al., "Change in Dietary Saturated Fat Intake Is Correlated with Change in Mass of Large Low-density Lipoprotein Particles in Men," *American Journal of Clinical Nutrition* 67, no. 5 (1998): 828–36.

7. D. M. Herrington, et al., "Dietary Fats, Carbohydrate, and Progression of Coronary Atherosclerosis in Postmenopausal Women," *American Journal of Clinical Nutrition* 80, no. 5 (2004): 1175–84.

8. Ibid.

9. R. H. Knopp and Barbara M. Retzlaff, "Saturated Fat Prevents Coronary Artery Disease? An American Paradox," *American Journal of Clinical Nutrition* 80, no. 5 (2004): 1102–3.

10. M. B. Katan et al., "Dietary Oils, Serum Lipoproteins, and Coronary Heart Disease," *American Journal of Clinical Nutrition* 61, no. 6 (1995): 1368S–73S.

11. S. Liu et al., "A Prospective Study of Dietary Glycemic Load, Carbohydrate Intake, and Risk of Coronary Heart Disease in U.S. Women," *American Journal of Clinical Nutrition* 71, no. 6 (2000): 1455–61.

12. M. U. Jakobsen et al., "Intake of Carbohydrates Compared with Intake of Saturated Fatty Acids and Risk of Myocardial Infarction: Importance of the Glycemic Index," *American Journal of Clinical Nutrition* 91, no. 6 (2010): 1764–68.

13. Ibid.

14. Ibid.

15. www.ncbi.nlm.nih.gov/pubmed/16904539.

16. R. S. Kuipers et al., "Saturated Fat, Carbohydrates, and Cardiovascular Disease," *Netherlands Journal of Medicine* 69, no. 9 (2011): 372–78.

17. A. P. Simopoulos,"Evolutionary Aspects of the Dietary Omega-6:Omega-3 Fatty Acid Ratio: Medical Implications," *World Review of Nutrition and Dietetics* 100 (2009): 1–21.

18. Ibid; A. P. Simopoulos, "Overview of Evolutionary Aspects of w3 Fatty Acids in the Diet," *World Review of Nutrition and Dietetics* 83 (1998): 1–11.

19. R. O. Adolf et al., "Dietary Linoleic Acid Influences Desaturation and Acylation of Deuterium-labeled Linoleic and Linolenic Acids in Young Adult Males," *Biochimica et Biophysica Acta* 1213, no. 3 (1994): 277–88; Ghafoorunissa and M. Indu, "N-3 Fatty Acids in Indian Diets—Comparison of the Effects of Precursor (Alpha-linolenic Acid) vs. Product (Long Chain N-3 Polyunsaturated Fatty Acids)," *Nutrition Research* 12, nos. 4–5 (1992): 569–82.

20. A. P. Simopoulos,"Evolutionary Aspects of the Dietary Omega-6:Omega-3 Fatty Acid Ratio: Medical Implications," *World Review of Nutrition and Dietetics* 100 (2009): 1–21.

21. A. P. Simopoulos, "Overview of Evolutionary Aspects of w3 Fatty Acids in the Diet."

22. P. Reaven et al., "Effects of Oleate-rich and Linoleate-rich Diets on the Susceptibility of Low-density Lipoprotein to Oxidative Modification in Mildly Hypercholesterolemic Subjects," *Journal of Clinical Investigation* 91, no. 2 (1993): 668–76.

23. L. G. Cleland, "Linoleate Inhibits EPA Incorporation from Dietary Fish Oil Supplements in Human Subjects," *American Journal of Clinical Nutrition* 55, no. 2 (1992): 395–99.

24. W. E. M. Lands, "Diets Could Prevent Many Diseases," *Lipids* 38. no. 4 (2003): 317–21.

25. Ibid.

26. W. E. M. Lands, "A Critique of Paradoxes in Current Advice on Dietary Lipids," *Progress in Lipid Research* 47, no. 2 (2008): 77–106.

CHAPTER 6

1. A. E. Dorr et al., "Colestipol Hydrochloride in Hypercholesterolemic Patients—Effect on Serum Cholesterol and Mortality," *Journal of Chronic Diseases* 31, no. 1 (1978): 5.

2. J. Stamler et al., "Effectiveness of Estrogens for the Long-Term Therapy of Middle-Aged Men with a History of Myocardial Infarction," *Coronary Heart Disease: Seventh Hahnemann Symposium*, eds. W. Likoff and J. Henry Moyer (New York: Grune & Stratton, 1963), 416.

3. D. Graveline, *Lipitor: Thief of Memory* (Duane Graveline, 2006), www.spacedoc.com/lipitor_thief_of_memory.html.

4. D. Kuester, "Cholesterol-Reducing Drugs May Lessen Brain Function, Says ISU Researcher," Iowa State University, last modified February 23, 2009, www2.iastate.edu/~nscentral/news/2009/feb/shin.shtml.

5. Ibid.

6. M. Beck, "Can a Drug That Helps Hearts Be Harmful to the Brain?" *Wall Street Journal*, February 12, 2008.

7. C. Iribarren et al., "Serum Total Cholesterol and Risk of Hospitalization and Death from Respiratory Disease," *International Journal of Epidemiology* 26, no. 6 (1997): 1191-1202; C. Iribarren et al., "Cohort Study of Serum Total Cholesterol and In-Hospital Incidence of Infectious Diseases," *Epidemiology and Infection* 121, no. 2 (1998): 335-47; J.D. Neaton and D. N. Wentworth, "Low Serum Cholesterol and Risk of Death from AIDS," AIDS 11, no. 7 (1997): 929-30.

8. D. Jacobs et al., "Report of the Conference on Low Blood Cholesterol: Mortality Associations," *Circulation* 86, no. 3 (1992): 1046-60.

9. C. Iribarren et al., "Serum Total Cholesterol"; C. Iribarren et al., "Cohort Study of Serum Total Cholesterol."

10. J. D. Neaton and D. N. Wentworth, "Low Serum Cholesterol and Risk of Death from AIDS."

11. J. Kantor, "Prevalence of Erectile Dysfunction and Active Depression: An Analytic Cross-Sectional Study of General Medical Patients," *American Journal of Epidemiology* 156, no. 11 (2002): 1035-42.

12. M. Kanat et al., "A Multi-Center, Open Label, Crossover Designed Prospective Study Evaluatiing the Effects of Lipid-lowering Treatment on Steroid Synthesis in Patients with Type 2 Diabetes (MODEST Study)," *Journal of Endocrinology Investigation* 32, no. 10 (2009): 852-56; R.D. Stanworth et al., "Statin Therapy is Associated with Lower Total but not Bioavailable or Free Testosterone in Men with Type 2 Diabetes," *Diabetes* Care 32, no. 4 (2009): 541-46; A. S. Dobbs et al., "Effects of High-Dose Simvastatin on Adrenal and Gonadal Steroidogenesis in Men with Hypercholesterolemia," *Metabolism* 49, no. 9 (2000): 1234-38; A. S. Dobs et al., "Effects of Simvastatin and Pravastatin on Gonadal Function in Male Hypercholesterolemic Patients," *Metabolism* 49, no. 1 (2000): 115-21; M. T. Hyyppä et al., "Does Simvastatin Affect Mood and Steroid Hormone Levels in Hypercholesterolemic Men? A Randomized Double-Blind Trial," *Psychoneuroendocrinology* 28, no. 2 (2003): 181-94.

13. B. Banaszewska et al., "Effects of Simvastatin and Oral Contraceptive Agent on Polycystic Ovary Syndrome: Prospective, Randomized, Crossover Trial," *Journal of Clinical Endocrinology & Metabolism* 92, no. 2 (2007): 456-61; T. Sathyapalan et al., "The Effect of Atorvastatin in Patients with Polycystic Ovary Syndrome: A Randomized Double-Blind Placebo-Controlled Study," *Journal of Clinical Endocrinology & Metabolism* 94, no. 1 (2009): 103-108.

14. C. Do et al., "Statins and Erectile Dysfunction: Results of a Case/Non-Case Study using the French Pharmacovigilance System Database," *Drug Safety* 32, no. 7 (2009): 591-97.

15. C. J. Malkin et al., "Low Serum Testosterone and Increased Mortality in Men with Coronary Heart Disease," *Heart* 96, no. 22 (2010): 1821-25.

16. S. Shrivastava et al., "Chronic Cholesterol Depletion Using Statin Impairs the Function and Dynamics of Human Serotonin (1A) Receptors," *Biochemistry* 49, no. 26 (2010): 5426-35; L.N. Johnson-Anuna et al., "Chronic Administration of Statins Alters Multiple Gene Expression Patterns in Mouse Cerebral Cortex," *Journal of Pharmacology and Experimental Therapeutics* 312, no. 2 (2005): 786-93. A. Linetti et al., "Cholesterol Reduction Impairs Exocytosis of Synaptic Vesicles," *Journal of Cell Science* 123, no. 4 (2010): 595-605.

17. T. B. Horwich et al., "Low Serum Total Cholesterol Is Associated with Marked Increase in Mortality in Advanced Heart Failure," *Journal of Cardiac Failure* 8, no. 4 (2002): 216-24.

18. S. Brescianini et al., "Low Total Cholesterol and Increased Risk of Dying: Are Low Levels Clinical Warning Signs in the Elderly? Results from the Italian Longitudinal Study on Aging," *Journal of the American Geriatrics Society* 51, no. 7 (2003): 991-96.

19. A. Alawi et al., "Effect of the Magnitude of Lipid Lowering on Risk of Elevated Liver Enzymes, Rhabdomyolysis, and Cancer," *Journal of the American College of Cardiology* 50, no. 5 (2007): 409-18.

20. D. Preiss et al., "Risk of Incident Diabetes with Intensive-Dose Compared with Moderate-Dose Statin Therapy," *Journal of the American Medical Association* 305, no. 24 (2011): 2556-64.

21. www.spacedoc.com, Statin Drugs, accessed May 2, 2012.

22. J. Graedon and T. Graedon, "Patients Find Statins Can Have Side Effects," *The People's Pharmacy*, April 18, 2005, accessed January 4, 2012, www.peoplespharmacy.com/2005/04/18/patients-find-s.

23. J. Graedon and T. Graedon, "Can Statins Cause Debilitating Muscle Pain," *The People's Pharmacy*, April 18, 2005, accessed January 4, 2012, www.peoplespharmacy.com/2007/09/12/can-statins-cau.

24. J. Graedon and T. Graedon, "Does Lipitor Affect Memory and Nerves," *The People's Pharmacy*, April 18, 2005, accessed January 4, 2012, www.peoplespharmacy.com/2007/06/20/does-lipitor-af/.

25. B. A. Golomb et al., "Physician Response to Patient Reports of Adverse Drug Effects," *Drug Safety* 30, no. 8 (2007): 669-75.

26. Ibid.

27. S. Jeffrey, "ALLHAT Lipid-Lowering Trial Shows No Benefit from Pravastatin," *Heartwire*, December 17, 2002, www.theheart.org/article/263333.do.

28. Heart Protection Study Collaborative Drug, "MRC/BHF Heart Protection Study of Cholesterol Lowering with Simvastatin in 20,536 High-Risk Individuals: A Randomised Placebo-Controlled Trial," *The Lancet* 360, no. 9326 (2002): 7-22.

29. U. Ravnskov, "Statins as the New Aspirin," *British Medical Journal* 324, no. 7340 (2002): 789.

30. S. Boyles, "More May Benefit from Cholesterol Drugs," *WebMD Health News*, January 13, 2009, www.webmd.com/cholesterol-management/news/20090113/more-may-benefit-from-cholesterol-drugs.

31. M. de Lorgeril et al., "Cholesterol Lowering, Cardiovascular Diseases, and the Rousuvastatin-JUPITER Controversy: A Critical Reappraisal," *Archives of Internal Medicine* 170, no. 12 (2010): 1032-36.

32. M. A. Hlatky, "Expanding the Orbit of Primary Prevention—Moving Beyond JUPITER," *New England Journal of Medicine* 359 (2008): 2280-82.

33. Ibid.

34. H. S. Hecht and S. M. Harman, "Relation of Aggressiveness of Lipid-Lowering Treatment to Changes in Calcified Plaque Burden by Electron Beam Tomography," *American Journal of Cardiology* 92, no. 3 (2003): 334-36.

35. W. A. Flegel, "Inhibition of Endotoxin-Induced Activation of Human Monocytes by Human Lipoprotein," *Infection and Immunity* 57, no. 7 (1989): 2237-45; W.A. Flegel et al., "Prevention of Endotoxin-Induced Monokine Release by Human Low- and High-Density Lipoproteins and by Apolipoprotein A-I," *Infection and Immunity* 61, no. 12 (1993): 5140-46; H. Northoff et al., "The Role of Lipoproteins in Inactivation of Endotoxin by Serum," *Beitr Infusionsther* 30 (1992): 195-97.

36. Jacobs et al., "Report of the Conference on Low Blood Cholesterol."

37. Iribarren et al., "Serum Total Cholesterol and Risk of Hospitalization"; Iribarren et al., "Cohort Study of Serum Total Cholesterol."

38. Neaton and Wentworth, "Low Serum Cholesterol and Risk of Death from AIDS."

39. A. C. Looker et al., "Vitamin D Status: United States, 2001-2006," Centers for Disease Control and Prevention, *NCHS Data Brief No. 59*, March 2011, www.cdc.gov/nchs/data/databriefs/db59.htm.

40. W. Faloon, "Startling Findings About Vitamin D Levels in Life Extension Members," *Life Extension Magazine*, January 2010, www.lef.org/magazine/mag2010/jan2010_Startling-Findings-About-Vitamin-D-Levels-in-Life-Extension-Members_01.htm.

41. "Health Conditions," Vitamin D Council, last modified September 27, 2011, www.vitamindcouncil.org/health-conditions.

42. "About Us," Therapeutics Initiative, http://ti.ubc.ca/about.

43. J. R. Downs et al., "Primary Prevention of Acute Coronary Events with Lovastatin in Men and Women with Average Cholesterol Levels: Results of AFCAPS/TexCAPS," *Journal of the American Medical Association* 279 (1998): 1615-22; J. Shepherd et al., "Prevention of Coronary Heart Disease with Pravastatin in Men with Hypercholesterolemia," *New England Journal of Medicine* 333 (1995): 1301-7.

44. Therapeutics Initiative, "Do Statins Have a Role in Primary Prevention?" *Therapeutics Letter #48*, April-June 2003, www.ti.ubc.ca/newsletter/do-statins-have-role-primary-prevention.

45. J. Abramson and J. M. Wright, "Are Lipid-Lowering Guidelines Evidence-Based?" *The Lancet* 369, no. 9557 (2007): 168-69.

46. M. Pignone et al., "Primary Prevention of CHD with Pharmacological Lipid-Lowering Therapy: A Meta-Analysis of Randomised Trials," *British Medical Journal* 321, no. 7267 (2000): 983-86.

CHAPTER 7

1. E. G. Campbell, "Doctors and Drug Companies—Scrutinizing Influential Relationships," *New England Journal of Medicine* 357 (2007): 1796-97; M. M. Chren, "Interactions Between Physicians and Drug Company Representatives," *American Journal of Medicine* 107, no. 2 (1999): 182-83.

2. "NYHA Classification—The Stages of Heart Failure," Heart Failure Society of America, last modified December 5, 2011, www.abouthf.org/questions_stages.htm.

3. P. H. Langsjoen , S. Vadhanavikit, and K. Folkers, "Response of Patients in Classes III and IV of Cardiomyopathy to Therapy in a Blind and Crossover Trial with Coenzyme Q10," *Proceedings of the National Academy of Sciences of the United States of America* 82, no. 12 (1985): 4240-44.

4. P. H. Langsjoen et al., "A Six-Year Clinical Study of Therapy of Cardiomyopathy with Coenzyme Q10," *International Journal of Tissue Reactions* 12, no. 3 (1990): 169-71.

5. F. L. Rosenfeldt et al., "Coenzyme Q10 in the Treatment of Hypertension: A Meta-Analysis of the Clinical Trials," *Journal of Human Hypertension* 21, no. 4 (2007): 297-306.

6. S. Hendler, PDR for *Nutritional Supplements*, 2nd ed. (Montvale, NJ: PDR Network, 2008), 152.

7. P. Davini et al., "Controlled Study on L-Carnitine Therapeutic Efficacy in Post-Infarction," *Drugs Under Experimental and Clinical Research* 18, no. 8 (1992): 355-65.

8. I. Rizos, "Three-Year Survival of Patients with Heart Failure Caused by Dilated Cardiomyopathy and L-Carnitine Administration," *American Heart Journal* 139, no. 2 (2000): S120-23.

9. L. Cacciatore et al., "The Therapeutic Effect of L-Carnitine in Patients with Exercise-Induced Stable Angina: A Controlled Study," *Drugs Under Experimental and Clinical Research* 17, no. 4 (1991): 225-35; G. Louis Bartels et al., "Effects of L-Propionyl-carnitine on Ischemia-Induced Myocardial Dysfunction in Men with Angina Pectoris," *American Journal of Cardiology* 74, no. 2 (1994): 125-30.

10. L. A. Calò et al., "Antioxidant Effect of L-Carnitine and Its Short Chain Esters: Relevance for the Protection from Oxidative Stress Related Cardiovascular Damage," *International Journal of Cardiology* 107, no. 1 (2006): 54-60.

11. M. J. Bolland et al., "Effects of Calcium Supplements on Risk of Myocardial Infarction and Cardiovascular Events: Meta-Analysis," *British Medical Journal* 341, no. c3691 (2010).

12. P. Raggi et al., "Progression of Coronary Artery Calcium and Risk of First Myocardial Infarction in Patients Receiving Cholesterol-Lowering Therapy," *Arteriosclerosis, Thrombosis, and Vascular Biology* 24, no. 7 (2004): 1272-77.

13. Ibid.

14. U. Hoffmann et al., "Use of New Imaging Techniques to Screen for Coronary Artery Disease," *Circulation* 108 (2003): e50-e53.

15. M. C. Houston and K. J. Harper, "Potassium, Magnesium, and Calcium: Their Role in Both the Cause and Treatment of Hypertension," *Journal of Clinical Hypertension* 10, no. 7 (2008): 3-11; L. Widman et al., "The Dose-Dependent Reduction in Blood Pressure Through Administration of Magnesium: A Double-Blind Placebo-Controlled Crossover Trial," *American Journal of Hypertension* 6, no. 1 (1993), 41-45.

16. P. Laurant and R. M. Touyz, "Physiological and Pathophysiological Role of Magnesium in the Cardiovascular System: Implications in Hypertension," *Journal of Hypertension* 18, no. 9 (2000): 1177-91.

17. R. Meerwaldt et al., "The Clinical Relevance of Assessing Advanced Glycation Endproducts Accumulation in Diabetes," *Cardiovascular Diabetology* 7, no. 29 (2008): 1-8; A. J. Smit, "Advanced Glycation Endproducts in Chronic Heart Failure," *Annals of the New York Academy of Sciences* 1126 (2008): 225-30; J. W. L. Hartog et al., "Advanced Glycation End-Products (AGEs) and Heart Failure: Pathophysiology and Clinical Implications," *European Journal of Heart Failure* 9, no. 12 (2007): 1146-55.

18. A. Sjögren et al., "Oral Administration of Magnesium Hydroxide to Subjects with Insulin-Dependent Diabetes Mellitus: Effects on Magnesium and Potassium Levels and on Insulin Requirements," *Magnesium* 7, no. 3 (1988): 117-22; L. M. de Lordes et al., "The Effect of Magnesium Supplementation in Increasing Doses on the Control of Type 2 Diabetes," *Diabetes Care* 21, no. 5 (1998): 682-86; G. Paolisso et al., "Dietary Magnesium Supplements Improve B-Cell Response to Glucose and Arginine in Elderly Non-Insulin Dependent Diabetic Subjects," *Acta Endocrinologica* 121, no. 1 (1989): 16-20.

19. F. Guerrero-Romero and M. Rodríguez-Morán, "Low Serum Magnesium Levels and Metabolic Syndrome," *Acta Diabetologica* 39, no. 4 (2002): 209-13.

20. "Magnesium, What Is It?" Office of Dietary Supplements, National Institutes of Health, http://ods.od.nih.gov/factsheets/magnesium-HealthProfessional.

21. S. Hendler, *PDR for Nutritional Supplements*, 2nd ed. (Montvale, NJ: PDR Network, 2008), 152.

22. E. S. Ford and A. H. Mokdad, "Dietary Magnesium Intake in a National Sample of U.S. Adults," *Journal of Nutrition* 133, no. 9 (2003): 2879-82.

23. R. Altschul et al., "Influence of Nicotinic Acid on Serum Cholesterol in Man," *Archives of Biochemistry and Biophysics* 54, no. 2 (1955): 558-59.

24. R. H. Knopp et al., "Contrasting Effects of Unmodified and Time-Release Forms of Niacin on Lipoproteins in Hyperlipidemic Subjects: Clues to Mechanism of Action of Niacin," *Metabolism* 34, no. 7 (1985): 642-50; J. M. McKenney et al., "A Comparison of the Efficacy and Toxic Effects of Sustained vs. Immediate-Release Niacin in Hypercholesterolemic Patients," *Journal of the American Medical Association* 271, no. 9 (1994): 672-77.

25. P. R. Kamstrup, "Genetically Elevated Lipoprotein(a) and Increased Risk of Myocardial Infarction," *Journal of the American Medical Association* 301, no. 22 (2009): 2331-39; M. Sandkamp et al., "Lipoprotein(a) Is an Independent Risk Factor for Myocardial Infarction at a Young Age," *Clinical Chemistry* 36, no. 1 (1990): 20-23; A. Gurakar et al., "Levels of Lipoprotein Lp(a) Decline with Neomycin and Niacin Treatment," *Atherosclerosis* 57, nos. 2-3 (1985): 293-301; L. A. Carlson et al., "Pronounced Lowering of Serum Levels of Lipoprotein Lp(a) in Hyperlipidaemic Subjects Treated with Nicotinic Acid," *Journal of Internal Medicine* 226, no. 4 (1989): 271-76.

26. J. Shepard et al., "Effects of Nicotinic Acid Therapy on Plasma High Density Lipoprotein Subfraction Distribution and Composition and on Apolipoprotein A Metabolism," *Journal of Clinical Investigation* 63, no. 5 (1979): 858-67; G. Wahlberg et al., "Effects of Nicotinic Acid on Serum Cholesterol Concentrations of High Density Lipoprotein Subfractions HDL2 and HDL3 in Hyperlipoproteinaemia," *Journal of Internal Medicine* 228, no. 2 (1990): 151-57.

27. Shepard et al., "Effects of Nicotinic Acid Therapy"; Wahlberg et al., "Effects of Nicotinic Acid on Serum Cholesterol."

28. A. Gaby, *Nutritional Medicine* (Concord, NH: Fritz Perlberg Publishing, 2011).

29. A. Hoffer, "On Niacin Hepatitis," *Journal of Orthomolecular Medicine* 12 (1983): 90.

30. McKenney et al., "A Comparison of the Efficacy and Toxic Effects of Sustained Vs. Immediate-Release Niacin"; J.A. Etchason et al., "Niacin-Induced Hepatitis: A Potential Side Effect with Low-Dose Time-Release Niacin," *Mayo Clinic Proceedings* 66, no. 1 (1991): 23-28.

31. Gaby, *Nutritional Medicine*.

32. E. Serbinova et al., "Free Radical Recycling and Intramembrane Mobility in the Antioxidant Properties of Alpha-Tocopherol and Alpha-Tocotrienol," *Free Radical Biology & Medicine* 10, no. 5 (1991): 263-75.

33. R. A. Parker et al., "Tocotrienols Regulate Cholesterol Production in Mammalian Cells by Post-Transcriptional Suppression of 3-Hydroxy-3-Methylglutaryl-Coenzyme A reductase," *Journal of Biological Chemistry* 268 (1993): 11230-38; B.C. Pearce et al., "Hypocholesterolemic Activity of Synthetic and Natural Tocotrienols," *Journal of Medicinal Chemistry* 35, no. 20 (1992): 3595-606; B.C. Pearce et al., "Inhibitors of Cholesterol Biosynthesis. 2. Hypocholesterolemic and Antioxidant Activities of Benzopyran and Tetrahydronaphthalene Analogues of the tocotrienols," *Journal of Medicinal Chemistry* 37, no. 4 (1994): 526-41.

34. S. G. Yu et al., "Dose-Response Impact of Various Tocotrienols on Serum Lipid Parameters in Five-Week-Old Female Chickens," *Lipids* 41, no. 5 (2006): 453-61; M. Minhajuddin et al., "Hypolipidemic and Antioxidant Properties of Tocotrienol-Rich Fraction Isolated from Rice Bran Oil in Experimentally Induced Hyperlipidemic Rats," Food and Chemical Toxicology 43, no. 5 (2005): 747-53; J. Iqbal et al., "Suppression of 7,12-Dimethyl-Benz[alpha]anthracene-Induced Carcinogenesis and Hypercholesterolaemia in Rats by Tocotrienol-Rich Fraction Isolated from Rice Bran Oil," *European Journal of Cancer Prevention* 12, no. 6 (2003): 447-53; A. A. Qureshi et al., "Novel Tocotrienols of Rice Bran Suppress Cholesterogenesis in Hereditary Hypercholesterolemic Swine," *Journal of Nutrition* 131, no. 2 (2001): 223-30; M. K. Teoh et al., "Protection by Tocotrienols against Hypercholesterolaemia and Atheroma," *Medical Journal of Malaysia* 49, no. 3 (1994): 255-62; A. A. Qureshi et al., "Dietary Tocotrienols Reduce Concentrations of Plasma Cholesterol, Apolipoprotein B, Thromboxane B2, and Platelet Factor 4 in Pigs with Inherited Hyperlipidemias," *American Journal of Clinical Nutrition* 53, no. 4 (1991): 1042S-46S; D. O'Byrne et al., "Studies of LDL Oxidation Following Alpha-, Gamma-, or Delta-Tocotrienyl Acetate Supplementation of Hypercholesterolemic Humans," *Free Radical Biology & Medicine* 29, no. 9 (2000): 834-45; A. A. Qureshi et al., "Lowering of Serum Cholesterol in Hypercholesterolemic Humans by Tocotrienols (Palm Vitee)," *American Journal of Clinical Nutrition* 53, no. 4 supplement (1991): 1021-26; Qureshi et al., "Response of Hypercholesterolemic Subjects to Administration of Tocotrienols," *Lipids* 30, no. 12 (1995): 1171-77; A. C. Tomeo et al., "Antioxidant Effects of Tocotrienols in Patients with Hyperlipidemia and Carotid Stenosis," *Lipids* 30, no. 12 (1995): 1179-83.

35. A. Stoll, *The Omega-3 Connection* (New York: Free Press, 2001).

36. J. Dyerberg et al., "Plasma Cholesterol Concentration in Caucasian Danes and Greenland West Coast Eskimos," *Danish Medical Bulletin* 24, no. 2 (1977): 52–55; H.O. Bang, et al., "The Composition of Food Consumed by Greenland Eskimos," *Acta Medica Scandinavica* 200, nos. 1–2 (1976): 69–73; H.O. Bang and J. Dyerberg, "Plasma Lipids and Lipoproteins in Greenlandic West Coast Eskimos," *Acta Medica Scandinavica* 192, nos. 1–2 (1972): 85–94; H.O. Bang et al., "Plasma Lipid and Lipoprotein Pattern in Greenlandic West Coast Eskimos," *The Lancet* 1, no. 7710 (1971): 1143–45; J. Dyerberg et al., "Fatty Acid Composition of the Plasma Lipids in Greenland Eskimos," *American Journal of Clinical Nutrition* 28, no. 9 (1975): 958–66.

37. D. Mozzafarian and J. H. Wu, "Omega-3 Fatty Acids and Cardiovascular Disease: Effects on Risk Factors, Molecular Pathways, and Clinical Events," *Journal of the American College of Cardiology* 58, no. 20 (2011): 2047–67.

38. GISSI-Prevenzione Investigators, "Dietary Supplementation with N-3 Polyunsaturated Fatty Acids and Vitamin E after Myocardial Infarction: Results of the GISSI-Prevenzione Trial," *The Lancet* 354, no. 9177 (1999): 447–55.

39. M. R. Cowie, "The Clinical Benefit of Omega-3 PUFA Ethyl Esters Supplementation in Patients with Heart Failure," *European Journal of Cardiovascular Medicine* 1, no. 2 (2010): 14–18.

40. "Clinical Guidelines, CG48," National Institute for Health and Clinical Excellence, last modified September 23, 2011, www.nice.org.uk/CG48.

41. Cowie, "The Clinical Benefit of Omega-3 PUFA Ethyl Esters."

42. D. Lanzmann-Petithory, "Alpha-Linolenic Acid and Cardiovascular Diseases," *Journal of Nutrition, Health & Aging* 5, no. 3 (2001): 179–83.

43. M. Yokoyama, "Effects of Eicosapentaenoic Acid (EPA) on Major Cardiovascular Events in Hypercholesterolemic Patients: The Japan EPA Lipid Intervention Study (JELIS)" presentation, American Heart Association Scientific Sessions, Dallas, Texas, November 13–16, 2005; Medscape, "JELIS–Japan Eicosapentaenoic Acid (EPA) Lipid Intervention Study," Medscape Education, www.medscape.org/viewarticle/518574.

44. G. Bon et al., "Effects of Pantethine on In Vitro Peroxidation of Low-Density Lipoproteins," *Atherosclerosis* 57, no. 1 (1985): 99–106.

45. A. C. Junior et al., "Antigenotoxic and Antimutagenic Potential of an Annatto Pigment (Norbixin) Against Oxidative Stress," *Genetics and Molecular Research* 4, no. 1 (2005): 94–99; G. Kelly, "Pantethine: A Review of its Biochemistry and Therapeutic Applications," *Alternative Medicine Review* 2, no. 5 (1997): 365–77; F. Coronel et al., "Treatment of Hyperlipemia in Diabetic Patients on Dialysis with a Physiological Substance," *American Journal of Nephrology* 11, no. 1 (1991): 32–36; P. Binaghi et al., "Evaluation of the Hypocholesterolemic Activity of Pantethine in Perimenopausal Women," *Minerva Medica* 81 (1990): 475–79; Z. Lu, "A Double-Blind Clinical Trial: The Effects of Pantethine on Serum Lipids in Patients with Hyperlipidemia," *Chinese Journal of Cardiovascular Diseases* 17, no. 4 (1989): 221–23; M. Eto et al., "Lowering Effect of Pantethine on Plasma Beta-Thromboglobulin and Lipids in Diabetes Mellitus," *Artery* 15, no. 1 (1987): 1–12; D. Prisco et al., "Effect of Oral Treatment with Pantethine on Platelet and Plasma Phospholipids in Type II Hyperlipoproteinemia," *Angiology* 38, no. 3 (1987): 241–47; F. Bellani et al., "Treatment of Hyperlipidemias Complicated by Cardiovascular Disease in the Elderly: Results of an Open Short-Term Study with Pantethine," *Current Therapeutic Research* 40, no. 5 (1986): 912–16; S. Bertolini et al., "Lipoprotein Changes Induced by Pantethine in Hyperlipoproteinemic Patients: Adults and Children," *International Journal of Clinical Pharmacology and Therapeutics* 24, no. 11 (1986): 630–37; C. Donati et al., "Pantethine Improves the Lipid Abnormalities of Chronic Hemodialysis Patients: Results of a Multicenter Clinical Trial," *Clinical Nephrology* 25, no. 2 (1986): 70–74; L. Arsenio et al., "Effectiveness of Long-Term Treatment with Pantethine in Patients with Dyslipidemia," *Clinical Therapeutics* 8, no. 5 (1986): 537–45; S. Giannini et al., "Efeitos da Pantetina Sobrelipides Sangineos," *Arquivos Brasileiros de Cardiologia* 46, no. 4 (1986): 283–89; F. Bergesio et al., "Impiego della Pantetina nella Dislipidemia dell'Uremico Cronico in Trattamento Dialitico," *Journal of Clinical Medicine and Research* 66, nos. 11–12 (1985): 433–40; G. F. Gensini et al., "Changes in Fatty Acid Composition of the Single Platelet Phospholipids Induced

by Pantethine Treatment," *International Journal of Clinical Pharmacology Research* 5, no. 5 (1985): 309-18; L. Cattin et al., "Treatment of Hypercholesterolemia with Pantethine and Fenofibrate: An Open Randomized Study on 43 Subjects," *Current Therapeutic Research* 38 (1985): 386-95; A. Postiglione et al., "Pantethine Versus Fenofibrate in the Treatment of Type II Hyperlipoproteinemia," *Monographs on Atherosclerosis* 13 (1985): 145-48; G. Seghieri et al., "Effetto della Terapia con Pantetina in Uremici Cronici Emodializzati con Iperlipoproteinemia di Tipo IV," *Journal of Clinical Medicine and Research* 66, nos. 5-6 (1985): 187-92; L. Arsenio et al., "Iperlipidemia Diabete ed Aterosclerosi: Efficacia del Trattamento con Pantetina," *Acta Biomed Ateneo Parmense* 55, no.1 (1984): 25-42; O. Bosello et al., "Changes in the Very Low Density Lipoprotein Distribution of Apolipoproteins C-III2, CIII1, C-III0, C-II, and Apolipoprotein E after Pantethine Administration," *Acta Therapeutica* 10 (1984): 421-30; P. Da Col et al., "Pantethine in the Treatment of Hypercholesterolemia: A Randomized Double-Blind Trial Versus Tiadenol," *Current Therapeutic Research* 36 (1984): 314-21; A. Gaddi et al., "Controlled Evaluation of Pantethine, a Natural Hypolipidemic Compound, in Patients with Different Forms of Hyperlipoproteinemia," *Atherosclerosis* 50, no. 1 (1984): 73-83; R. Miccoli et al., "Effects of Pantethine on Lipids and Apolipoproteins in Hypercholesterolemic Diabetic and Non-Diabetic Patients," *Current Therapeutic Research* 36 (1984): 545-49; M. Maioli et al., "Effect of Pantethine on the Subfractions of HDL in Dyslipidemic Patients," *Current Therapeutic Research* 35 (1984): 307-11; G. Ranieri et al., "Effect of Pantethine on Lipids and Lipoproteins in Man," *Acta Therapeutica* 10 (1984): 219-27; A. Murai et al., "The Effects of Pantethine on Lipid and Lipoprotein Abnormalities in Survivors of Cerebral Infarction," *Artery* 12, no. 4 (1983): 234-43; P. Avogaro et al., "Effect of Pantethine on Lipids, Lipoproteins and Apolipoproteins in Man," *Current Therapeutic Research* 33 (1983): 488-93; G. Maggi et al., "Pantethine: A Physiological Lipomodulating Agent in the Treatment of Hyperlipidemia," *Current Therapeutic Research* 32 (1982): 380-86; K. Hiramatsu et al., "Influence of Pantethine on Platelet Volume, Microviscosity, Lipid Composition and Functions in Diabetes Mellitus with Hyperlipidemia," *Tokai Journal of Experimental and Clinical Medicine* 6, no. 1 (1981): 49-57.

46. M. Houston et al., "Nonpharmocologic Treatment of Dyslipidemia," *Progress in Cardiovascular Disease* 52, no. 2 (2009): 61-94.

47. R. Pfister et al., "Plasma Vitamin C Predicts Incident Heart Failure in Men and Women in European Prospective Investigation into Cancer and Nutrition–Norfolk Prospective Study," *American Heart Journal* 162, no. 2 (2011): 246-53.

48. W. Wongcharoen and A. Phrommintikul, "The Protective Role of Curcumin in Cardiovascular Diseases," *International Journal of Cardiology* 133, no. 2 (2009): 145-51.

49. M. Houston, *What Your Doctor May Not Tell You About Heart Disease* (New York: Grand Central Life & Style, 2012).

50. G. Ramaswami, "Curcumin Blocks Homocysteine-Induced Endothelial Dysfunction in Porcine Coronary Arteries," *Journal of Vascular Surgery* 40, no. 6 (2004): 1216-22.

51. H. Sumi et al., "Enhancement of the Fibrinolytic Activity in Plasa by Oral Administration of Nattokinase," *Acta Haematologica* 84, no. 3 (1990): 139-43.

52. Houston, *What Your Doctor May Not Tell You.*

53. M. A. Carluccio et al., "Olive Oil and Red Wine Antioxidant Polyphenols Inhibit Endothelial Activation: Antiatherogenic Properties of Mediterranean Diet Phytochemicals," *Atherosclerosis, Thrombosis, and Vascular Biology* 23, no. 4 (2003): 622-29.

54. "Study Shows Chocolate Reduces Blood Pressure and Risk of Heart Disease," *European Society of Cardiology*, March 31, 2010, www.escardio.org/about/press/press-releases/pr-10/Pages/chocolate-reduces-blood-pressure.aspx.

55. M. Houston et al., "Nonpharmologic Treatment for Dyslipideia," *Progress in Cardiovascular Disease* 52, no. 2 (2009), 61-94.

CHAPTER 8

1. R. Relyea, "Predator Cues and Pesticides: A Double Dose of Danger," *Ecological Applications* 13, no. 6 (2003): 1515-21.

2. J. C. Buck, "The Effects of Multiple Stressors on Wetland Communities: Pesticides, Pathogens, and Competing Amphibians," *Freshwater Biology* 57, no. 1 (2012): 61-73; Q. Guangqiu et al., "Effects of Predator Cues on Pesticide Toxicity: Toward an Understanding of the Mechanism of the Interaction," *Environmental Toxicology and Chemistry* 30, no. 8 (2011): 1926-34; M. L. Groner and R. Relyea, "A Tale of Two Pesticides: How Common Insecticides Affect Aquatic Communities," *Freshwater Biology* 56, no. 11 (2011): 2391-404; A. Sih et al., "Two Stressors Are Far Deadlier than One," *Trends in Ecology and Evolution* 19, no. 6 (2004): 274-76.

3. R. Sapolsky, "Stress and Your Body," Lecture 3, The Great Courses: Teaching Company.

4. "Hypertension," World Heart Federation, www.world-heart-federation.org/cardiovascular-health/cardiovascular-disease-risk-factors/hypertension.

5. R. Sapolsky, "Stress and Your Body" (Lecture 3, The Great Courses: Teaching Company).

6. "Mental Stress Raises Cholesterol Levels in Healthy Adults," *Medical News Today*, November 23, 2005, www.medicalnewstoday.com/releases/34047.php.

7. M. Hitti, "Cut Stress, Help Your Cholesterol," *WebMD Health News*, November 22, 2005, www.webmd.com/cholesterol-management/news/20051122/cut-stress-help-your-cholesterol.

8. A. H. Glassman et al., "Psychiatric Characteristics Associated with Long-Term Mortality Among 361 Patients Having an Acute Coronary Syndrome and Major Depression: Seven-Year Follow-Up of SADHART Participants," *Archives of General Psychiatry* 66, no. 9 (2009): 1022-29.

9. A. H. Glassman, "Depression and Cardiovascular Comorbidity," *Dialogues in Clinical Neuroscience* 9, no. 1 (2007): 9-17.

10. S. Sinatra, *Heart Break and Heart Disease* (Chicago: Keats Publishing, 1996).

11. R. Foroohar, "The Optimist: Why Warren Buffet Is Bullish on America," *Time*, January 23, 2012.

12. Ibid.

CHAPTER 9

1. Johns Hopkins Medicine, "The New Blood Lipid Tests—Sizing Up LDL Cholesterol," *Johns Hopkins Health Alerts*, last modified on June 13, 2008, www.johnshopkinshealthalerts.com/reports/heart_health/1886-1.html.

2. J. J. Stec et al., "Association of Fibrinogen with Cardiovascular Risk Factors and Cardiovascular Disease in the Framingham Offspring Population," *Circulation* 102, no. 14 (2000): 1634-38.

3. Ibid; L. Nainggolan, "Fibrinogen Tests Should Be Used for Additional Information when Assessing Cardiovascular Disease," *Heartwire*, October 3, 2000, www.theheart.org/article/180167.do.

4. Stec et al., "Association of Fibrinogen with Cardiovascular Risk Factors."

5. J. T. Salonen et al., "High Stored Iron Levels Are Associated with Excess Risk of Myocardial Infarction in Eastern Finnish Men," *Circulation* 86, no. 3 (1992): 803-11; L. K. Altman, "High Level of Iron Tied to Heart Risk," *New York Times*, September 8, 1992.

6. Salonen et al., "High Stored Iron Levels."

7. "Statins Can Damage Your Health," Vitamin C Foundation, www.vitamincfoundation.org/statinalert.

8. H. Refsum et al., "The Hordaland Homocysteine Study: A Community-Based Study of Homocysteine, Its Determinants, and Associations with Disease," *Journal of Nutrition* 136, no. 6 (2006): 1731S-40S; Homocystein Studies Collaboration, "Homocysteine and Risk of Ischemic Heart Disease and Stroke: A Meta-Analysis," *Journal of the American Medical Association* 288, no. 16 (2002): 2015-22; D.S. Wald et al., "Homocysteine and Cardiovascular Disease: Evidence on Casualty from a Meta-Analysis," *British Medical Journal* 325, no. 7374 (2002): 1202.

9. D. S. Wald et al., "The Dose-Response Relation Between Serum Homocysteine and Cardiovascular Disease: Implications for Treatment and Screening," *European Journal of Cardiovascular Prevention and Rehabilitation* 11, no. 3 (2004): 250-53.

10. M. Haim et al., "Serum Homocysteine and Long-Term Risk of Myocardial Infarction and Sudden Death in Patients with Coronary Heart Disease," *Cardiology* 107, no. 1 (2007): 52-56.

11. M. Houston, *What Your Doctor May Not Tell You About Heart Disease* (New York: Grand Central Life & Style, 2012).

12. S. Seely, "Is Calcium Excess in Western Diet a Major Cause of Arterial Disease?" *International Journal of Cardiology* 33, no. 2 (1991): 191-98.

13. U. Hoffmann, T. J. Brady, and J. Muller, "Use of New Imaging Techniques to Screen for Coronary Artery Disease," *Circulation* 108 (2003): e50-e53

14. Ibid.

15. K. L. Stanhope et al., "Consumption of Fructose and High-Fructose Corn Syrup Increase Postprandial Triglycerides, LDL-Cholesterol, and Apolipoprotein-B in Young Men and Women," *Journal of Clinical Endocrinology & Metabolism* 96, no. 10 (2011): E1596-605; "Fructose Consumption Increases Risk Factors for Heart Disease: Study Suggests US Dietary Guideline for Upper Limit of Sugar Consumption Is Too High," *Science Daily*, July 28, 2011, www.sciencedaily.com/releases/2011/07/110728082558.htm; K. L. Stanhope and P. J. Havel, "Endocrine and Metabolic Effects of Consuming Beverages Sweetened with Fructose, Glucose, Sucrose, or High-Fructose Corn Syrup," *American Journal of Clinical Nutrition* 88, no. 6 (2008): 1733S-37S.

16. S. Sieri et al., "Dietary Glycemic Load and Index and Risk of Coronary Heart Disease in a large Italian Cohort: The EPICOR Study," *Archives of Internal Medicine* 12, no. 170 (2010): 640-47.

17. Tel Aviv University, "How High Carbohydrate Foods Can Raise Risk For Heart Problems," *Science Daily*, June 25, 2009, retrieved February 8, 2012, from www.sciencedaily.com/releases/2009/06/090625133215.htm

18. "How High Carbohydrate Foods Can Raise Risk for Heart Problems," *Science Daily*, June 25, 2009, retrieved February 8, 2012, www.sciencedaily.com/releases/2009/06/090625133215.htm.

19. S. Liu et al., "Relation Between a Diet with a High Glycemic Load and Plasma Concentrations of High-Sensitivity C-Reactive Protein in Middle-Aged Women," *American Journal of Clinical Nutrition* 75, no. 3 (2002): 492-98.

20. Ibid.

21. C. Laino, "Trans Fats Up Heart Disease Risk," *WebMD Health News*, November 15, 2006, www.webmd.com/heart/news/20061115/heart-disease-risk-upped-by-trans-fats.

22. F. B. Hu et al., "Dietary Fat Intake and the Risk of Coronary Heart Disease in Women," *New England Journal of Medicine* 337, no. 21 (1997): 1491-99.

23. Institute of Medicine of the National Academies, *Dietary Reference Intakes for Energy, Carbohydrate, Fiber, Fat, Fatty Acids, Cholesterol, Protein, and Amino Acids* (Washington, D.C.: The National Academies Press, 2005), 504.

24. Harvard School of Public Health, "Eating Processed Meats, but Not Unprocessed Red Meats, May Raise Risk of Heart Disease and Diabetes," news release, May 17, 2010, www.hsph.harvard.edu/news/press-releases/2010-releases/processed-meats-unprocessed-heart-disease-diabetes.html.

25. Ibid.

26. J. Bowden, *The 150 Healthiest Foods on Earth* (Beverly, MA: Fair Winds Press, 2007).

27. L. Zhang et al., "Pterostilbene Protects Vascular Endothelial Cells Against Oxidized Low-Density Lipoprotein-Induced Apoptosis In Vitro and In Vivo," *Apoptosis* 17, no. 1 (2012): 25-36.

28. H. C. Ou et al., "Ellagic Acid Protects Endothelial Cells from Oxidized Low-Density Lipoprotein-Induced Apoptosis by Modulating the PI3K/Akt/eNOS Pathway," *Toxicology and Applied Pharmacology* 248, no. 2 (2010): 134-43.

29. H. C. Hung et al., "Fruit and Vegetable Intake and Risk of Major Chronic Disease," *Journal of the National Cancer Institute* 96, no. 21 (2004): 1577-84.

30. Ibid.

31. F. J. He et al., "Increased Consumption of Fruit and Vegetables Is Related to a Reduced Risk of Coronary Heart Disease: Meta-Analysis of Cohort Studies," *Journal of Human Hypertension* 21, no. 9 (2007): 717-28.

32. F. J. He et al., "Fruit and Vegetable Consumption and Stroke: Meta-Analysis of Cohort Studies," *The Lancet* 367, no. 9507 (2006): 320-26.

33. H. C. Hung et al., "Fruit and Vegetable Intake and Risk of Major Chronic Disease," *Journal of the National Cancer Institute* 96, no. 21 (2004): 1577-84.

34. Bowden, *The 150 Healthiest Foods on Earth*.

35. D. Mozaffarian et al., "Changes in Diet and Lifestyle and Long-Term Weight Gain in Men and Women," *New England Journal of Medicine* 364, no. 25 (2011): 2392-404.

36. M. Burros, "Eating Well; Pass the Nuts, Pass Up the Guilt," *New York Times*, January 15, 2003.

37. O. H. Franco et al., "The Polymeal: A More Natural, Safer, and Probably Tastier (than the Polypill) Strategy to Reduce Cardiovascular Disease by More Than 75%," *British Medical Journal* 329, no. 7480 (2004): 1447.

38. D. M. Winham et al., "Pinto Bean Consumption Reduces Biomarkers for Heart Disease Risk," *Journal of the American College of Nutrition* 26, no. 3 (2007): 243-49.

39. E. K. Kabagambe et al., "Decreased Consumption of Dried Mature Beans Is Positively Associated with Urbanization and Nonfatal Acute Myocardial Infarction," *Journal of Nutrition* 135, no. 7 (2005): 1770-75.

40. Bazzano et al., "Legume Consumption and Risk of Coronary Heart Disease in U.S. Men and Women," *Archives of Internal Medicine* 161, no. 21 (2001): 2573-78.

41. A. Buitrago-Lopez et al., "Chocolate Consumption and Cardiometabolic Disorders: Systematic Review and Meta-Analysis," *British Medical Journal* 343 (2011): d4488.

42. S. Desch et al., "Effect of Cocoa Products on Blood Pressure: Systemic Review and Meta-Analysis," Abstract, *American Journal of Hypertension* 23, no. 1 (2010): 97-103.

43. B. Buijsse et al., "Cocoa Intake, Blood Pressure, and Cardiovascular Mortality," *Archives of Internal Medicine* 166, no. 4 (2006): 411-17.

44. M. Aviram et al., "Pomegranate Juice Consumption Reduces Oxidative Stress, Atherogenic Modifications to LDL, and Platelet Aggregation: Studies in Humans and in Atherosclerotic Apolipoprotein E-Deficient Mice," *American Journal of Clinical Nutrition* 71, no. 5 (2000): 1062-76; M. Aviram et al., "Pomegranate Juice Flavonoids Inhibit Low-Density Lipoprotein Oxidation and Cardiovascular Diseases: Studies in Atherosclerotic Mice and in Humans," *Drugs Under Experimental and Clinical Research* 28, no. 2-3 (2002): 49-62.

45. M. Aviram et al., "Pomegranate Juice Consumption for 3 Years by Patients with Carotid Artery Stenosis Reduces Common Carotid Intima-Media Thickness, Blood Pressure and LDL Oxidation," *Clinical Nutrition* 23, no. 3 (2004): 423-33.

46. L. J. Ignarro et al., "Pomegranate Juice Protects Nitric Oxide Against Oxidative Destruction and Enhances the Biological Actions of Nitric Oxide," *Nitric Oxide* 15, no. 2 (2006): 93-102.

47. D. K. Das et al., "Cardioprotection of Red Wine: Role of Polyphenolic Antioxidants," *Drugs Under Experimental and Clinical Research* 25, nos. 2-3 (1999): 115-20.

48. V. Ivanov at al., "Red Wine Antioxidants Bind to Human Lipoproteins and Protect them from Metal Ion-Dependent and Independent Oxidation," *Journal of Agriculture and Food Chemistry* 49, no. 9 (2001): 4442-49; M. Aviram and B. Fuhrman, "Wine Flavonoids Protect Against LDL Oxidation and Atherosclerosis," *Annals of the New York Academy of Sciences* 957 (2002): 146-61.

49. A. Lugasi et al., "Cardio-Protective Effect of Red Wine as Reflected in the Literature," Abstract, Orvosi Hetilap 138, no. 11 (1997): 673-78; T.S. Saleem and S.D. Basha, "Red Wine: A Drink to Your Heart," *Journal of Cardiovascular Disease Research* 1, no. 4 (2010): 171-76.

50. D. B. Panagiotakos et al., "Mediterranean Diet and Inflammatory Response in Myocardial Infarction Survivors," *International Journal of Epidemiology* 38, no. 3 (2009): 856-66.

51. J. Sano, "Effects of Green Tea Intake on the Development of Coronary Artery Disease," *Circulation Journal* 68, no. 7 (2004): 665-70.

52. S. L. Duffy, "Short- and Long-Term Black Tea Consumption Reverses Endothelial Dysfunction in Patients with Coronary Artery Disease," *Circulation* 104 (2001): 151-56.

53. Medscape, "Black Tea Shown to Improve Blood Vessel Health," *Medscape News*, July 17, 2001, www.medscape.com/viewarticle/411324.

54. A. Trichopoulou et al., "Mediterranean Diet and Survival Among Patients with Coronary Heart Disease in Greece," *Archives of Internal Medicine* 165, no. 8 (2005): 929-35.

55. A. Ferrera et al., "Olive Oil and Reduced Need for Antihypertensive Medications," *Archives of Internal Medicine* 160, no. 6 (2000): 837-42.

56. "Olive Oil Contains Natural Anti-Inflammatory Agent," *Science Daily*, September 6, 2005, www.sciencedaily.com/releases/2005/09/050906075427.htm.

57. American Botanical Council, "Garlic," *Herbalgram*, http://cms.herbalgram.org/expandedE/Garlic.html.

58. J. Bowden, *The Most Effective Natural Cures on Earth* (Beverly, MA: Fair Winds Press, 2008).

59. J. W. Pennebaker, *Opening Up: The Healing Power of Expressing Emotions* (New York: Guilford Press, 1997); J. Frattaroli, "Experimental Disclosure and Its Moderators: A Meta-Analysis," *Psychological Bulletin* 132, no. 6 (2006): 823-65.

ABOUT THE AUTHORS

Jonny Bowden, Ph.D., C.N.S., is a nationally known expert on weight loss, nutrition, and health. He is a board-certified nutritionist with a master's degree in psychology and the author of twelve books on health, healing, food, and longevity, including the best-sellers, *The 150 Healthiest Foods on Earth,* and *Living Low Carb*. A frequent guest on television and radio, he has appeared on CNN, MSNBC, Fox News, ABC, NBC, and CBS as an expert on nutrition, weight loss, and longevity. He is the nutrition editor for *Pilates Style* and is a regular contributor to *Clean Eating, Better Nutrition*, and *Total Health Online*.

He has contributed to articles for dozens of print and online publications, including *The New York Times, The Wall Street Journal, Forbes, O (The Oprah Magazine), The Daily Beast, The Huffington Post, Vanity Fair Online, Time, Oxygen, Marie Claire, Diabetes Focus, GQ, US Weekly, Cosmopolitan, Self, Fitness, Family Circle, Allure, Men's Heath, Prevention, InStyle,* and *Natural Health*. He appears regularly as an expert on ABC-TV Los Angeles. He is a member of the American College of Nutrition and the American Society for Nutrition. He lives in the Topanga Canyon section of Southern California with his dogs, Lucy and Emily. Follow him at www.jonnybowden.com and @jonnybowden.

Stephen T. Sinatra, M.D., F.A.C.C., F.A.C.N., C.N.S., C.B.T., is a board-certified cardiologist and assistant clinical professor of medicine at the University of Connecticut School of Medicine. He is the author of many books, including *The Sinatra Solution: Metabolic Cardiology, Earthing: The Most Important Health Discovery Ever, Reverse Heart Disease Now*, and *Lower Your Blood Pressure in Eight Weeks*. Certified as a bio-energetic psychotherapist and nutrition and antiaging specialist, Dr. Sinatra integrates psychological, nutra-ceutical, and electroceutical therapies in the matrix of healing. He is the founder of www.heartmdinstitute.com, an informational website dedicated to promoting public awareness of integrative medicine. He is a fellow in the American College of Cardiology and the American College of Nutrition. His websites include www.drsinatra.com.

Deirdre Rawlings holds a Ph.D. in holistic nutrition, a master's degree in herbal medicine, and is a naturopathic doctor. She is the founder of Nutri-Living, is a healthy cooking coach, and designs condition-specific meal plans and recipes. She is the author of *Foods That Fight Fibromyalgia, Fermented Foods for Health*, and coauthor of *Beat Sugar Addiction Now! Cookbook*. She lives in Atlanta.

INDEX

B

H

M

N

O

Y

Z

DON'T MISS THESE OTHER TITLES FROM FAIR WINDS PRESS

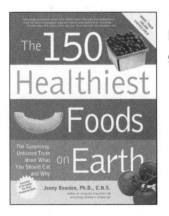

150 HEALTHIEST FOODS ON EARTH

978-1-59233-228-1

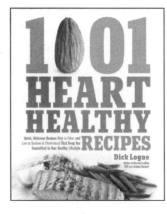

1,001 HEART HEALTHY RECIPES

978-1-59233-540-4

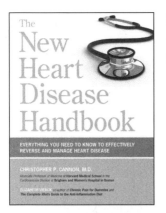

NEW HEART DISEASE HANDBOOK

978-1-59233-381-3

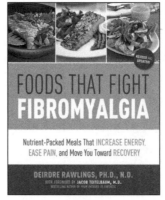

FOODS THAT FIGHT FIBROMYALGIA

978-1-59233-539-8

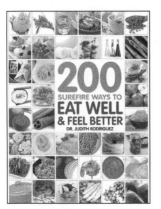

200 SUREFIRE WAYS TO EAT WELL AND FEEL BETTER

978-1-59233-653-1